Written By
Cameron McCluskie

Designed By
Sterling Vanderhoof

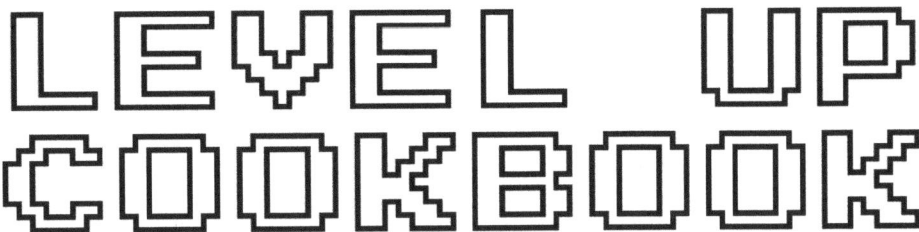

LEVEL UP COOKBOOK

A Guide to Epic Culinary Adventures

NEW GAME

LOAD GAME

SETUP

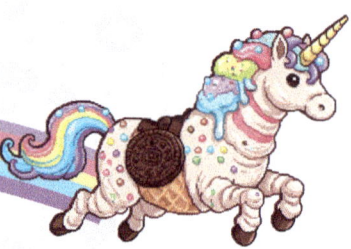

Introduction

Recipes, in a way, are like puzzles. When you first begin your cooking journey, your puzzles have just a few pieces; as you grow and get better at putting those together, the puzzles grow in size and complexity. You start by forming the frame and then filling out the middle. Soon, you have a puzzle that looks just like the picture on the box. However, with cooking, you'll learn that there's more than one way to fit the pieces together and some of the fun is seeing what can fit where. But that takes time and practice, and a willingness to try new things. That's part of what you'll learn as you progress through this book.

I'm very happy that you chose to open up this book and that you share my interest in cooking. I'm a professional, well-educated chef with many years of experience, and I love to cook. It's my life's work and I've been cooking since my teen years. With this book, my goal is to share what I know with you in a broad but detailed way, and I would love to see young people, as well as my contemporaries, get into cooking the way I have. Cooking your own food means both eating better and saving money, something that's good for all of us especially during tough economic times. Fast food, and even the food at many restaurants, can take a toll on your wallet and your health. Cooking at home gives you the power to control your budget better, and know exactly what you're eating. This book will also give insight on shopping practices and setting up your fridge, freezer, and pantry effectively.

Within this book is a curated list of some my favorite recipes. My personal creations which I have tested, re-tested, and transcribed for you: an eager explorer into the world of culinary arts. Whether you're an excited beginner, an experienced home cook, or even a professional chef, I hope this book provides both insight and knowledge to serve you well on your journey. I've done my best to provide not only guidance on the cooking of delicious dishes, but also a helpful reference for anyone wishing to gain a deeper understanding of the culinary world. While cooking may seem daunting for some people, I believe completely that "Anyone can cook"; but I prefer to amend that to say:

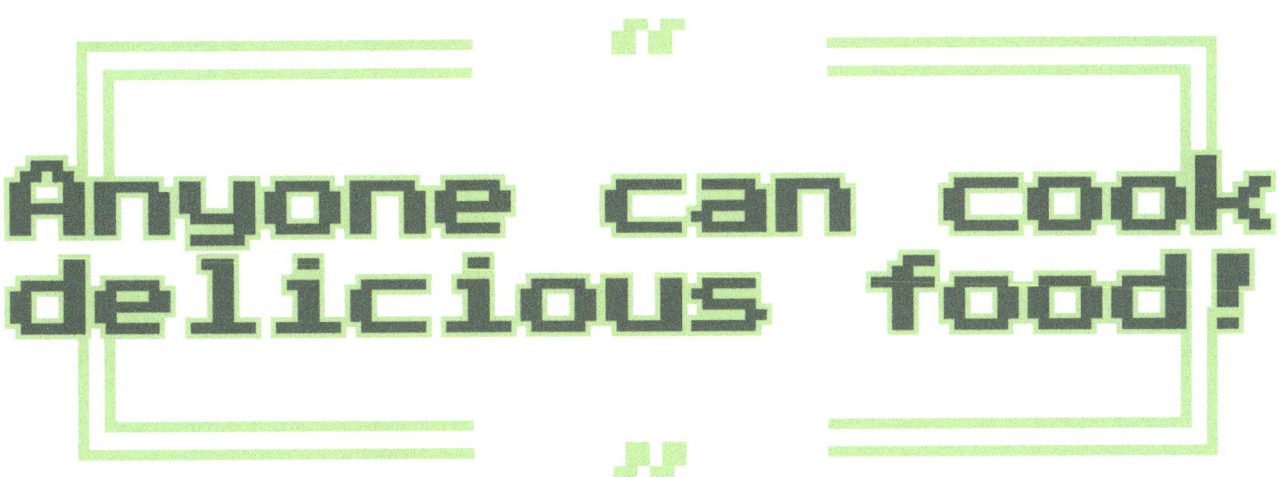

Why this book is different

Most cookbooks will give you a recipe to follow and include a beautiful photo of the menu item perfectly plated, well lit, in full color next to the list of ingredients and directions. You won't find that in this book. While plating is important and yes, we eat with our eyes first, I don't think setting the expectation that your meal will look just like a perfectly presented and professionally photographed image is reasonable. Instead, I want to help you increase your skills, ensure that you have the basics under your belt, and that you move fluidly from one level of cooking to the next. The art of plating your food will come naturally over time, and will be varied and expressive; unique to you and you alone. Thus, I present to you a unique and playful approach on food representation in this book.

I've broken down my recipes into four skill levels:

Novice
Apprentice
Adept
Expert

- Do you like having total control of every aspect of the food you cook?

- Do you want to cook great meals for yourself, for a significant other, or someone you want to impress with your culinary skills?

- Do you want to cook for parties, friends and family events or intimate gatherings with small groups?

- Do you want to get better at utilizing leftovers in creative ways?

They are color coded to make it easy for you to find them when you need them, and to help you work your way through the book. Some of you have limited knowledge about cooking; others may have years of experience under their belts. Wherever you are on the scale, I have recipes and lessons that'll help you grow as a cook. I love beginners who have a passion for food and cooking; if that's you, you're right at home. For those who've been cooking for a long time, I believe you'll find things in this book that you hadn't tried or considered to make cooking easier and more enjoyable.

I've always held a love for Fantasy, both in books and games. From table tops to gaming consoles, Fantasy RPGs have had a profound impact on my life. It's with this love and passion in mind that I have assembled this book for your enjoyment, and to help you Level Up into the best cook you can be! To this end, I have assembled a list of cooking styles which I have affectionately labeled as "Classes". We all have unique personality traits and desires, and those help shape the way we eat and cook.

There are lots of ways to approach cooking and everyone has their own reasons for cooking in the ways that suit their lifestyles. Thus, choosing your Class is an important first step on your culinary journey.

The main thing I want for you as you use this book is to have fun when you cook, even if it's just a meal for one. My Class System and Skill Trees make it fun and easy to progress through the book. They'll help you understand how you learn, and help you Level Up to become a more skilled cook. There are links to videos I've made for visual instruction, and clear steps to move you from rank to rank. I want you to create great food to eat, share, and fully enjoy.

Food is life. Learning to make delicious food is a way to connect with others and increase your own joy. So, let's figure out where you are on this journey and get started cooking!

Dedication

I want to first thank my family, my lifelong friends, and my wife, Julia. Their support and love gave me the courage to persevere no matter how difficult or obstructed my path became.

Secondly, I need to thank my High School Culinary Arts instructor, Chef Roger. He was the man who introduced me to the world of professional cooking and provided the firm foundation of knowledge upon which I built my career and philosophy of life.

Without any of these wonderful people in my life, I cannot imagine where I would be today.

Table of Contents

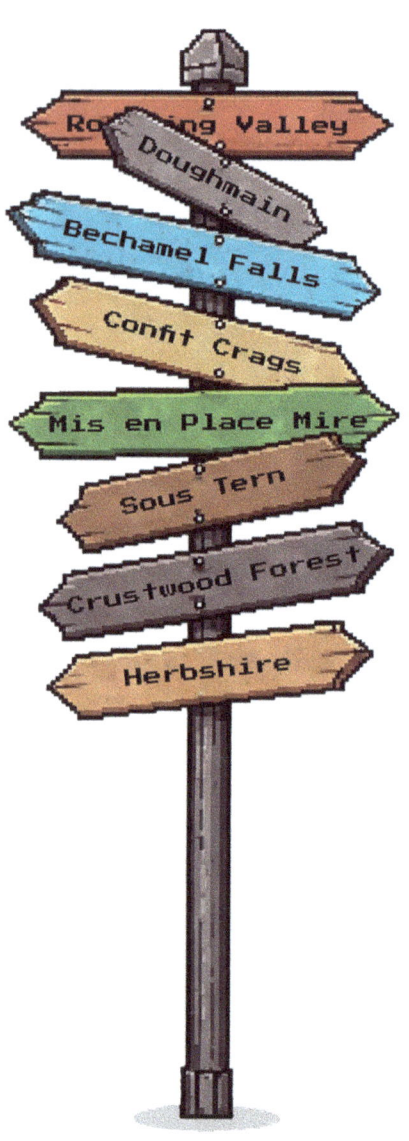

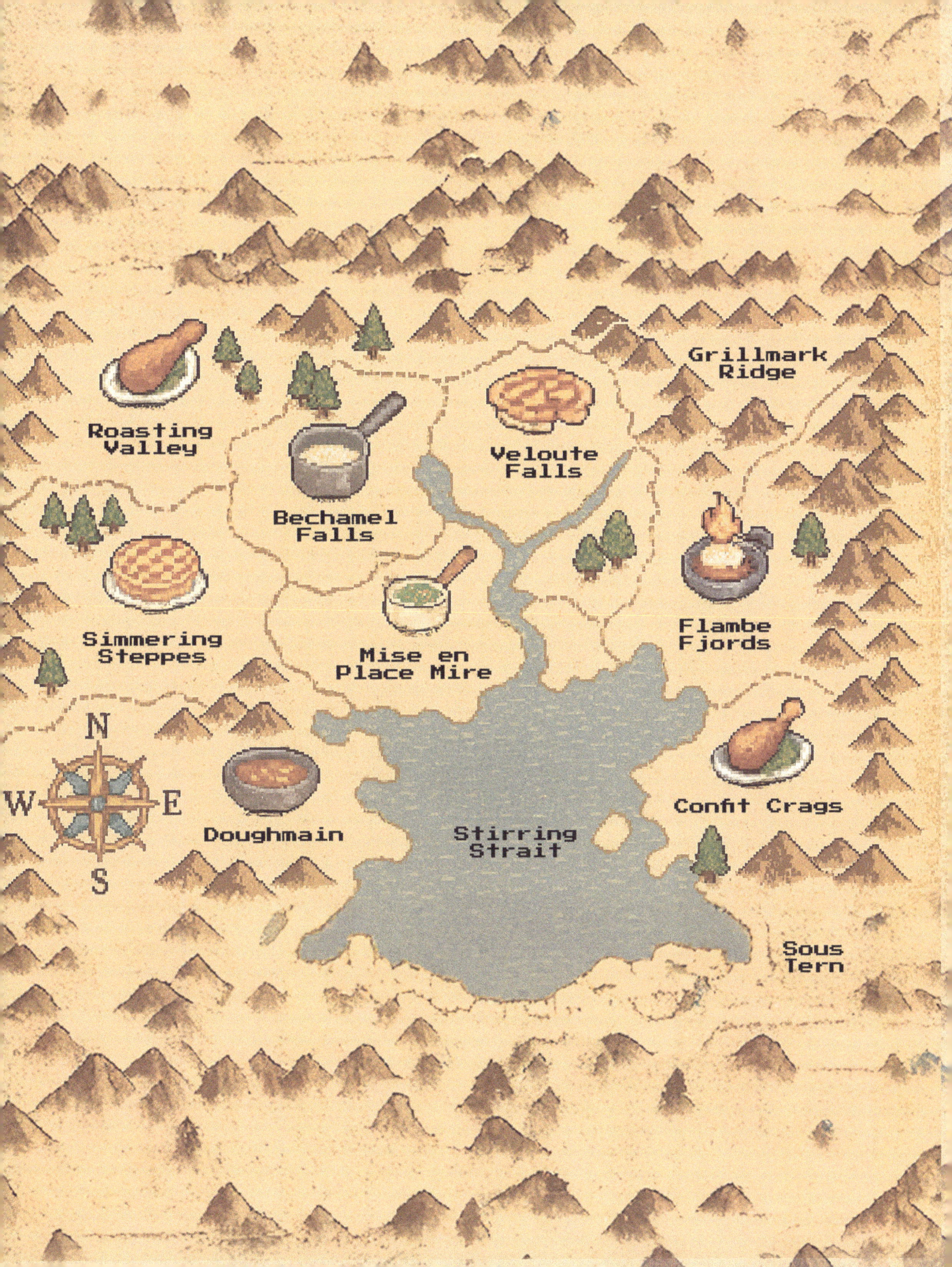

Roasting
Valley

Grillmark
Ridge

Bechamel
Falls

Veloute
Falls

Simmering
Steppes

Mise en
Place Mire

Flambe
Fjords

N
W E
S

Doughmain

Stirring
Strait

Confit Crags

Sous
Tern

Philosophy & Advice

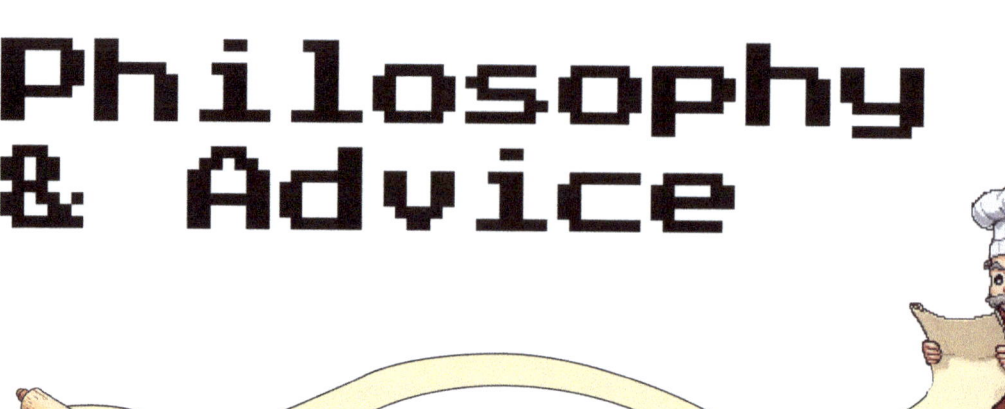

Cooking isn't a science. It's a form of art that relies on science. So, recipes are simultaneously formulae and guidelines for cooking. That being said, there's still a set of principles and methods to help make cooking simpler, easier, and more streamlined. This section will outline these in a clear way. It's an invaluable tool for anyone looking to really Level Up their cooking skills. Think of this as an instruction manual outlining the basics and principles of the levels you'll be rising through on your journey. And don't forget the guideline aspect of recipes and methods. Take these words and use them to form your own unique styles and practices that make cooking fun and enjoyable for you. All of these things will help you build up "Experience Points."

As an art, cooking food is a subjective expression of yourself and your feelings toward both food and the people you're feeding. The old adage "The secret ingredient is love" may be a bit corny, but it's true. Without the love for food, for the people you'll be feeding, and for yourself, the finished product will always be less than what it could be. So when you pick up your knife, your spatula, or your pots and pans, hold onto the feelings that drove you to begin your culinary adventure. Whether you are seeking to improve your skills at home, have aspirations to work in a fast-paced professional environment, or are working toward being the source of joy and enjoyment at social gatherings, don't lose sight of what brought you to take your first steps.

Now, we'll move away from my philosophy on cooking and into the more solid grounds of practice, technique, and the methods for creating delectable dishes. Here are some tips, advice, and techniques developed through my own experience that'll illuminate the paths you walk as you craft, alter, and perfect your own personal methodology. There's one aspect of this section that is most important: Mis en Place. So, let's tackle that subject first.

Most of the recipes in this book are complimentary; be creative and combine them in exciting new ways!

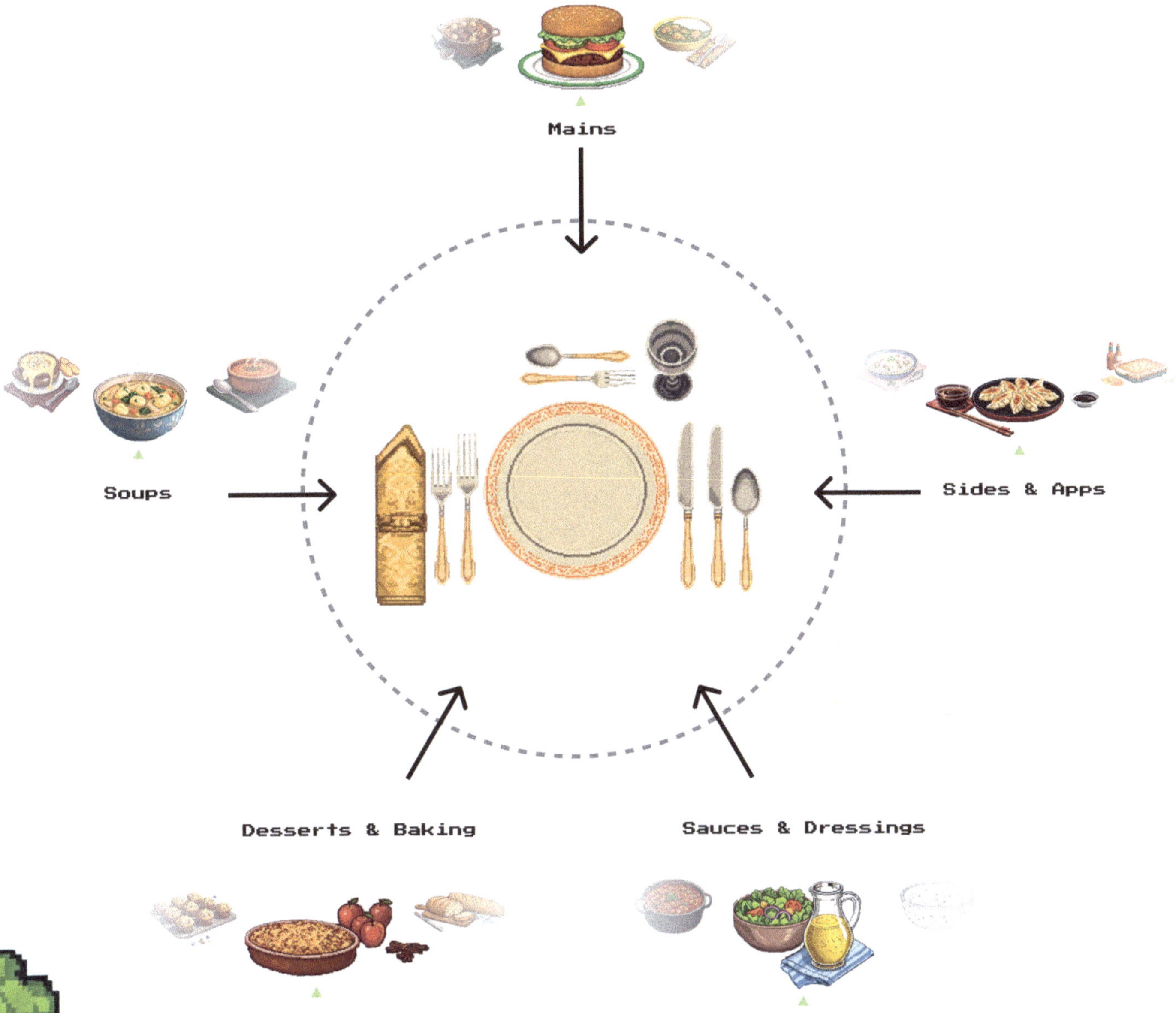

Mains

Soups

Sides & Apps

Desserts & Baking

Sauces & Dressings

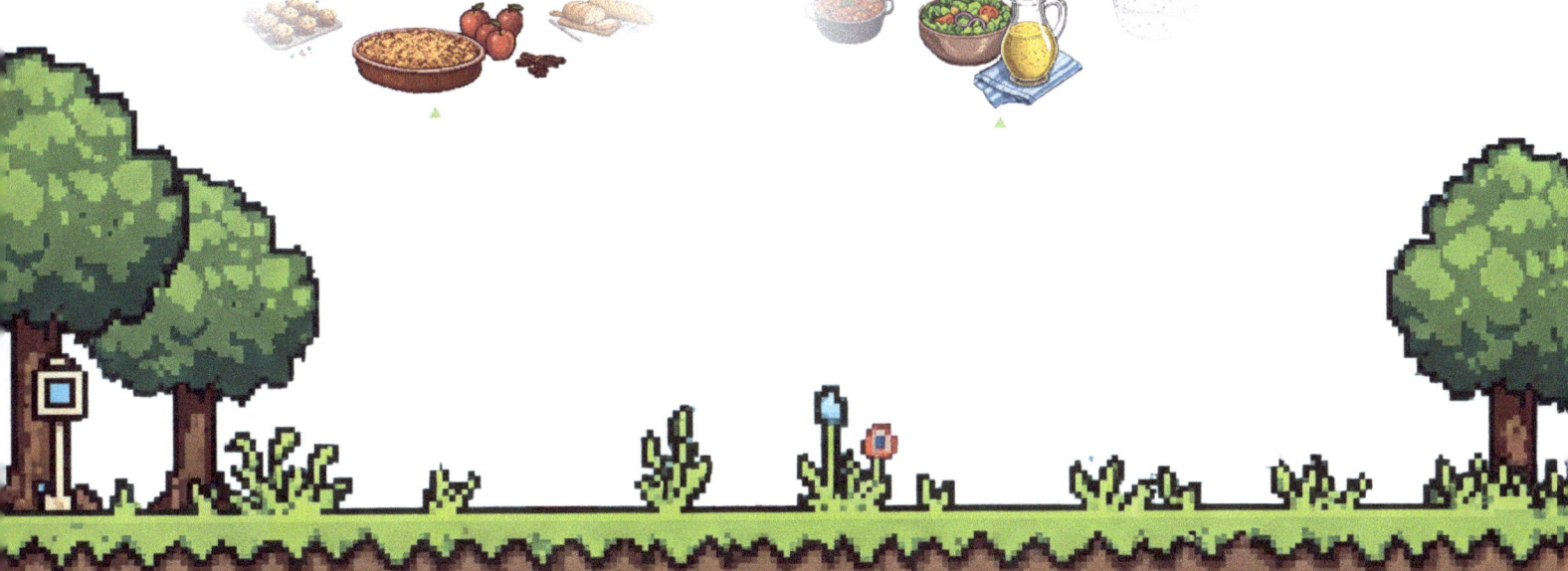

The Concept of

"Mis en Place"

"Mis en Place" (pronounced Mees-in-plaas) is a French culinary term. It translates to "set up" or "put in place." The practice of Mis en Place, at its most basic, is to read through the recipe several times so that you are familiar with its components, required techniques, and the process it outlines. Then you gather all your ingredients and cut, measure, and portion them before moving on to the actual cooking steps.

- Need diced bell pepper? Make sure you know the dimensions of the cut you'll be using.

- Does the recipe require multiple pots and pans? Have them ready to be accessed.

- Does the recipe require you to incorporate a component made from a separate recipe? Make it before you begin.

Going through these steps will guarantee a smooth and simpler cooking experience. Mis en Place is like reading the map before setting out on an adventure. It's important to have a good idea of what paths you'll take and what your destination will be. These paths are hardly ever the same from person to person, so it's important to remember two things:

1 These are all guidelines

They are made to be altered, reformed, and customized to fit your own style and way of doing things. While it's true there are certain aspects of cooking that cannot be left open to interpretation (proper cooking temperatures, the way to make a roux, the definition of searing) there's a lot of them that are unique to each person. What is spicy? What is the best way to organize your kitchen? What is the ideal amount of salt? These are subjective by nature and must be taken into account in your own Mis en Place.

2 Everything is Mis en Place

Reframing your thought process around this concept will make you a better and more organized cook and a more organized and prepared individual. Any obstacle can be broken down into its composite parts, and plans can be made for dismantling each aspect. There's no mountain too high, no river too deep, and no forest too dense when you have preparation and understanding. This same concept in life applies to cooking. There'll be no recipe beyond your grasp if your Mis en Place is in order.

Now that I've waxed poetic on my philosophy of this process, let's move on to the concrete aspects of Mis en Place. Here are the key elements and methods that'll help you on your way to success in crafting your ideal dishes.

Reading the Recipe

This seems like an obvious step, but it's a bit more involved than you might think. Reading the recipe isn't just reading through it, getting an overview, and jumping into the action. It involves taking in the ingredient list, visualizing how you think the ingredients should be cut, what the proteins should look and smell like, and what the composed dish will look like. Take in the whole list and think of how those ingredients would best interact with one another. Let's use a pan of fajitas as an example.

- How thick would you like the peppers and onions to be cut?
- How would that thickness effect the overall cooking time?
- How large do you want your protein to be in relation to your vegetables?

Visualize these things, and use that mental image to inform your decision on how to prepare your ingredients. After the ingredients list, read through the directions. These are important, not just for actually cooking, but also for preparing. There are three key things to take away here:

- How long things should take to cook
- What utensils, pots, and pans you will require
- What you envision the end result looking and tasting like

This is why you should read through the recipe completely at least twice when you choose it, and once more before beginning your prep work. This'll help you familiarize yourself with the ingredients and tools required, as well as your own method of preparation. As time goes on, this'll become easier to do. In the case of recipes you enjoy cooking regularly, soon you won't even have to do it! You'll be so familiar with the method, it'll become second nature.

Setting Up

Now that you've read through the recipe multiple times, it's time for you to set up your work area. This is all about utilizing your space effectively and asking yourself some simple questions to help you decide how best to use that space.

- How large of a cutting board will you need?

- How many different pots and pans will you need?

- What sizes of your available equipment would be best for cooking this recipe?

- How many bowls/containers will you need to hold your various ingredients?

- What variety of measuring tools will you need?

- What kind of knife will be best for your cutting needs?

- Speaking of which, when was the last time you honed/ sharpened your knife?

All of these questions are examples of the things you should consider and be familiar with when setting up. Save anything to do with your knives until the very end of this step. Moving around and setting up with a sharp knife sitting on the counter is an accident waiting to happen.

If your recipe is fast-paced and doesn't allow time to gather and set up the things you'll need for serving, now's the time for that too. Make sure your plates, bowls, platters, and eating utensils are out, or at least easily accessible now to save you time and worry later. If your recipe does allow for time to do this later, do yourself a service and use that time effectively.

Don't overcrowd yourself, if you can help it.

Preparation

You've set up your cooking station. You have your pots and pans selected. You have any specialty equipment in its place and ready to use. Your vessels for holding ingredients are organized. Your knife's honed and ready. The oven is preheated.

Now you need to start cutting and measuring ingredients. Begin with washing fruits and vegetables first to prevent cross contamination, always. This is very important. Even if it comes prewashed, wash it anyway. It doesn't take long, and it ensures your food is safe to eat. Also, it gives you one final opportunity to examine your produce and make sure it passes quality control. Cutting fruits and vegetables first prevents cross-contamination on one of the most overlooked spots when cooking: your cutting board. Since almost everything during the prep stage will be done on this surface, it's important to be mindful of what you place on it and to clean it off regularly when it becomes too messy. Learning the proper sizes for different cuts seems daunting, but once you get the feel for your knife and have done a little slicing and dicing, you'll see that it's not too hard. You'll develop your own techniques and methods for achieving your goals with your knife, and soon it'll be a reflex. If you have a garnish in mind, prepare that as well.

After the produce is cut, measured, and placed in the vessels set aside for it, you can move onto measuring and portioning your herbs, spices, and miscellaneous ingredients. Things such as rice, breadcrumbs, flour, butter, and oil. Can all the seasonings of your recipe be added at the same time? Place them all in one vessel. If not, be sure to set them aside in separate containers for use. This step can get a bit messy, so either measure over your cutting board or do it over the sink. Remember, you can always add things to a blend or recipe, but once they're in, it's impossible to remove them. Be gentle when moving these ingredients around.

Finally, you move onto the proteins (if there are any). You always want to save protein, raw or cooked, until the end of your prep phase. This way no cross-contamination can happen, and you'll have the space needed to prepare it properly. There are cases where no cutting is required, but it's still a good idea to bring your protein out of the fridge and let it rest on the counter. Don't worry, letting raw proteins sit on the counter for 30-40 minutes won't keep it from being safe to eat, provided it's not seafood. Those should not be out of the fridge for more than five minutes before cooking. Doing this helps the food cook more evenly, and gives you another chance to inspect it. Always prepare your protein by dabbing it dry with paper towels. No matter how you are cooking it, this will help with forming good color and texture, especially when searing.

Method

You've read your recipe thoroughly, you've set up your cooking area, and you've prepared the various ingredients. Now it's time to begin the real action!

Follow the steps as directed; this is why reading through the recipe multiple times comes in handy. You'll avoid wasting time and potentially making errors since you won't be checking the recipe every step. You need to know, at a minimum, the first four steps in a recipe by heart before starting. This'll give you the time to check back if there's something you can't quite remember, and the focus needed to start off on the right foot. Everyone's stove top and oven is different, so take the advised heat settings with a grain of salt. If you know that your stove eyes run hot, then adjust your temperature accordingly.

You don't always want to blindly follow the recipe when it comes to subjective terms such as "Medium Low" or "High." Know your equipment, understand the desired result, and you'll do well.

It's a good idea, when you aren't cooking, to take a pot filled with a pint of water and time how long it takes each eye to bring it to a boil. Take notes of the settings that hold a boil well, and what settings hold a simmer well, both covered and uncovered. This easy test will give you a better understanding of how your equipment works, so you can make it work best for you. Also, getting an oven thermometer so you can regularly check how your oven holds temperature isn't a bad idea.

I'm sure you're thinking "When are we going to talk about the actual cooking?" Well, that's the thing, isn't it? Beyond knowing your recipe and equipment, and visualizing your desired outcome, there isn't much more to this part of the process. You know your steps, you have a firm understanding of what you are trying to accomplish, and you can be decisive with your actions. You've come too far to second guess yourself; besides, you're prepared.

You can do this!

Tasting & Temping

This is an often overlooked aspect to preparing food. It's important to regularly taste your food as you cook, and when nearing completion, testing the temperature (temping) with a thermometer. I suggest having a small ramekin or other dish on hand so you can separate a small amount of what you are taste testing to prevent contamination. In a professional kitchen, it's not uncommon for there to be a large pan full of spoons and forks for the purpose of testing taste. However, in a professional kitchen, a utensil is used once then thrown into a pile to be washed. This is not ideal for your home (who wants to wash 20 spoons every time they cook?) so having a separate small dish specifically for this purpose is needed. As you cook, you are examining the color, texture, and aroma of the food. It's silly not to also be monitoring and examining the flavors.

As for temping, this is usually done both in the middle and at the end of the process. You need to make sure that your food is at the desired or required temperature, and not using a thermometer is like turning off the lights before opening a book. Temping helps ensure you are delivering the desired result every time and is a sign that you truly care about your food. Also, it helps make sure you know the food is safe to eat . . . which is really important.

Serving

You've made the food. The smell has drawn in you and everyone around and the look of it is captivating. It's time to plate up. Get creative with your expression. This food is yours after all, so make it yours. Unless you're confident in the stability of your food, avoid precarious positioning on a plate. Resting your protein on your starch or vegetables, getting creative with the application of sauces, experimenting with angles and juxtaposition, and adding that little touch of garnish right at the end convey the thought and care you have been pouring into this meal right from the start.

For basic plating techniques, there are three things that are helpful to keep in mind.

1. **Angles are your Friend** - Positioning food so that it contrasts is a simple way to make the whole plate look more appetizing. This doesn't have to be fancy; something as simple as laying a pan-seared pork chop at a 45-degree angle against the roasted potatoes with the vegetables filling the space between them. Little things like this show your mindfulness and make the dish really sing.

2. **Mindful Application** - Keep in mind what sort of dish you are serving when applying sauces and gravies. Is it the kind of dish that benefits from being smothered, or will a "less is more" approach be better? A chicken fried steak deserves to be covered in your pepper gravy, but a roasted chicken thigh would benefit more from the sauce being drizzled sparsely on the piece, with more resting on the plate. Think of how you will be eating the food; by hand, or with utensils? You can always have more sauce in a separate vessel but taking it off the plate is messy.

3. **Garnish with Purpose** - Don't garnish a plate with something that adds nothing to the dish or isn't edible. There's a reason you rarely see that superfluous piece of kale sitting on one end of a plate anymore. It's pointless and brings down the whole dish. When sprinkling things like herbs and spices on a plate, the goal is to give it the appearance that those ingredients magically fell down from the heavens. So, do just that. Hold your hand eight to ten inches away from the food when applying a garnish like say, parsley, and you will notice that there is no bunching or extreme concentration of it anywhere on the plate. If you're feeling very artistic, more complex garnishes can be prepared, just make sure that they elevate and complement your dish; no random slap-shots allowed.

Cleaning

Ah yes, the part that nobody enjoys. Cleaning's a necessary part of the cooking process. As I once told a group of students I was teaching during a volunteer program in Providence, Rhode Island, "Everyone cleans. If you want to cook, you've got to accept that. You can't cook if you don't clean, so let's make this as simple as we can."

Cleaning as you work isn't as difficult as it sounds. Obviously when you've got food actively cooking on the stovetop, that's where your focus should be.

However there are always little pockets of time that need to be filled and that's when the cleaning happens. Be mindful of your dishwasher, if you've got one. Try to begin the prep process with an empty or partially full washer. When you're all done with your prep work, take a few minutes to wash any equipment, utensils, and of course your knife. Rinse them off at least, if you don't feel you have the time to actually wash them or load them into the dishwasher.

You should always make time to wash and dry your knife. Don't wash it with hot water, and never put it in the dishwasher. That is the fastest way to ruin the edge on your knife, and it also causes the handle to dry out over time. Using soap and cold water, wash your knife immediately after you are done using it, dry it off with a towel, and place it back in your knife stand. This'll be talked about further in the "Concerning Knives" section.

If your recipe calls for "occasional" stirring while the food cooks for five minutes or more, you just found a little window to get some cleaning done. Just make sure to set some timers! When you transfer ingredients from their vessels into the pan or pot, give the vessels a quick rinse when you drop them in the sink. When you transfer food from one pan to another, set the pan to the side on a heat-safe trivet to let cool. Never take a hot pan or pot from the stove and put it under running water. The rapid temperature change will warp them immediately, and they'll no longer heat evenly.

When done with the meal, it's understandable to not want to clean. But taking certain measures will make your job that much easier. Once you've moved the leftovers into their containers, rinse the pots and pans out. If they need to soak to help remove stuck on food, start that now. Leaving dishes in the sink overnight is not usually ideal, but if you must leave them to soak, be sure to cover them properly to avoid spillage and attracting insects. If you have a system in your home where one person cooks and the other cleans, be considerate of them. Try to make their life easier when the dishes need to be done, so that both of you have a better time of it.

Following this advice will help speed up this aspect of the cooking process and, like most things with cooking, become second nature after a little time.

Storage

The opinion on leftovers varies from person to person. If you know that you don't really care for eating leftovers, downsize the recipe to closer fit your projected needs. If you love having leftovers in the fridge, all the better. When cooling food, it's important to remember the Temperature Danger Zone: 40-140 degrees. This is the temperature at which bacteria grows best in cooked food and liquids. Keeping food in this range for an extended period of time (over 4 hours) is asking for trouble. That's the window of time you have to get the food down below 40 for storage or above 140 for reheating. So when you are done eating, it is not necessary to immediately get up and rush to the fridge, but be mindful of your time window.

You should, when possible, cool your food to room temperature before putting it in the fridge. Remember, you have four hours to work with for safety, so maximize that schedule. If the item is too large or dense to cool to room temperature before putting in the fridge, there's a solution. Let's use a pot of stock you just finished straining into a large bowl as an example.

- If you have a heat-safe (stainless steel or properly graded plastic) vessel that will fit even a quarter of the stock, transfer some into it. Even better, if you have vessels already in mind for the stock, get those out and ready. The act of pouring hot liquid reduces the temperature by roughly 20 degrees almost at once, so that right there has moved you closer to your goal. If you don't have a vessel large enough or don't want to make any more dirty dishes, make sure to stir your stock every 15 minutes as it cools on the counter. Agitation allows heat to escape, which is what we are looking for.

- When cooling, utilize your thermometer. You don't want to place items over 120 degrees in the fridge. That throws off the equilibrium of the temperature zones inside. Once the stock is below 100, it's safe to move it into your separate vessels for storage, or move the whole pot into the fridge. Separating it into different containers will allow for more heat to be released and also makes for quicker cooling times overall.

- Even below 100 degrees, don't cover food until it has sufficiently chilled. If you place a lid on your storage container and the interior fogs up and condensation occurs, it is too hot. Remove the lid and let it cool more. This will ensure that your food does not remain in the Danger Zone any longer than necessary.

- Utilizing your freezer is an option, but it's risky. Without frequent agitation, the food will cool at an uneven rate, and may impact its overall quality in the future. If you are looking to freeze the items right away, place in a freezer-safe container or bag once below 100 degrees, and you are good to go.

Allocating Experience Points

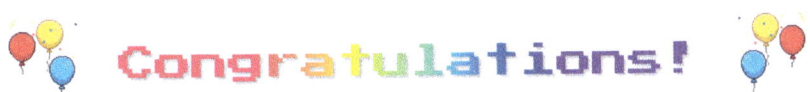 **Congratulations!**

You've followed all the steps, stayed mindful and organized, and have just enjoyed a delicious homemade meal! You should be proud of yourself, and take time to think about how things turned out. Never be afraid to think of what you might do differently, how you can improve even in small ways, and what you really liked about the process that you want to make sure to do again.

Right after eating is the best time to alter a recipe you're working on or trying for the first time. Being mindful of the previous steps is important, but this step is crucial for improvement. This is where those "Experience Points" we talked about at the start of this section come into play. Think about how you could do things differently, how you could make the process smoother, and how you'd like to tweak your recipe. As you do this, you'll find your skills will grow, your understanding of food and cooking will deepen, and your culinary reflexes will sharpen.

In short, you are Leveling Up!

It'll happen when you create a triumph of a meal, and it'll happen when you make a grievous mistake. The important thing is to keep your mind open, taking in the good and the bad so that both can be used to better inform your decisions in the future. Everyone starts out as a Novice in the beginning, but everyone also has the potential to rise through the ranks as high as they wish to go.

From Novice, to Apprentice, to Adept, to Expert; anyone can cook delicious food. I hope this outline of my core philosophies and guidelines will help you grow and Level Up at whatever pace suits you best!

Crafting & Stockpiling

Shoring up equipment and ingredients, creating your own stocks, and freezing meats properly are great ways to help control your budget and also reduce your intake of processed foods. While processed foods, like everything else, have their place in the kitchen, we've come to understand that a whole-foods-based diet is healthier for your body overall. While crafting and storing your own stocks and broths requires more time and space, the impact it will have on the taste of your food (and your wallet) is well worth the effort. Properly wrapping or vacuum sealing meats for freezing will ensure you have a ready supply when meal time comes.

There's nothing wrong with purchasing stocks, broths, and premade sauces from the store. However, making the time to prepare them yourself is a wise decision; not only for the flavor enhancement, but also for the Experience Points.

As with all things, Mis en Place plays an integral role in the process of making your own stocks, broths, and sauces. It's important to sit down and take a minute to decide what sorts of flavors you are looking for, what sorts of flavors you enjoy often when cooking, and what your needs for the coming week's meal schedule will be. You'll want to go online and purchase a quantity of either one-quart or one-pint plastic containers (the kind that you receive when getting soup to-go from a restaurant). Both options are affordable, come in large quantities, and are dishwasher safe so they can be used over and over again.

I also recommend getting some funnels of various sizes (for measuring and transferring stocks and sauces), a large colander, and bowl to match if you're planning on making your own stocks and broths regularly. Finally, do your research on where you can get good deals on the herbs and spices you plan to purchase, as well as the vegetables and any bones you'll need.

Taking the time to go through these steps and making sure you have the right equipment for your needs will save you money, time, and effort.

Let's begin by talking about stocks and broths. The primary difference between the two is a simple one. Stock is made with the roasted bones of an animal; the fat and meat are cooked off in the oven. Broth incorporates raw, uncooked bones with small amounts of meat and fat on them. As such, stocks will generally be darker and will be less opaque after straining than broths. Both are nutritious and yield delicious flavor when made properly.

Whether you use stock or broth in a recipe will be decided by what you are looking for in your finished product. For dishes like pot roast, beef stew, and chili, broths will serve you just as well as stock. When making most soups and sauces, use stock, as the flavor is usually deeper and the mouthfeel is lighter. Ultimately, it all comes down to what you prefer and desire for your dishes; this is another example of guidelines rather than rules.

Purchasing meat from the store when it's on sale and then properly wrapping or vacuum sealing it for freezing is a great way to stretch your budget as far as it can go. When preparing your meats for freezing, you'll want to wrap them tightly in plastic wrap, then again in aluminum foil to ensure there's as little excess air in the wrapping as possible. Air pockets contain moisture, and those lead to freezer burn when stored for over two weeks. Vacuum sealers can be a bit of a large investment upfront, but the cost is justified in comparison to the ease of use and the quality control it allows for your frozen goods. Always write the date of freezing on the package and make sure to use the product within four months of freezing.

I have many sauce recipes in this book, as well as a whole section outlining the different kinds of roux, their applications, and what sauces pair well with them. I'll also outline the principles of making a quality stock or broth from home, along with a table giving values for various ingredients and cooking times.

Take these tools, get creative, and most of all have fun!

Crafting

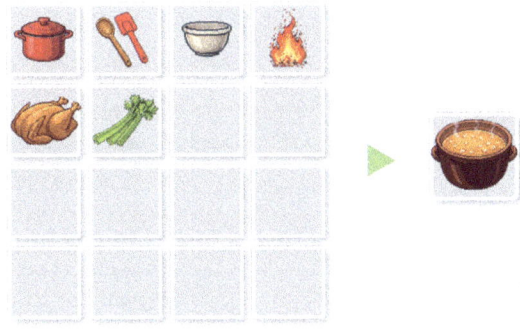

Stockpiling

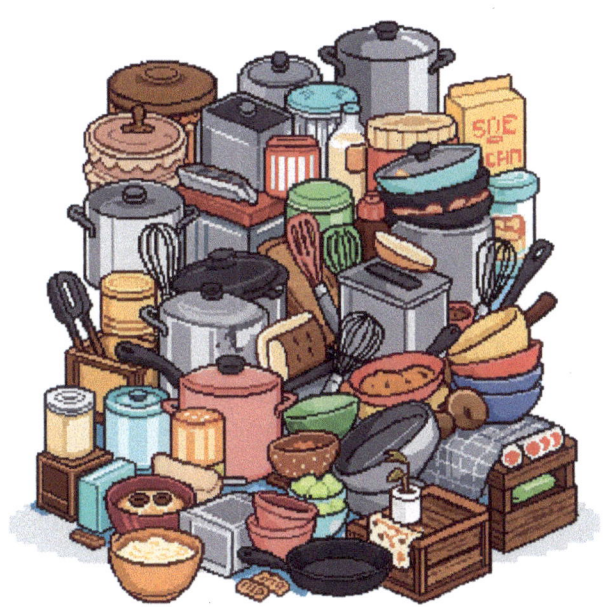

Concerning Roux

Roux is a mixture of equal parts All Purpose (AP) flour and oil. Melted butter can also be used, as butter is considered an oil in the context of the cooking. The type of oil used not only changes the flavor of your roux subtly, but also has an effect on its consistency when being held for future use. Roux is one of the most basic and essential elements of good cooking, which is why it gets a whole section of this book.

Knowing the proper types of roux and how to craft them is required for making quality sauces, gravies, soups, stews, and even pie fillings. I'll be breaking down the names of each type, their identifying characteristics, their method of preparation, and how to store roux in large quantities for later use. All of this is important, so I advise familiarizing yourself with this information and committing it to memory.

While my recipes contain instructions on how to make any roux you'll need during the cooking process, knowing how to make it ahead of time and store it properly will make a noticeable difference. Let's get into it then, shall we?

Roux Reference Chart

Type	Color	Average Cook Time	Volume/Weight Needed per 8 Fl. Oz.
Blanc (White)	Off White/Pale White	2 - 3 minutes over Medium Heat	1 - 1½ Tbsp. or ½ - ¾ oz.
Blond (Blonde)	Buttery Yellow	4 - 5 minutes over Medium Heat	2 - 2½ Tbsp. or 1 - 1¼ oz.
Brun (Brown)	Light Brown/Peanut Butter	6 - 8 minutes over Medium Heat	3 - 3½ Tbsp. or 1½ - 1¾ oz.
Bien Colorè (Dark Brown/Black)	Milk Chocolate/Cacao Powder	10 - 15 minutes over Medium Heat	6 - 8 Tbsp. or 3 - 4 oz.

Starting Point

Every roux begins the same way: reading the recipe to see what kind you need to make, how many ounces are required, and then portioning out your amounts of flour and oil. Since one tablespoon equals half an ounce in volume, and roux is equal parts flour and oil, one ounce of roux will require one tablespoon each of flour and oil. The ideal mixture will look like very watery sand when you stir it.

You start by placing the oil in your pot or pan and heating it over Medium Low to Medium heat. At this stage, it's important to know how your stovetop cooks and start on the side of lower heat. If the oil is too hot, it'll burn the flour. You're looking to gently cook the flour, not burn it.

Once the oil is gently shimmering (if using butter, wait until the bubbling is soft and almost stopped), you add your flour. It's important while making roux to stir it very often, nearly constantly. The higher the heat you are cooking it over, the more frequently it must be stirred. If the flour settles in the pan, there will be a slight separation and layers will form. The bottom layers will cook faster than the upper layers, and the potential for burning increases. And once the flour becomes burnt, even if it's less than half of it, the roux becomes useless.

Stirring very often or constantly, you cook the flour in the oil and watch as it changes color and aroma. The darker the color, the more intense the flavor and the lesser the thickening power. This may seem counter-productive for creating a thickening agent, but understanding this fact helps you understand the applications of different types of roux.

Your desired product will determine what kind of roux you should be using and how much. Obviously, the more thickening power the roux has, the less of it you'll need. This understanding is key as well, and is why I've given the descriptions of the four different types of roux that are used in cooking.

Roux Blanc (White Roux)

This is the first stage of roux development. Roux Blanc is the essential ingredient to making the delicious breakfast gravies that go over biscuits and fried steaks. Roux Blanc is achieved after two to three minutes of cooking. The mixture will be an off-white color, and the aroma will be slightly nutty, like opening a can of cashews. This is the sign that your flour has begun to cook, and for Roux Blanc, this is the point when it's done cooking. It has the most thickening power of all types of roux, so you generally only need 1 - 1½ tablespoons (½ - ¾ oz.) of Roux Blanc for each 8 oz. cup of liquid you are trying to thicken. Obviously, if you are using half and half or heavy cream, you'll need even less for thickening. It's used to create the Mother Sauce Bechamel, and is the secret behind the velvety texture of sausage, bacon, and black pepper gravies most commonly used for breakfast dishes. Of course, those gravies can be used for any meal...

Roux Blond (Blonde/Yellow Roux)

This is the second stage of roux development. It's achieved after four to five minutes of cooking. The mixture will have gone beyond the off-white color and will move into a buttery, yellow color and the aroma given off will be of a deep, almost toasted nut quality. Think toasted pecans or pine nuts. Typically, you'll require 2 - 2½ tablespoons (1 - 1¼ oz.) of Roux Blond for each 8 oz. cup of liquid you are thickening. Roux Blond is most often used for thickening soups and stew liquids, as well as making the Mother sauce Veloutè.

Roux Brun (Brown Roux)

The third stage of roux development is achieved after six to eight minutes of cooking. The mixture will move past the buttery color of Roux Blond, and begin to take on a light brown color. It will resemble the color of peanut butter, and the aroma will begin to smell less nutty, leaning toward the bitter side, like toasted almonds. This is when the needed values become less concrete; you may require more or less depending on your desired product. If you're seeking a looser consistency, then you'll usually require 3 - 3½ tablespoons (1½ - 1¾ oz.) of Roux Brun, while a thicker consistency will require 4 - 5 tablespoons (2 - 2½ oz.) for each 8 oz. cup of liquid. This roux is used to thicken sauces and looser gravies. Think of your classic turkey and beef gravies, as well as the Mother sauces Espagnole and Demi-Glace.

Roux Bien Colorè (Dark Brown/Black Roux)

The fourth and final stage of roux development. It's achieved after ten to fifteen minutes of cooking and near constant stirring. This roux is the trickiest to get right, as the line between properly darkened and burnt is as thin as a frog hair split sideways. Therefore, it's advised to lower the temperature slightly after the roux enters the Brun phase, since roux does not cool quickly, and the temperature adjustment will take time to come into effect. This roux will take on the appearance of melted milk chocolate, and have an almost earthy aroma to it. Think roasted mushrooms or charred beef. It has the least amount of thickening power, so recipes using it will require a lot of it. Typically, anywhere from 6 - 8 tablespoons (3 - 4 oz.) for each 8 oz. cup of liquid being used.

This roux is most commonly used in Cajun and Creole cuisine. Its distinct flavor and color are the reason that Gumbo and Jambalaya are so unique and delicious. However, it can also be used to make other sauces and stews if you are looking to impart the specific, deeply unctuous flavor it possesses into your recipe.

Using Premade Roux

About 30-60 minutes before you begin setting up to cook, remove the roux from the fridge and place on the counter. If frozen, remove the cubes you'll require from the freezer, place in a small bowl, and let rest on the counter for 1 - 1½ hours before starting the cooking process. When adding them to a recipe, at whichever point you would normally add your flour to start making a roux, just add a small amount (1 teaspoon is usually enough) of oil or butter to the pan and place your roux on top of that. Stir thoroughly until it has completely melted back into a liquid, and proceed to the next step of the recipe. Doing things this way makes recipes that involve either large amounts of roux, or roux that takes a longer time to cook, much simpler and faster to prepare.

Storage for Later Use

Making your roux ahead of time is a great way to cut down on cooking times. Roux can be held on the counter for up to three hours before refrigeration, and can be stored in an airtight container in the fridge for up to seven days before use. Another method is to freeze the roux, but this requires a bit more time, so it's up to you to decide which is best.

To store in the fridge, transfer the roux from your pan/pot into a heat-safe vessel (stainless steel, ceramic, or glass) and place it on the counter. Let it rest for an hour or so, until the roux has cooled enough so it can be placed in an airtight container and held in the fridge.

If freezing the roux, you'll need a tablespoon for measuring and an ice cube tray. The roux should be cooled, very thick, and easily scooped. Using your tablespoon stir the roux well and measure out the desired volume. You can make each cube one, two, or even three tablespoons, depending on the size of your tray. The volume you need is determined by the type of roux. If you're freezing Roux Blanc, for instance, you'll probably want to keep each cube at one tablespoon, as this is close to the measurement for how much you need for 8 oz. of liquid.

Place the filled tray in the fridge for at least eight hours, pop the cubes out, and place them in a labeled freezer bag. Now you can make a large batch of roux all at once, and then have your portioned cubes ready to go whenever you need them.

Stocks & Broths

Making your own stock or broth is very simple and rewarding. Not only for the additional flavor, but also for those valuable Experience Points you can allocate to help you Level Up! There are four components to every stock: the mirepoix (meer-pwah), the substance, aromatics, and reduction. Depending on the type of product you are making, the substance and aromatics will change, as will whether or not you use a traditional mirepoix. One thing that does not change, however, is the importance of reducing your stock/broth. Let's break down the importance of each component, and see how they all come together so you can get started on making and storing your own homemade stocks and broths.

This chart gives suggested values for the various ingredients needed to make 8 Cups (2 Qt.) of the desired product, so before reduction you will need 16 Cups (4 Qt./1 Gal.) of water. These values can be divided or multiplied freely to suit your needs.

Stock & Broths Chart

Desired Product	Mierpoix	Substance	Aromatics	Cooking Time
Vegetable Stock	Same as Substance	2 Lb. Onion, 1 Lb. Celery, 1 Lb. Carrot, ½ Lb. Leeks, Large Dice	-3 ea. Thyme, Rosemary, Sage Sprigs -6 ea. Parsley Sprigs -1 tsp. Whole Peppercorns -4 ea. Garlic Cloves	1½ - 2 Hours for full extraction
Seafood Stock	½ Lb. Onion, ½ Lb. Celery, ¼ Lb. Carrots, Large Dice	1 Lb. Shrimp Shells/Heads or 1½ Lb. Fish Bones	-4 ea. Thyme Sprigs -2 ea. Sage Sprigs -8 ea. Parsley Sprigs -1 tsp. Whole Peppercorns -3 ea. Garlic Cloves	2 - 2½ Hours for full extraction
Poultry Stock	½ Lb. Onion, ¼ Lb. Celery, ¼ Lb. Carrots, Large Dice	2½ Lb. of Roasted Chicken/Duck/Turkey Bones	-3 ea. Thyme, Rosemary Sprigs -4 ea. Sage Sprigs -4 ea. Parsley Sprigs -1½ tsp. Whole Peppercorns -3 ea. Garlic Cloves	3½ - 4 Hours for full extraction
Poultry Broth	½ Lb. Onion, ¼ Lb. Celery, ¼ Lb. Carrots, Large Dice	2½ Lb. Raw Chicken/Duck/Turkey Bones, meat and fat attached	3 ea. Thyme, Rosemary Sprigs -4 ea. Sage Sprigs -4 ea. Parsley Sprigs 1½ tsp. Whole Peppercorns -3 ea. Garlic Cloves	3½ - 4 Hours for full extraction
Beef/Lamb/Pork Stock	¾ Lb. Onion, ½ Lb. Celery, ¼ Lb. Carrots, Large Dice	3 Lb. of Roasted Beef/Lamb/Pork Bones	-4 ea. Rosemary Sprigs -3 ea. Thyme, Sage Sprigs -6 ea. Parsley Sprigs -1½ tsp. Whole Peppercorns -4 ea. Garlic Cloves	6 - 8 Hours for full extraction
Beef/Lamb/Pork Broth	¾ Lb. Onion, ½ Lb. Celery, ¼ Lb. Carrots, Large Dice	3 Lb. of Raw Beef/Lamb/Pork Bones, meat and fat attached	-4 ea. Rosemary Sprigs -3 ea. Thyme, Sage Sprigs -6 ea. Parsley Sprigs -1½ tsp. Whole Peppercorns -4 ea. Garlic Cloves	6 - 8 Hours for full extraction

Mirepoix

Classic mirepoix is a mix of diced vegetables consisting of onions, carrots, and celery with the onion having a 2:1 ratio in relation to the others. So if you have a ½ cup of onion, you would require a ¼ cup of both carrots and celery. This mix is used in a wide range of recipes, most of them French in origin. However, in the context of making your stock/broth, the mirepoix refers to the vegetables that will be used to balance the flavor of your product. Onions add acid and tang, carrots add sweetness, and celery adds a savory depth of flavor. You can use other vegetables than those three, just be mindful of the flavors they'll impart. Not all vegetables are meant to go into a stock/broth though. Until you have a firm understanding of the ways various foods interact and affect each other, stick to a classic mirepoix for your homemade stock/broth. This is an excellent chance to practice any knife cuts you want to improve on since the shape of the vegetables won't change the quality of your stock/broth!

Aromatics

The aromatics are the ingredients that impart more subtle flavors than the substance of your stock/broth. They're the herbs and spices used to add flavor to your stock/broth, along with garlic (or ginger, depending on the stock/broth). The aromatics are all bundled up in cheesecloth and tied off with butchers twine, creating a pouch called a "Bouquet Garni." The traditional blend is equal amounts of rosemary, thyme, and sage, with twice as much parsley, as well as whole peppercorns added. I have provided a chart with some guidelines for the values of traditional ingredients that would go into your stock/broth. Depending on what you are using the stock/broth for, your types of aromatics and their values will vary. Some specialty stocks/broths may not even include any of the ingredients of the traditional aromatics blend. This is an area ripe for experimentation, as the imparted flavors are not as intense as those produced by your mirepoix or substance ingredients.

Substance

The substance of your stock/broth is the primary flavor you are looking to impart, and this will tell you what type of stock/broth you are making. This is where the knowledge of that one key difference between stocks and broths is essential. If you are looking to make beef stock, you'll need roasted beef bones. If you are making chicken broth, however, the bones need to be raw with some skin and meat on them. If using only vegetables, it's always a stock, regardless of if they are roasted beforehand or not; vegetables have no fat and therefore, do not produce a broth. If using shellfish carapaces or fish bones, it's seafood stock, as those should have very little to no flesh on them. Make the product best suited for your needs and desires.

Reduction

Reduction is the act of using heat to evaporate water in order to concentrate flavors and thicken a product; however, thickening is not the goal of reduction with stocks/broths. It's important to keep an eye on your stock/broth as it cooks to make sure it doesn't reduce lower than your desired volume. Typically, you want to reduce your stock/broth by ½ for optimal flavor development and concentration. For example, if you are looking to make 2 Qt. (8 cups) of stock/broth, you should start with 4 Qt. of cold water (always start with cold water, that's a firm rule). Without proper reduction, your stock/broth will be less flavorful and intense than it should be. Of course, you can reduce it by more than ½ but more isn't always better, so exercise caution when making this decision.

Concerning the Mother Sauces

In the world of Culinary Arts, there are six sauces known as the "Mother Sauces." The legendary French Chef Georges Auguste Escoffier categorized five of the six Mother Sauces in the late 19th Century, with the inclusion of the sixth still being debated by some. They're so named because the vast majority of sauces that are made in a kitchen are derivatives of them. They're basic and can be used by themselves but adding various ingredients will alter them, giving them different profiles and names. I'll be providing the names, pronunciation, and several derivatives of these sauces. An understanding of these sauces will develop a deeper understanding of the more complex sauces you'll be making from this book or developing on your own. This is culinary knowledge at its most basic level, right next to making roux and knowing your measurement values, so study this section and learn it well.

Bechamel (bay-sha-mell)

A Bechamel sauce consists of milk, half and half, or heavy cream thickened with Roux Blanc. It's traditionally made by cutting an onion in half, piercing it with cloves, and stewing it along with bay leaves in the milk for 20 - 30 minutes. However, in modern times, it's most commonly just milk thickened with roux and nutmeg or all spice added. It has a lightly sweet, slightly unctuous flavor. This sauce is the base for sauces made when creating Mornay (a thickened cheese sauce) and Breakfast Gravies (sausage, bacon, black pepper), among others.

Espagnole (ess-pan-yoll)

An Espagnole sauce is a dark brown sauce, made with Beef Stock or Broth. Traditionally, it also includes tomato paste, but that's not necessary. This rich, velvety sauce is the basis for beef gravies, but is also the principle behind the thickened broth found in the best soups and stews. It's thickened with Roux Brun or Roux Bien Colorè, and as such plays a heavy role in making Gumbo, or the near gravy needed for a classic Roast Beef Debris Po' Boy, among other Cajun and Creole dishes. The beef stock/broth is the distinguishing ingredient of this sauce. So even if a sauce is made using Roux Brun or Bien Colorè, without beef stock/broth, it is not a derivation of Espagnole.

Tomato

It may seem surprising to see Tomato sauce on this list; the modern idea of a tomato sauce is one that comes from a jar and is used almost exclusively for Italian cooking. However, there's a whole catalog of sauces that stem from this Mother Sauce made from diced, pureed, or sieved tomatoes. That is all there is to a tomato sauce: simply prepare your tomatoes, add water, vegetable, or even chicken stock, and cook over a gentle simmer for 30 - 45 minutes until reduced and thickened. The value of this sauce is its versatility. Add basil, oregano, and garlic to create Pomodoro, from which a whole litany of Italian sauces can be made by adding different ingredients. Or take it down a French path by instead adding thyme, rosemary, and garlic to create the distinct flavor of the sauce required for the well-known Ratatouille. Or maybe instead head over to Africa and add cinnamon, turmeric, and mace to make a Tagine sauce, used in a variety of braised and stewed protein dishes. Even America has its own derivations of this sauce. There is Sauce Creole from Louisiana, utilizing chicken or seafood stock, thyme, and Worcestershire. And Cincinnati Chili, using cinnamon, nutmeg, and cumin to create a truly unique topping for spaghetti. There's no limit on the ways to augment this Mother Sauce, and that's what makes it so special and useful.

Veloutè (vel-OO-tay)

This is a light sauce made by thickening chicken, seafood, veal, or vegetable stock/broth with Roux Blond, and adding white pepper and salt. It's the sauce found in Chicken Pot Pies, and is used to make velvety, rich sauces paired with chicken, pork, and seafood. Add tomato paste to make sauce Aurore. Cook minced shallots with white wine and add that mixture to your Veloutè to create Sauce Bercy. Add Dijon Mustard to your Bercy to turn it into Ravigote. Any flavors that are delicate and acidic will pair well with this Mother Sauce.

Hollandaise (hall-un-days)

This Mother Sauce is made by whisking egg yolks (just the yolks, no whites) with melted butter and a small amount of lemon juice or vinegar in a metal or glass bowl set over a simmering pot of water. This is made challenging due to the fact that temperature control is paramount to successfully making the sauce. Too hot and the egg yolk scrambles; too cool and the yolks won't bind with the butter and acid. The egg yolks and butter provide fat that blends with the acid in the lemon juice/vinegar to create a temporary emulsion, and as such does not reheat well. It has a delicate, but rich and decadent flavor and a velvety texture. It is used primarily in French cooking; most will immediately think of the dishes Eggs Benedict or Asparagus Hollandaise. However, you can augment the sauce in various ways to adapt it for different purposes. Add a tarragon reduction to create Béarnaise, a sauce commonly served with grilled and broiled steaks. Or, use orange juice instead of lemon juice and create Maltaise, a sauce that pairs wonderfully with chicken or duck. Or, if you are feeling up to the task, reduce some Espagnole sauce with brandy and mix that in to create Foyot, a decadent and potent sauce that complements nearly any protein it is paired with.

Demi-Glace (dem-ee glaas)

The most recent Mother Sauce to be added to the list. Whether or not it belongs on the list is controversial. Traditionally speaking, Demi-Glace is made by first creating an Espagnole sauce and then reducing it by 50%. Hence the term 'Demi' (French for half) being in the title. When prepared this way, it's considered a secondary or derivative sauce of Espagnole. However, I was taught (and believe) that in the modern world of cooking, Demi-Glace deserves its own spot on this list for one primary reason: reducing any stock, broth, or sauce creates a product that is distinct in flavor, appearance, aroma, and texture totally different from the original. This reduction can then be augmented to make a wide range of new sauces. To make Demi-Glace, either make your sauce and reduce it, or reduce the base liquid for the sauce by 50% and then thicken it. Using red wine and beef stock when making your reduction results in a Bordelaise sauce. Adding fruit to the liquid as it reduces brings out deeper and richer flavors, like in my recipe for a Cherry Bordelaise (see Pg 321). Being a "newer" mother sauce, a lot of recipes utilizing it are not classically named. This is an opportunity for experimentation and discovery; just remember to use red wine with dark-colored stocks, and white wine with light-colored stocks. The ways this sauce can be altered are nearly limitless, and for this reason, I hold that Demi-Glace deserves a place on this list.

Honorable Mention: Mayonnaise

Mayonnaise is not a sauce; it is an emulsion. However, it's the basis for many salad dressings and dips, and understanding its properties will help you utilize it to the fullest. An emulsion is a stabilized mixture of two or more substances that don't normally mix, such as oil and vinegar. There are two types: Temporary and Permanent.

Temporary - An emulsion that holds its stability for only a short time and must be mixed thoroughly before use. Think of Vinaigrette Dressings used for salad; the water, oil, and vinegar separate into distinct layers and must be remixed before use.

Permanent - This is a bit of a misnomer, as there is no such thing as a completely permanent emulsion. Given enough time, every emulsion will separate into its distinct parts eventually. However, a "permanent" emulsion holds its stability for much longer than temporary ones.

I have included a recipe for Mayonnaise in this book on Pg. 145 detailing the various ingredients and their ratios needed to make this delicious condiment. Because of the variety of things that Mayonnaise can be altered into, it receives an honorary place on this list. You can change it into all sorts of things, but it's great on its own. If you've never had homemade Mayonnaise, do yourself a service and try it, just once. There's nothing wrong with sticking to your preferred store-bought mayo, but homemade mayo is on a different level for sure. From salad dressings to aiolis, get creative and enjoy this "Sauce" to its fullest.

Your Supply Chest & Equipment

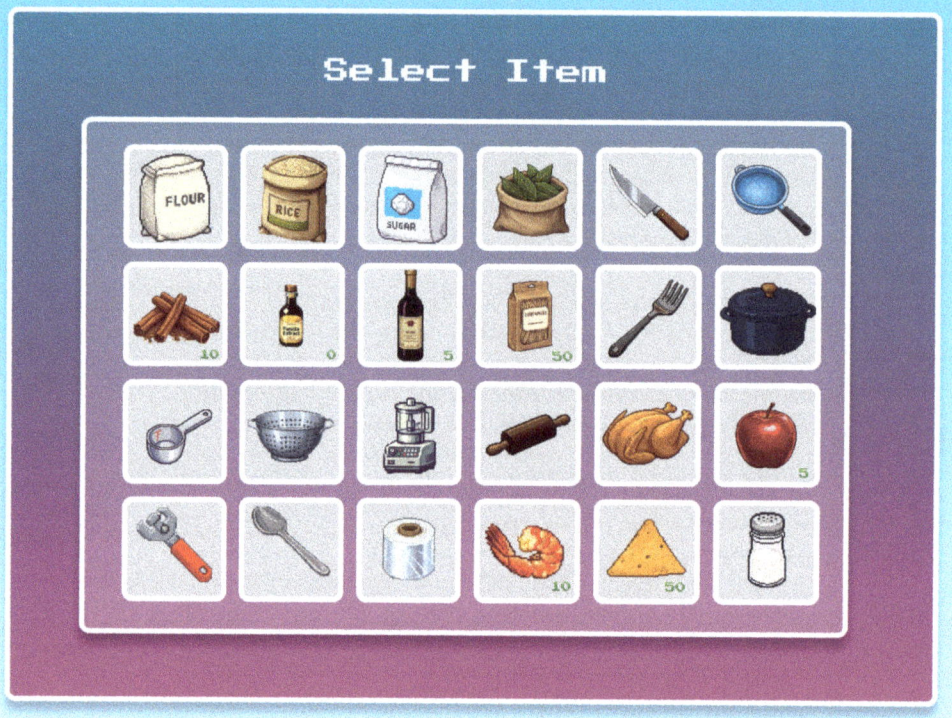

Select Item

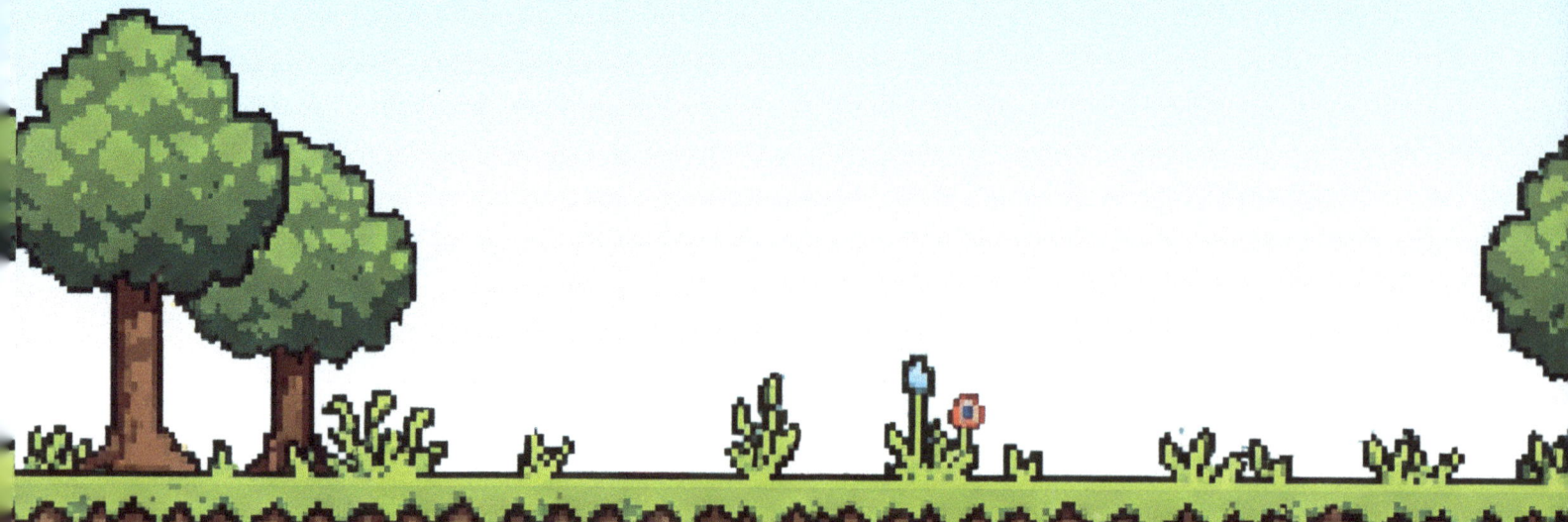

Pantry Staples

Here's a list of the most commonly used items in the pantry (Supply Chest) of a dedicated home cook. Like with most things in this book, these are guidelines more than rules. Keeping these supplies well stocked will reduce your time in the grocery store and keep many options open for menu items available in the long run. Having to buy specialty ingredients can be costly, so keep costs down by making sure your supply chest is well provisioned and ready for any dish you want to create. Not only will this help with your meal planning, but it also allows for action when inspiration strikes, you want to try something new, or make an old favorite quickly to provide comfort. As always, these lists are guidelines and are meant to be tools to help you decide what you'd like to keep stocked in your supply chest. These lists are large, and you don't need to have everything on them.

Dry Goods

These ingredients do not need to be refrigerated and have expiration dates that are far in the future, making it easy to keep them stocked in your supply chest. This is a basic list made from the ingredients that not only appear often in the recipes in this book, but in recipes in general. If you keep them well stocked and buy in bulk, you'll be ready for almost any recipe.

- AP Flour
- Baking Powder
- Baking Soda
- Basil, dry
- Bay leaves, dry
- Black Pepper, ground & whole
- Cayenne
- Cheap Wine for cooking
- Cinnamon, ground
- Coriander, ground
- Cumin, ground
- Dark Brown Sugar
- Garam Masala/Curry
- Garlic Powder
- Ginger Powder
- High Smoke Point Oil
- Long Grain Rice

- Mustard Powder
- Nutmeg, ground
- Olive Oil
- Oregano, dry
- Paprika
- Parsley, dry
- Red Pepper Flakes
- Red Wine Vinegar
- Rosemary, dry
- Sage, ground
- Salt
- Soy Sauce
- Thyme, dry
- Tomato Paste
- Toothpicks
- Vanilla Extract
- White Sugar

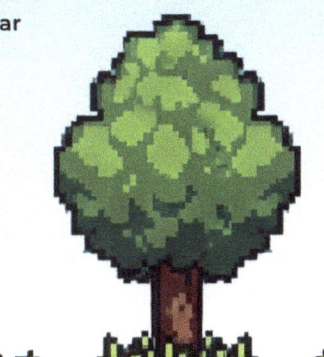
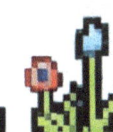
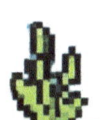
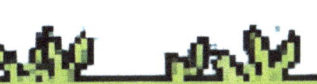

Refrigerated Goods

These ingredients require space in the fridge, so take the list with a grain of salt. Pick and choose the items you feel will be the most useful for you to keep ready at all times. Some items may appear to be obvious, but they're there because they're still useful to have on hand, and not everyone buys the same items regularly. There will be limited inclusion of ingredients such as onions, potatoes, carrots, etc. because there may be a whole week that goes by where those ingredients are not used in your recipes, and quality control is important.

- Bacon
- Butter, Salted
- Dijon Mustard
- Fish Sauce
- Garlic, whole or minced
- Ginger Root
- Green or Red Curry Paste
- Heavy Cream
- Hot Sauce
- Ketchup
- Lard or Tallow
- Large Eggs
- Mayo
- Milk

Frozen Goods

This section is entirely optional, as everyone uses their freezer for different purposes. Perhaps you prefer to have your freezer stocked with prepared items that help you manage time easier, or you like to devote room to storing meats for future use. Use it to give you inspiration and help you outline what would work best for you. Utilize the sale papers from the stores, and when a good deal on a certain product comes around, buy in bulk and store the excess in the freezer for later. Also, making large amounts of stock/broth and freezing it is a good way to make sure you always have some on hand. Making and freezing things like Gyoza, Spring Rolls, and cut vegetables for stock/broth is a good way to help save time and have snacks at the ready. All this makes sure you have food that holds for a long time at the ready, and it also helps control budget expenses.

- Already Cut Vegetables for Stock/Broth
- Bone-In Chicken Thighs
- Chicken Breasts
- Extra Butter
- Frozen Vegetable Medley
- Ground Beef
- Gyoza & Spring Rolls
- Pork Chops
- Rack of Rib Sections
- Stock/Broth
- Various Roux Cubes

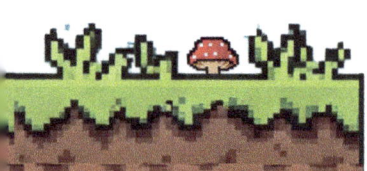

Suggested Cooking Equipment

Choosing cooking equipment can seem daunting, but it's a simple process if you approach it with an organized mind. Everyone starts out at the beginning, and everyone will start their journey with different equipment already in their inventory. When choosing equipment, versatility is paramount. Purchasing pots and pans of multiple sizes is always helpful and having at least one non-stick skillet is extremely useful. When purchasing non-stick cookware, it's important to remember that you need to take care of it; avoid placing it in the dishwasher, and never use metal utensils on it. Protecting that non-stick coating is vital, and proper care will save you money and frustration. This list will encompass the variety of pots and pans that are used regularly, and while it seems intimidating to have all these things at home, room can usually be made and you don't have to break the bank to have good and useful cookware. Shopping around in both second-hand stores and stores that specialize in selling the overstock of larger chain stores is a great way to save money. Good deals on quality products can be found in these places. Knives will be getting their own section and won't be included in this part.

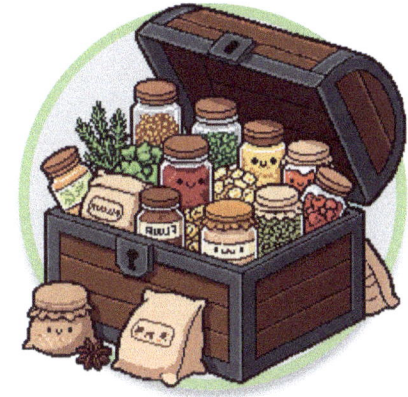

- 1 Qt. Sauce Pot, with lid
- 10" Skillet x1
- 10-12 Qt. Crock Pot Cooker
- 12 C Muffin Tin, nonstick x1
- 12" Cast Iron Skillet
- 12-14" Skillet, with lid x1
- 13"x 9" Baking Tray x1
- 13"x 9" Casserole Dish
- 13"x 9" Wire Rack x1
- 13"x 9"x 2" Roasting Pan x1
- 14"x 16" Baking Sheet
- 15" x 10" Baking Tray x1
- 17" x 11" Baking Tray x1
- 2 Qt. Sauce Pot, with lid x2

- 6 C XL Muffin Tin x1
- 8" Skillet, non-stick x1
- 8" Square Baking Pan
- A 2-3 Qt. Pot, with lid
- A 4-6 Qt. Pot, with lid
- Heat Safe Rubber Spatula x2
- Large Ladle x1
- Large Plastic Spoon x2
- Lg. Colander x1
- Lg. Mesh Strainer x1
- Metal Tongs x1
- Potato Masher x1
- Rubber Tipped Tongs x1
- Rubber Whisk x1

Suggested Prep Equipment

Having versatile prep equipment will help your cooking journey go smoothly from the first step you take. A variety of cutting boards, bowls, vessels for storage, and measuring spoons/cups are all very useful to have on hand. These things do take up space, so be mindful of your kitchen and think of the best way to organize it before making any purchases. The plastic to-go soup containers are excellent for prep work at home, are easy to find online, and cheap.

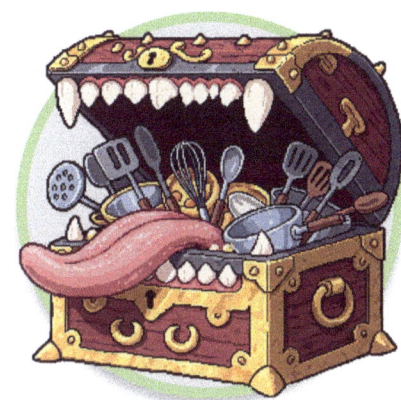

- 1 C Liquid Measuring Cup x1 (Glass Preferred)
- 1 Pt. Food Processor x1
- 1 Pt. Plastic Containers x4
- 1 Qt. Plastic Containers x4
- 15"x 11" Cutting Board x1 (Plastic Preferred)
- 18"x 12" Cutting Board x1
- 2 C Liquid Measuring Cup x1
- 2 Qt. Plastic Containers x2
- 4 C Liquid Measuring Cup x1
- 8 Qt. Bowl x1

- 8 Qt. Stand Mixer, Y-Paddle and Whisk x1
- Can Opener x1
- Cheese Cloth
- Cheese Grater x1
- Immersion Blender/Standing Blender x1
- Salad Spinner x1
- Set of Dry Measuring Cups (¼ C through 1 C)
- Set of Measuring Spoons (⅛ tsp through 1 Tbsp.)
- Variety Set of Metal/Glass   Bowls x1
- Variety Set of Plastic/Glass Airtight Containers x1
- Vegetable Peeler x1

Concerning Knives

There are many types of knives and the quality of them varies. A good knife set is imperative for any home chef, and choosing the right knives for yourself can be tricky. You have to consider how large your hands are, how comfortable the handle is in your hand, and how comfortable you are with various lengths. This section will cover the different types of knives, their typical dimensions and applications, and the variety of materials they can be made from. Use this information to inform your decisions on what kind of knives would suit you best. It may not be necessary for you to have a large knife set. Thankfully, they are usually sold in a uniform set, and you don't need to break the bank to get a good set of knives.

When selecting your knives, there are some very important things to keep in mind. The first of these are the three parts to each knife: The Blade, the Tang, and the Handle.

Knife Materials Chart

Blade Material	Wear Resistance	Corrosion Resistance	Dent/Chip Resistance	Edge Retention
Carbon Stainless Steel	High	High	Low	High
Ceramic	Very High	Very High	Very Low	Moderate
Damascus Steel	High	Low	High	Very High
High Carbon Steel	High	Very Low	Moderate	Very High
Stainless Steel	Very High	Very High	Low	Moderate
Tool Steel	High	Low	High	Very High

The Blade

This is the part of knife that cuts through food. It has a sharpened edge and a flat side. The edge is usually double beveled, comprised of 25 - 35 degree angles meeting at a point. Some knives are single beveled, with only one 25 - 35 degree angle meeting to a point with a flat side. Double-beveled knives are what I recommend for home chefs and beginners, as they're easier to sharpen and maintain. There are knife sets that are comprised of only serrated blades, and I advise strongly against using those. Serrated blades do hold an edge longer, but they are impossible to sharpen without specialty equipment, and they cut food by tearing, rather than slicing. This makes them unsuitable for preparing most foods, apart from slicing bread.

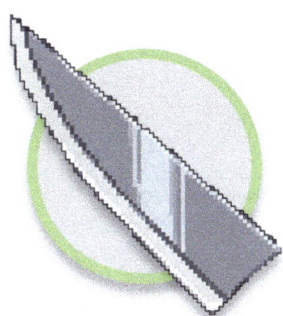

The Handle

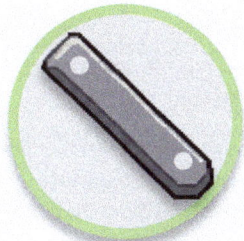

The handle is where you hold the knife, and finding one that fits your hand comfortably is important. Some handles are overly contoured, while others have little to no contouring to the shape of a hand. It's entirely subjective what kind of handle fits your hand best and can only be discovered by trying multiple styles in-person at a kitchen store. This isn't to say that the only place you can buy your knives from is a specialty kitchen store; quality knives are sold in all kinds of stores, and a higher price doesn't necessarily mean a perfect fit for your hands and needs.

The Tang

The tang is the metal that the blade is attached to and is wrapped up in the handle. Knives come in two varieties: Half and Full Tang. Half-tang knives have a shorter tang encased in the handle and are cheaper to manufacture. Full-tang knives have a tang that runs the full length of the handle and are usually held in place with several rivets. Solid metal knifes, where one piece of metal is used to form the blade, tang, and handle are my personal preference, as they're the easiest to clean and maintain. If solid metal isn't an option, I recommend knives that have both a full tang and rivets holding the handle to it. This style of knife handle is longer lasting and easier to keep clean.

Knife Block

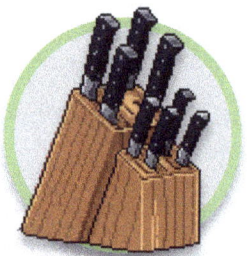

This block is where your knives are stored on the counter and is typically made of wood. If you have the counter space, I highly recommend having one of these, and there are multitudes of knife sets that come with a knife block for storage. They make organizing and storing your knives very easy, and help reduce the risk of injuries that can happen when storing knives in a drawer. There are also magnetic bars that can be mounted on a wall which serve a similar purpose, but this leaves your knives (and their blades) exposed to humidity and other airborne contaminants, so they are not suited for every kitchen.

Chef's Knife

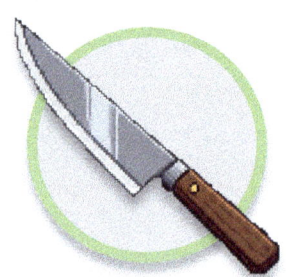

The most versatile knife in the block, this is the instrument used for all your chopping, dicing, and slicing needs. They come in a variety of sizes, with the most common being eight, ten, and twelve inches in length. Figuring out the length of knife that fits your arm is a simple matter. Just go to a kitchen store and talk with the employees there about your needs and ask to try out various sizes and shapes. They should have a cutting board you can use to practice chopping on. Focus on two things: the feel of the handle and the easy of movement with the length of the blade. The handle should fit your hand comfortably, not too small or large, and not overly contoured. The ease of movement is tested by going through various dicing, chopping, and cutting motions. You need a blade length that fits your arm well, and is not cumbersome to make room for or maneuver.

Carving Knife

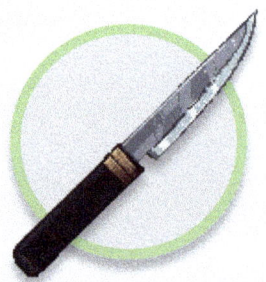

This knife is longer than almost any other in the block. It's made for slicing large pieces of meat, usually cooked, into smaller serving portions. Its utility is limited to that function since the blade is usually thinner and less curved than a Chef's Knife. This knife has its place in the kitchen, but is not a requirement to have in your block as your Chef's Knife can also perform this function. If you want to have a Carving Knife, I advise against choosing a serrated blade, as it will tear your meat instead of slicing it.

Bread Knife

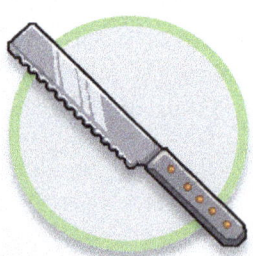

This is a knife with a serrated blade, made for slicing bread. They come in a variety of sizes, ranging from 7" - 14", typically. Bigger isn't always better, however, and a 10" - 12" blade provides enough length to slice through most loaves of bread. However, a shorter blade will still get the job done, so think of how comfortable it is to hold and handle the knife when you purchase one.

Paring Knife

The definition of paring is trimming an object (food) by removing its outer edges. This knife is short, typically 4" - 6" in length, with a smaller handle than the others. It's used for more precise work, such as trimming large cuts of meat, or removing small parts of food product for quality control or aesthetic reasons. It's a useful tool to have in your inventory, and I advise selecting one which has a handle that fits comfortably in your hand and is not too thin or short.

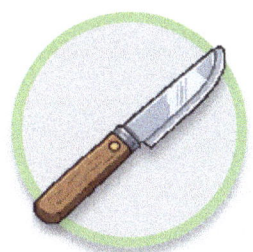

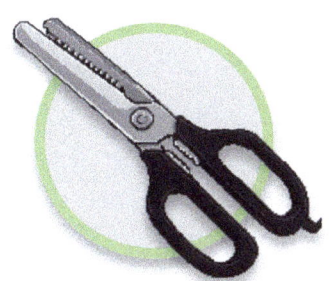

Kitchen Shears

While not actually a knife, they're usually included in knife sets when purchased and are extremely useful. They're heavy-duty, very sharp scissors that are versatile in their application. I recommended that every home chef has a pair of kitchen shears in their inventory. They're easier to clean and hold an edge much better than traditional scissors.

Honing Steel

This is the textured rod of steel with a handle attached that comes with knife sets. The definition of "Hone" (in this context) is to smooth and remove the burs that form on a blade to maintain sharpness. Honing your knife before using it helps keep the blade sharp and cut your food cleanly. To hone your blade, hold the knife in your dominant hand and the steel in your other. Place the base of the blade against the steel about two inches from the tip. Hold the knife so the blade is against the steel at the same angle which your blade is beveled. Holding the steel stationary and firmly in your other hand, carefully draw the blade across the steel while simultaneously moving it slightly down the steel When the whole blade has been drawn across the steel, move it back into position and repeat the process, drawing the other side of your double-beveled blade against the steel. If you have a single-bevel blade, you only need to hone the side the bevel is on, so knowing that is important. Start off slowly, being careful not to cut yourself. As you practice, this motion will become familiar, and in no time at all, you'll be moving quickly and efficiently. It's always better to do something slower and properly than to move quickly and make mistakes.

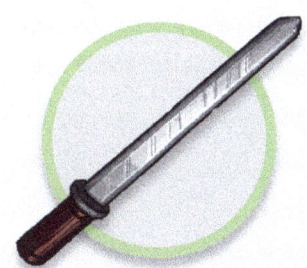

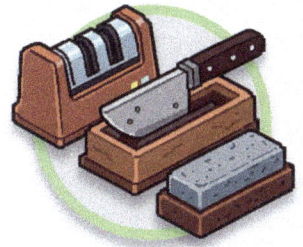

Sharpening Tools

There are a wide variety of implements that can be used to sharpen your blade. While honing is helpful in maintaining your blade, it's not enough to keep your knife sharp. I advise sharpening your blades every two to four weeks, depending on how often you use your knives. When selecting a sharpening tool, do a little research and pick one that fits your space and needs well. Whether electric, hand held, or a set of stones, pick the style that fits you best and can be stored in your home so you can make sure your knives are always sharp and ready for use.

Knife Care and Maintenance

As a cook, there's nearly no other piece of your equipment that's more important to care for than your knife. If your knife isn't properly maintained, the effects will ripple out into every aspect of the food you prepare. This isn't to say that your other equipment is unimportant, but your knife should always be the first thing on your list for cleaning and maintenance. Knowing what type of material your knife is made of will help you determine the proper method of care. For example, if you have High Carbon steel for your knife, it'll hold an edge for a long time, but is more susceptible to corrosion, meaning that it must be treated regularly with mineral oil to keep it from rusting. Inversely, if you have a Stainless Steel knife, it'll require sharpening and honing more often, but needs minimal care to prevent corrosion.

Most knives sold for home use are Stainless or Carbon-Stainless steel, and if you're purchasing an artisanal knife, then the specifics of the type of steel will be made clear to you. I've provided a chart to help you understand the commonly used materials, and how they vary from one another. This will help you be informed when purchasing a new knife or knife set.

There's one aspect of knife care that's universal, and that's how to wash and store it. A knife should never be placed in a dishwasher or washed with extremely hot water. The edge of a knife blade is a delicate thing, and water that's too hot will dull it quickly. A knife blade, on a microscopic level, is a series of juxtaposed ridges that over time form steeper and steeper angles opposite from one another. When you hone and sharpen a knife, you're removing any micro burs that form on the edge, and you work those opposing ridges back into a more uniform line. Very hot water from a sink or a dishwasher causes those micro ridges to become soft and meld together, thus reducing the cutting ability of your blade.

Washing your knife in cold or lukewarm water with soap and drying immediately after is sufficient to keep your knife free from bacteria and contamination. Drying immediately after is essential as well, especially for steel that is susceptible to corrosion. Once dry, the knife should be returned to the knife block or the interior of your kit for both safety and preservation.

Never use your knife on a surface that's not meant for cutting. Doing so can not only damage the surface you use it on, but also your knife. A chip or dent in the blade of a knife is difficult to mend, and will require special equipment and knowledge to repair it. Following these simple rules will help keep your knives sharp and useful for a very long time.

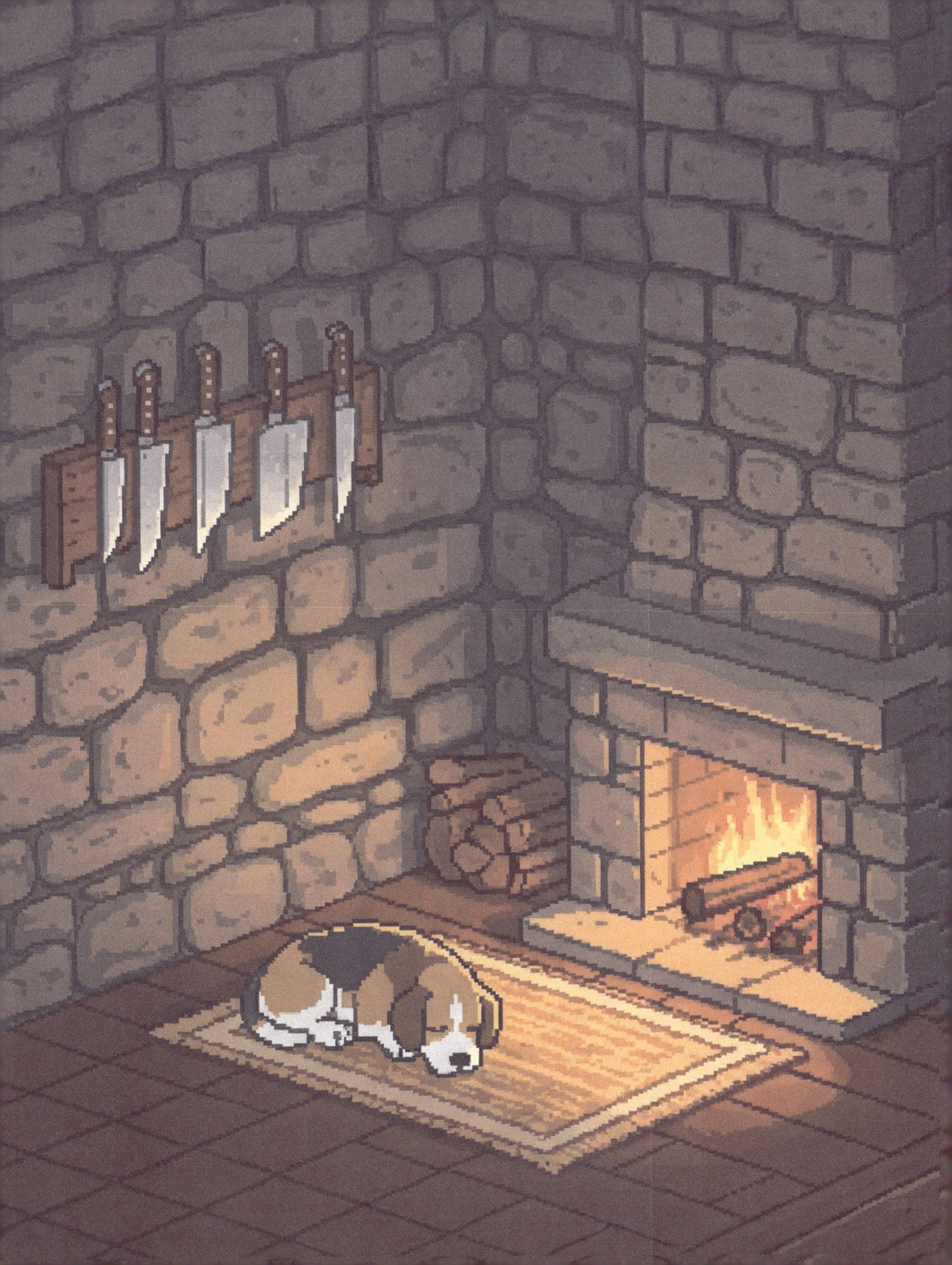

Meal Planning

Let's Eat!

One of the biggest obstacles to cooking regularly at home is planning what to cook and when. Going into a grocery store or market without a list is like exploring a cave without a lantern. Unless you went in with one specific item in mind, you'll probably end up finding things you weren't looking for. Taking the time to plan out meals for the coming week is important not only for your budget, but also for time management. Sitting down on a Saturday and taking just 30 minutes to review the sale papers from local stores along with your recipes to form a meal plan is a simple and fun thing to do!

When choosing recipes, it's best to focus on finding one or two ingredients on sale at the stores you most often like to shop at, or are interested in trying out, and then use those as the base for choosing other recipes.

Cross-utilization of ingredients, pre-made sauces, and leftovers are important for saving time and money. This might seem difficult to plan out and follow through with, but it's actually very simple. This methodology is one I apply every week, and you can too with a little determination. Before you know it, you'll be looking forward to doing this every week, and you'll see the benefits in both your home life and your wallet!

Cross-utilization means purchasing one ingredient and using it in multiple recipes. You can weave together a more cohesive menu, opening doors to trying multiple cuisines in a week. It also helps you better understand the ingredients you choose. I provide an example of proper cross-utilization with recipes from this book, along with a list of recommended pantry staples and cooking gear.

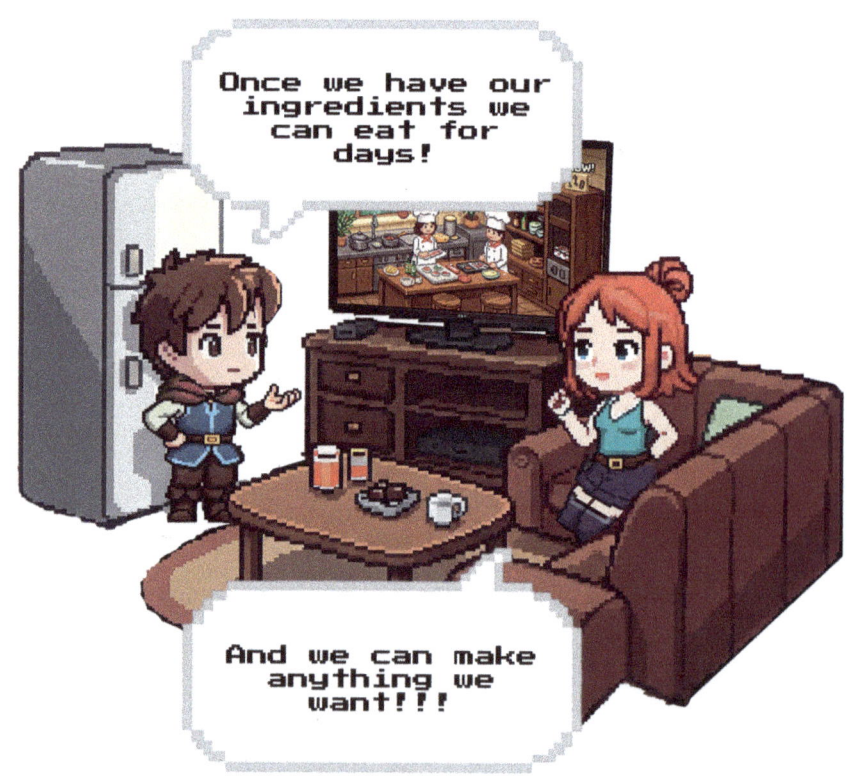

Once we have our ingredients we can eat for days!

And we can make anything we want!!!

Having a supply of commonly used ingredients will make your life easier in both planning and cooking. Tackle it a little at a time, slowly building up your reserves in your Supply Chest. Before you know it, you'll have a dragon's hoard of options to choose from! As for proper cooking equipment, this is very important. The gear you have will determine what recipes are within your grasp and what items you can search out for in your journey to help you try new recipes.

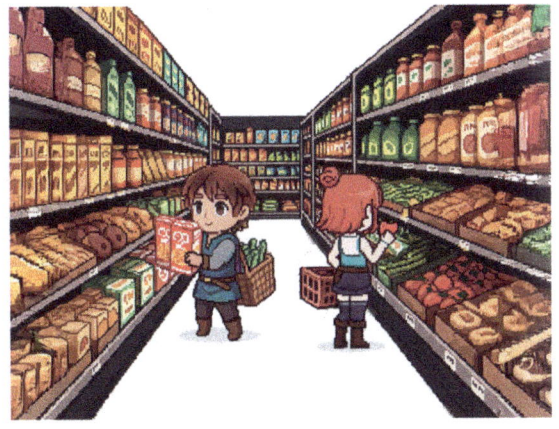

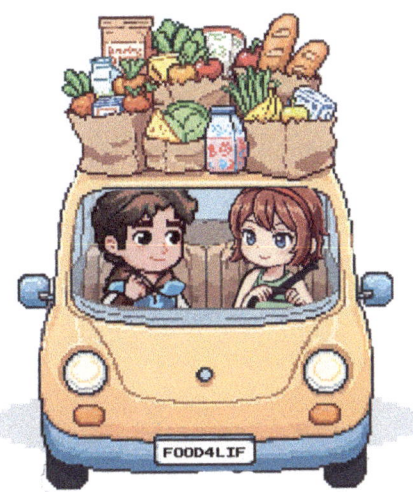

Meal Planning is a great way to get in touch with your food preferences, as well as the preferences of your family, friends, and others you enjoy cooking for. Looking over your supplies at home, the sale papers of local stores, and surveying the local farmers markets will flood your mind with so many ideas it might be hard to choose! But this is a good thing; it shows you're excited about this part of your journey! Making a meal plan on Saturday for your meals from Sunday through Thursday is a great way to begin. It gives you the time to go shopping on Sunday and gather all your ingredients for the coming week, and you can reward yourself on Friday and Saturday with unusual meals that might require going out of your way for ingredients, or taking the night off and using some of the money you've been saving to go out and treat yourself.

Planning more than five days in advance makes sticking to the schedule difficult and doesn't always guarantee your food will stay fresh in the fridge. Don't be afraid of your freezer either. Properly wrapping raw proteins, or vacuuming sealing them, and utilizing the space you have is a great way to stock up on meat when you get it on a good sale. This will save you money and open the doors for a wider variety of recipes for weeks to come!

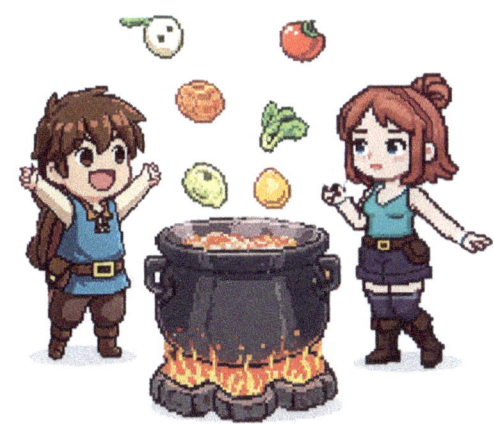

Meal Schedule Examples

Just ahead are two separate examples of how you can structure your meal planning on a week-to-week basis. If typing or writing it out in a different format is easier for you, develop that style to the fullest. The important thing is that you make a meal plan, stick to purchasing just those ingredients, and then follow through with the plan throughout the week. Hold yourself accountable to the meal schedule, and do your best not to deviate from the plan you put together.

It's fun to get take-out or go out for a meal, but it's not always fun for your budget or your health. Make sure to treat yourself every now and then by making room for getting take-out or going out to eat in your meal schedule to help prevent random alterations. The examples given will not only show you how to structure your grocery list, but will also be for two consecutive weeks, to show how to plan ahead and make time for long-term meal planning.

Each week will be Sunday through Thursday, with Friday being open for going out to eat and Saturday being open for a more elaborate dish, along with prep work for the next week's meals. The shopping takes place on Sunday; this is the most commonly available day to make time for it. Everyone's schedule is different, so those may not be the days you choose to do shopping and prepping. Find the best days for you to make and execute your meal plans!

Every dish in the example is a recipe that's in this book. This style of planning may seem restrictive to your schedule, but keep in mind this is just an example for you to form your own schedules. Develop a system that works best for you and enjoy the time you spend in the kitchen to the fullest! These menu examples are made with the frame of a well-stocked supply chest, so items needed for the recipes that appear in the Supply Chest section won't be listed.

Before making your own meal schedules, always take a minute to view your inventory, and make note of any staples that are running low.

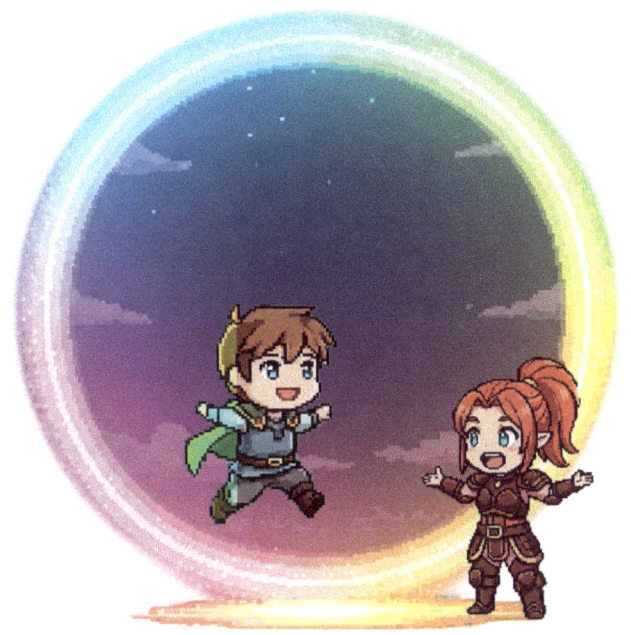

You will notice that the protein purchases made each week are utilized to make two or more different meals each. And the dry goods, along with almost all the vegetables, are used in multiple meals as well. This is cross-utilization in action. Purchase as few single-use ingredients as possible, and when you do purchase them, make sure you make a meal large enough to ensure leftovers. Every time you eat leftovers for a separate meal, you are dividing the cost of the meal in half. If you do it twice, the impact on your budget is divided by four. This is the key to maintaining a healthy budget and keeping food cost down.

Use this method along with the weekly sale papers at your preferred grocery stores to maximize the value of the food you buy. The sale papers and your arsenal of recipes are your best tools for saving money and never growing bored of the food you cook at home. Looking over the sale papers and using them as the inspiration for what meals you'll cook that coming week is both a way to save money and give yourself a fun challenge. Saving your large meals that involve a lot of work for the weekend, or your days off will also maximize your time management and help you choose recipes you are really excited about!

WEEK 1 MENU PLAN

Sunday

Lunch

Leftovers from last week, Make Summer Chicken Salad for the coming week, freeze one Chicken Breast and 1Lb. of Ground Beef

Dinner

Classic Burgers, leftovers planned

Monday

Lunch

Summer Chicken Salad Sandwich with Chips

Dinner

Old School Pot Roast, start cooking in crock pot in the morning

Tuesday

Lunch

Leftover Burger with Vegetables or Chips

Dinner

Turmeric Chicken Soup with Buffalo Cauliflower (leftovers planned)

Wednesday

Lunch

Summer Chicken Salad Sandwich with Chips

Dinner

Kefta Kebabs with Rice and Roast Vegetables (leftovers planned)

Thursday

Lunch

Leftover Pot Roast, make Ranch Dressing

Dinner

Fettucine Alfredo with Chicken, Side Salad & Ranch

Friday

Lunch

Go out and treat yourself, or Turmeric Chicken Soup

Dinner

Go out and treat yourself, or Turmeric Chicken Soup

Saturday

Lunch

Leftover Kefta Kebabs, prep for dinner and make 2 Qt. Beef Stock at home

Dinner

Roasted Buffalo Wings with Crudité

Advice

Take time on Friday to do prep work for Saturday's meals and place 1 Lb. Ground Beef in fridge to thaw for use in the next week.

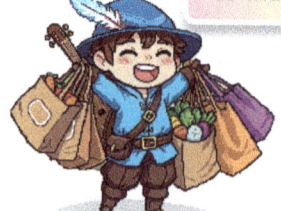

Grocery List for Week 1

Produce
- Apple x1
- Baby Carrots, 24 oz.
- Celery x1 Bunch
- Ginger Root, 1" piece
- Green Bell Pepper x1
- Iceberg Lettuce Head x1
- Lemon x2
- Lg. Yellow Onion x4
- Med. Red Potatoes, 6 - 7 ea.
- Mushrooms 10 oz.
- Tomato x2
- Zucchini x1

Meat/Seafood
- Beef Soup Bones x1 Package
- Chicken Wings, whole, 3 Lb.
- Chuck Roast, 3 - 4 Lb.
- Ground Beef, 3 Lb.
- Lg. Chicken Breasts x4

Dairy
- Heavy Cream, 16 oz.
- Parmesan Cheese, 3 oz.

Bread
- Fettucine Pasta x1 Box
- Hamburger Buns x8
- Lg. French Bread Loaf x1

Dry Goods
- Beef Stock, 1 Qt.
- Chicken Stock, 2 Qt.
- Hot Sauce x1 Bottle
- Mayo (if not homemade)
- Potato Chips x2 Bags

WEEK 2 MENU PLAN

Sunday

Lunch

Lunch- Ham & Turkey Sandwich with Potato Chips. Make Sweet Heat BBQ Sauce, Enchilada Sauce, Pomodoro Sauce, and Fluffy Ground Beef for Bolognese

Dinner

Fettucine with Bolognese Sauce and Side Salad with Ranch

Monday

Lunch

Leftover Buffalo Wings

Dinner

Dinner- Roasted ½ Pork Loin with Cinnamon Apples, Sweet and Sour Green Beans (leftovers planned)

Tuesday

Lunch

Ham & Turkey Sandwich with Chips

Dinner

BBQ Pulled Pork Sandwiches and Nanny's Coleslaw

Wednesday

Lunch

Leftover Pulled Pork Sandwiches. Place Frozen Chicken Breast in fridge to thaw

Dinner

Roasted Pork Loin with Braised Cabbage & Mashed Potatoes

Thursday

Lunch

Leftovers from last week, Make Summer Chicken Salad for the coming week, freeze one Chicken Breast and 1Lb. of Ground Beef

Dinner

Classic Burgers, leftovers planned

Friday

Lunch

Leftover Braised Cabbage and half of the Andouille Sausage, pan

Dinner

Go out and treat yourself

Saturday

Lunch

Leftover Enchiladas

Dinner

Chicken and Sausage Gumbo with Creole Rice, use the beef stock you made last week.

Grocery List for Week 2

Produce
- Apple x1
- Green Beans, 16 oz.
- Green Bell Pepper x2
- Green Cabbage x 1 Head
- Russet Potatoes, 24 oz.
- White Onion x2

Meat/Seafood
- Andouille Sausage x1
- Bacon, 12 oz.
- Deli Cut Ham & Turkey
- Pork Loin, 3 - 4 Lb.
- Pork Shoulder, 3 - 4 Lb.

Bread
- White Bread x ½ Loaf
- White Corn Tortillas, 18 ct.

Dry Goods
- Canned Red Beans, 15 oz.
- Cheap White Wine, 16 oz.
- Potato Chips x1 Bag
- Whole Canned Tom. 28 oz.

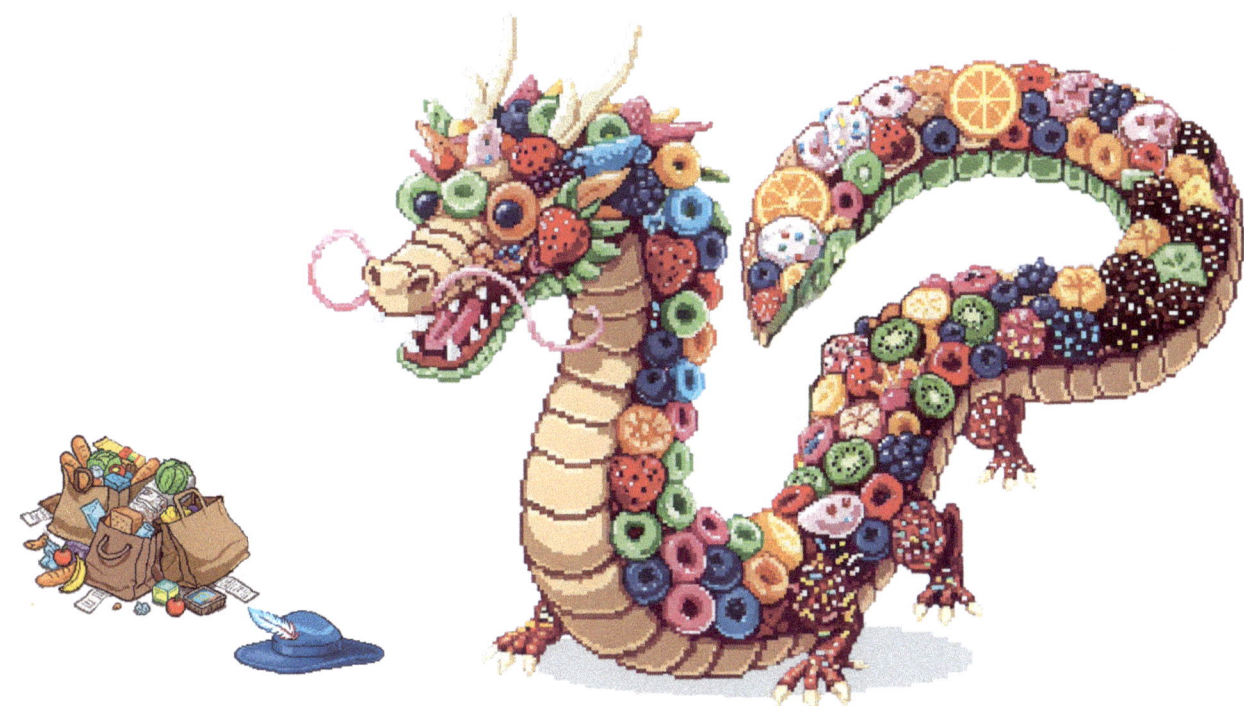

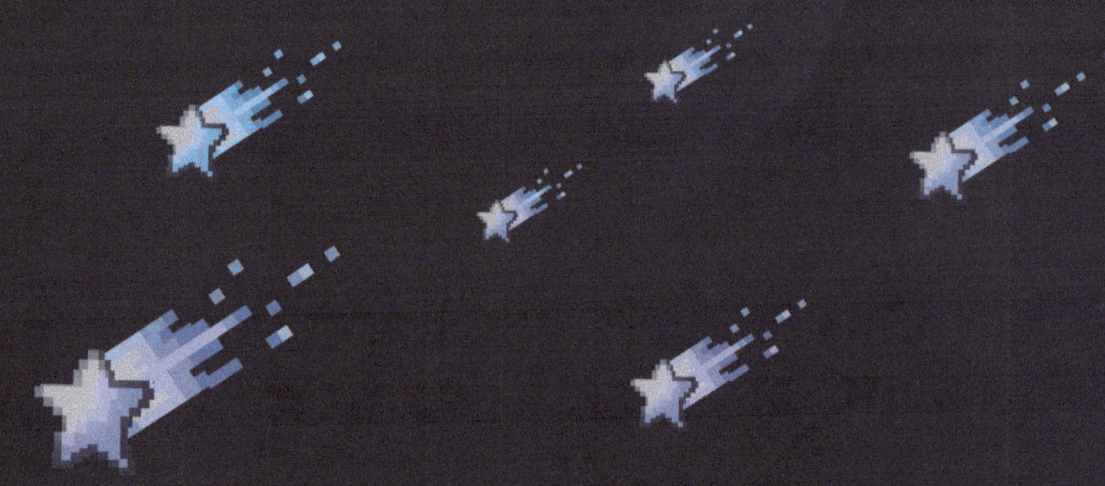

NEW HORIZONS
BECKON...

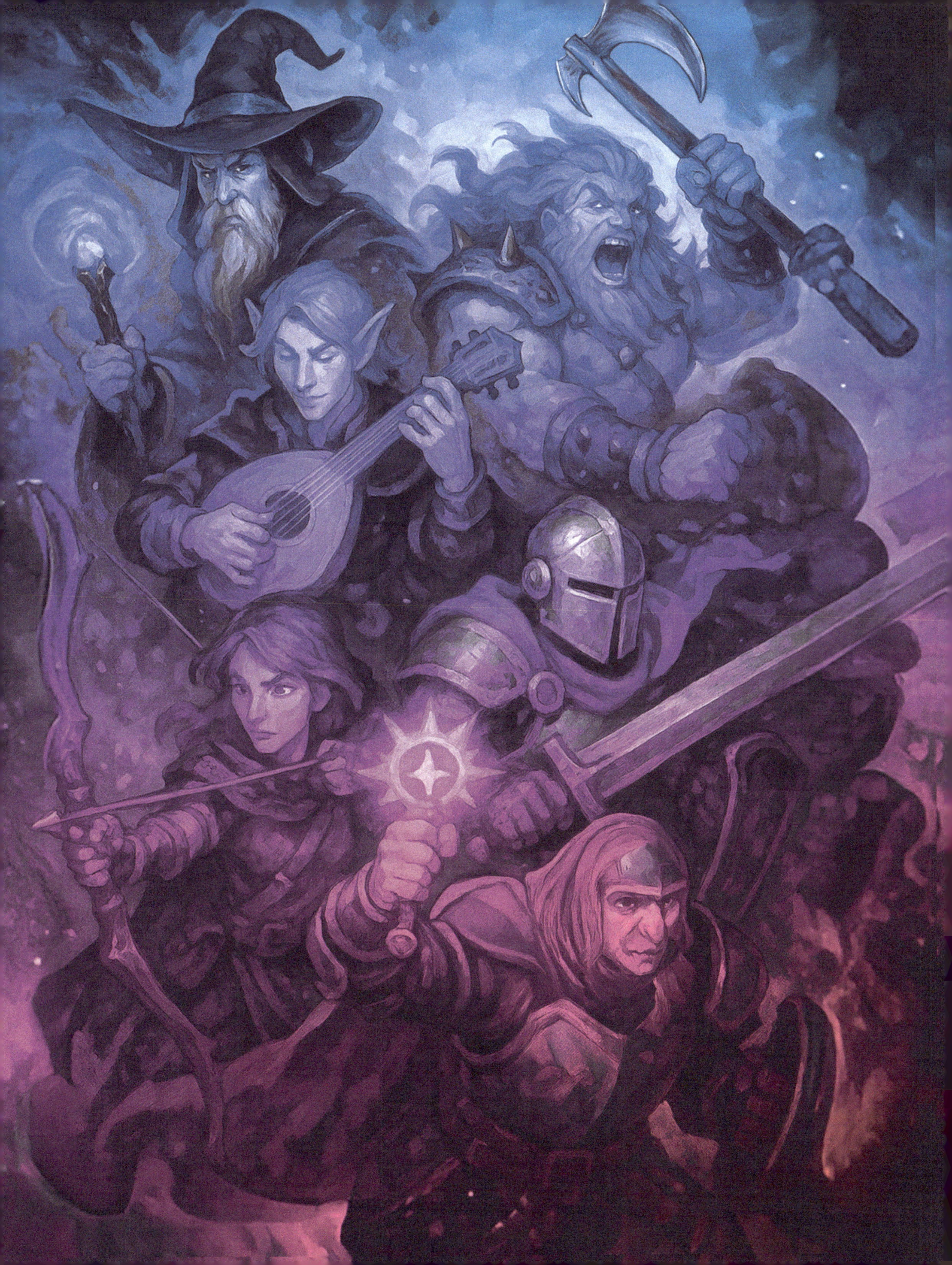

Choose Your Class

Everyone has their own unique approach to cooking; each style is their own. Think about what kinds of food you like eating, and what kinds you would like to get better at preparing. Knowing what style fits your personality best is the first step in your culinary journey. I've assembled a list of different "Classes" with descriptors that I hope can help you figure out what style you enjoy most. Then we can determine what skills you're going to need to help you become the best chef you can and make the kind of food you'll want to be a pro at creating.

The Skill Trees included in this book are going to help you focus your efforts on developing the specific skills you need to create the food you want to eat and share with your friends and family. Following these steps will help keep track of your progress as you develop your skills and Level Up.

Ideally, you'll pick your Class and focus on completing the Skill Tree for that Class before choosing a new one to develop your skills with. But if you want to jump around and develop a wider range of skills from various Classes that works too! You might fit into one or more categories in the way you feel about food. These Classes can be combined and adapted for your personal tastes and lifestyle. You don't have to travel down only one specific path. I encourage you to take the time to seriously consider which Class (or Classes) fit your personality best and then use that knowledge to set out on your own journey into the world of culinary arts!

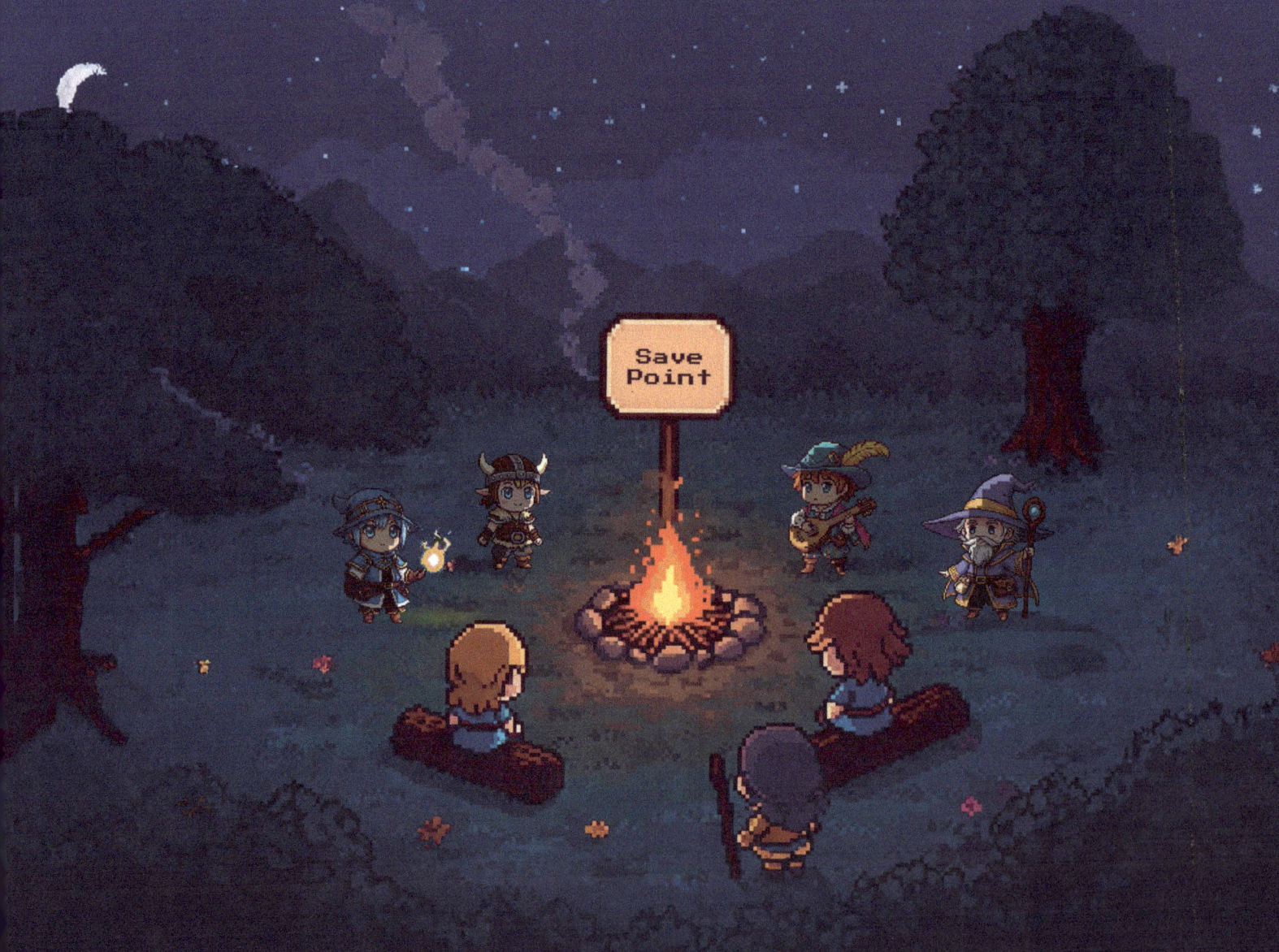

Barbarian

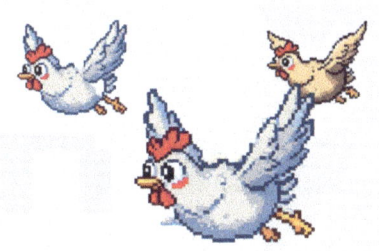

The Barbarian is all about large portions, robust flavors, and making sure no one walks away hungry and have leftovers to spare. If you enjoy large, hearty, stick to your ribs meals, the Barbarian Class is the path to walk. Cooking meals with a focus on making the protein component shine, the sides are chosen not just for their added nutrition, but also to complement the main item to the utmost.

You don't shy away from extra seasoning, adding sauces, or cramming your plate as full as you can. The large recipes you make are not only enjoyed that meal, but in future meals as well. All that extra food means your table is always filled, and you never have to ask yourself "Do I have anything to eat?" You find yourself drawn to the more traditional recipes with little extra flair and embellishment needed. Intense flavors and a focus on making sure no one walks away hungry sets this Class apart.

This Class can grow quickly, due to the nature of the food you enjoy creating and eating. It pairs well with The Ranger and The Bard Classes.

Cooking Style

Rustic, Protein-Centric, Large Portions

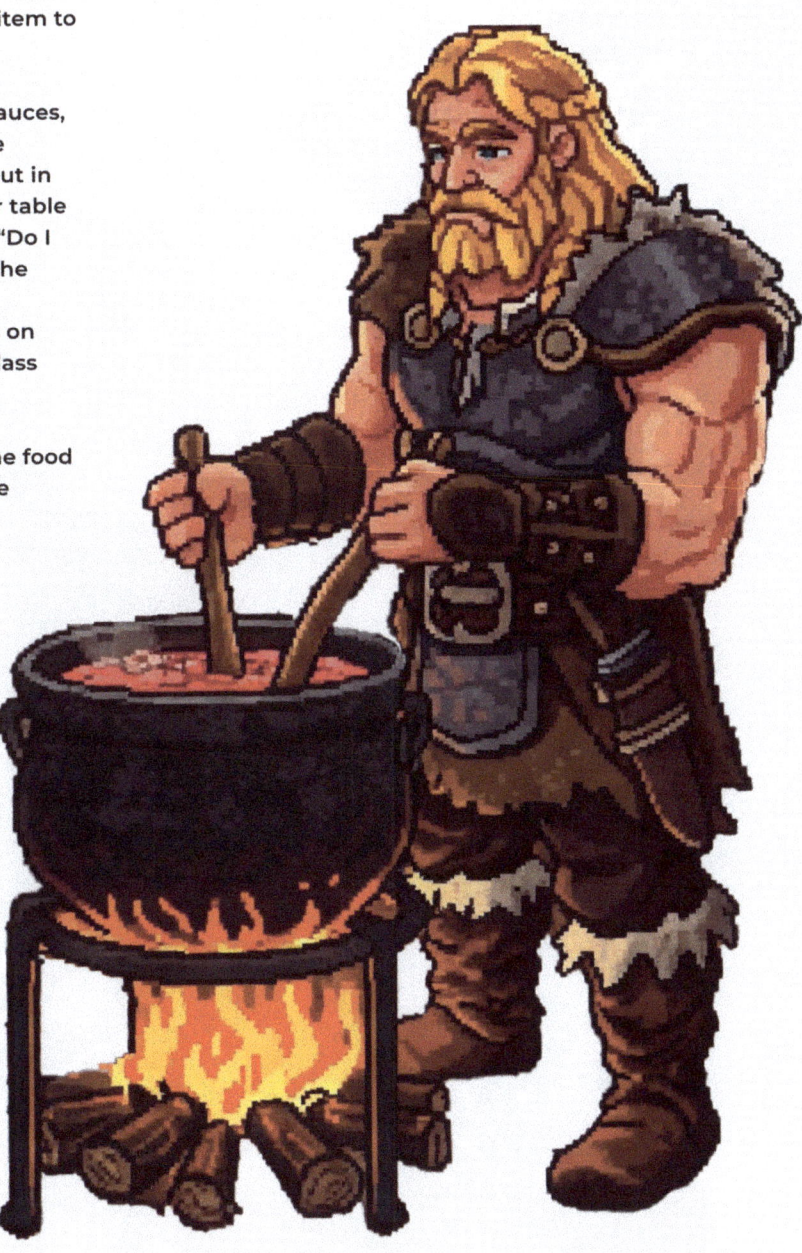

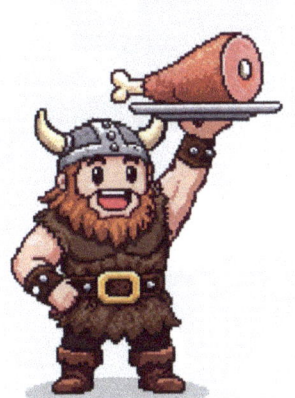

Bard

The Bard is the party member who lifts the spirts of others, using their skills to bolster the spirit and create an environment of success. If you enjoy being the source of entertainment and joy throughout an evening, then The Bard is your Class of choice. When you cook for yourself, it's usually to practice and develop new recipes that you hope to cook for your family and friends. You enjoy making large amounts of food to feed crowds, and pairing your foods with a unique atmosphere and music brings you a sense of accomplishment. The extra work required to make these large amounts of food, and the clean up afterward, is a small price to pay when you compare it to the satisfaction you feel when you see people enjoying the experience you've crafted. Using your talents to lift the spirits and fill the bellies of those around you is your focus. This Class is a bit slower to grow than the others, so it pairs well with faster growing Classes, such as The Knight or the Ranger.

Cooking Style

Group-Minded, Lively, Fashionable

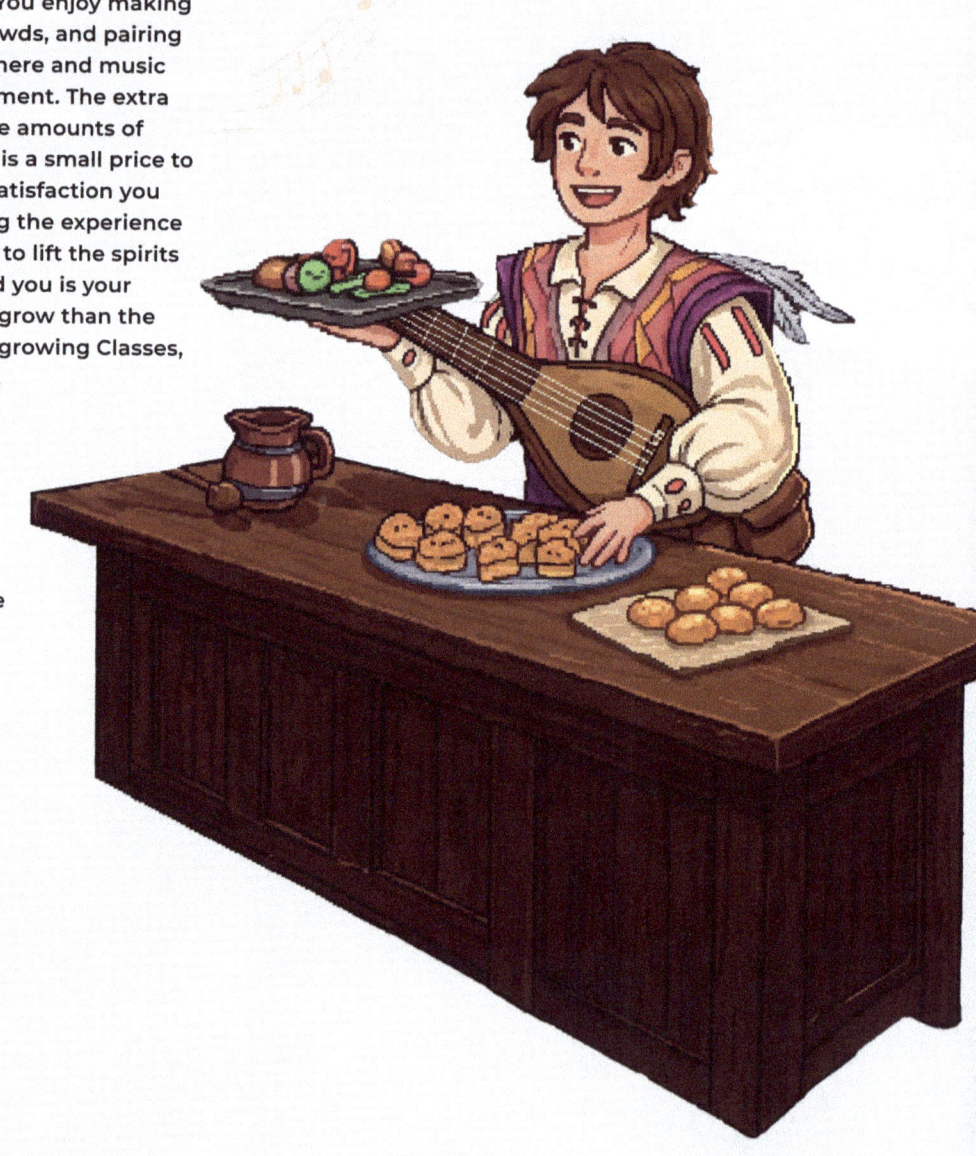

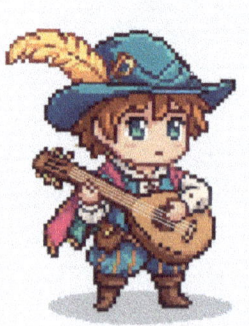

Cleric

The Cleric works tirelessly to keep those they adventure with and live beside healthy and feeling good. If you enjoy knowing that the food you are preparing and serving is healthy and conscious of nutritional needs, The Cleric may be the Class you choose. Clerics enjoy knowing what effects the food they prepare will have on the body and want to utilize that to the fullest. A focus on reducing unhealthy components and finding healthier alternatives to use in recipes is your passion. To you, there is no better feeling than when you prepare a dish that both tastes delicious and is good for you. Using food to aid in a diner's health is a passion you have. There may be people in your life who have dietary restrictions for health reasons, and they are the ones you Level Up for. A detailed study of foods, spices, and herbs (and their effects on the body) is imperative for this Class, so it requires a bit more effort than some of the others, but that is no obstacle for the committed Cleric. This Class grows moderately, and by its nature pairs well with The Ranger Class.

Cooking Style

Health-Conscious, Mindful, Adaptive

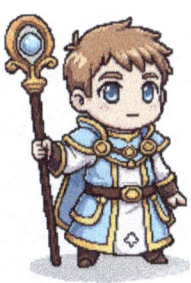

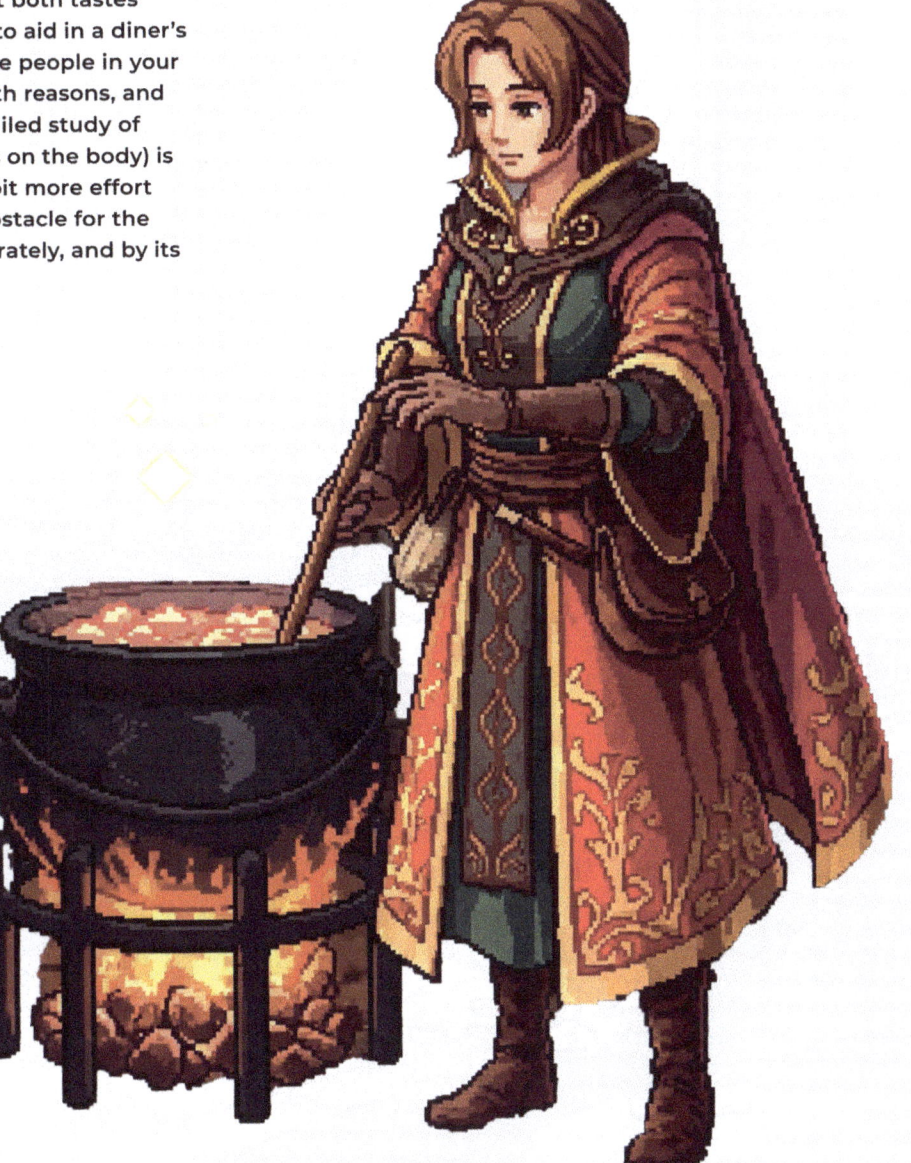

Knight

The Knight is dedicated and orderly, enjoying the regiments and well-learned courses of action needed for consistency. You don't seek intensive and complicated recipes until you are sure of your skill, and when moving into uncharted territory, you do so with a prepared mind and a set of well-maintained equipment. The Knight enjoys finding recipes they think they and others will enjoy and following the recipe to the letter, honing their skills so that they can advance in level at a respectable rate. Experimentation is not something you pursue, and instead, you seek to establish a regiment when making recipes that allows you to consistently prepare the same dish time and again. Your list of tried-and-true standbys will grow as you Level Up, the recipes becoming second nature to you when mealtime comes, and memorizing the methods to create them will come naturally to you. This Class is one that's well-suited for those taking their first journey into the culinary world. This is a quick growing Class, as it applies skills that are utilized by nearly all the others, and pairs with any other Class, and especially well with The Bard Class.

Cooking Style

Organized, Prepared, Dedicated

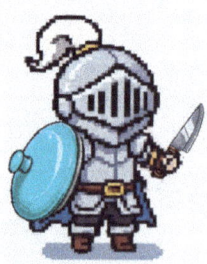

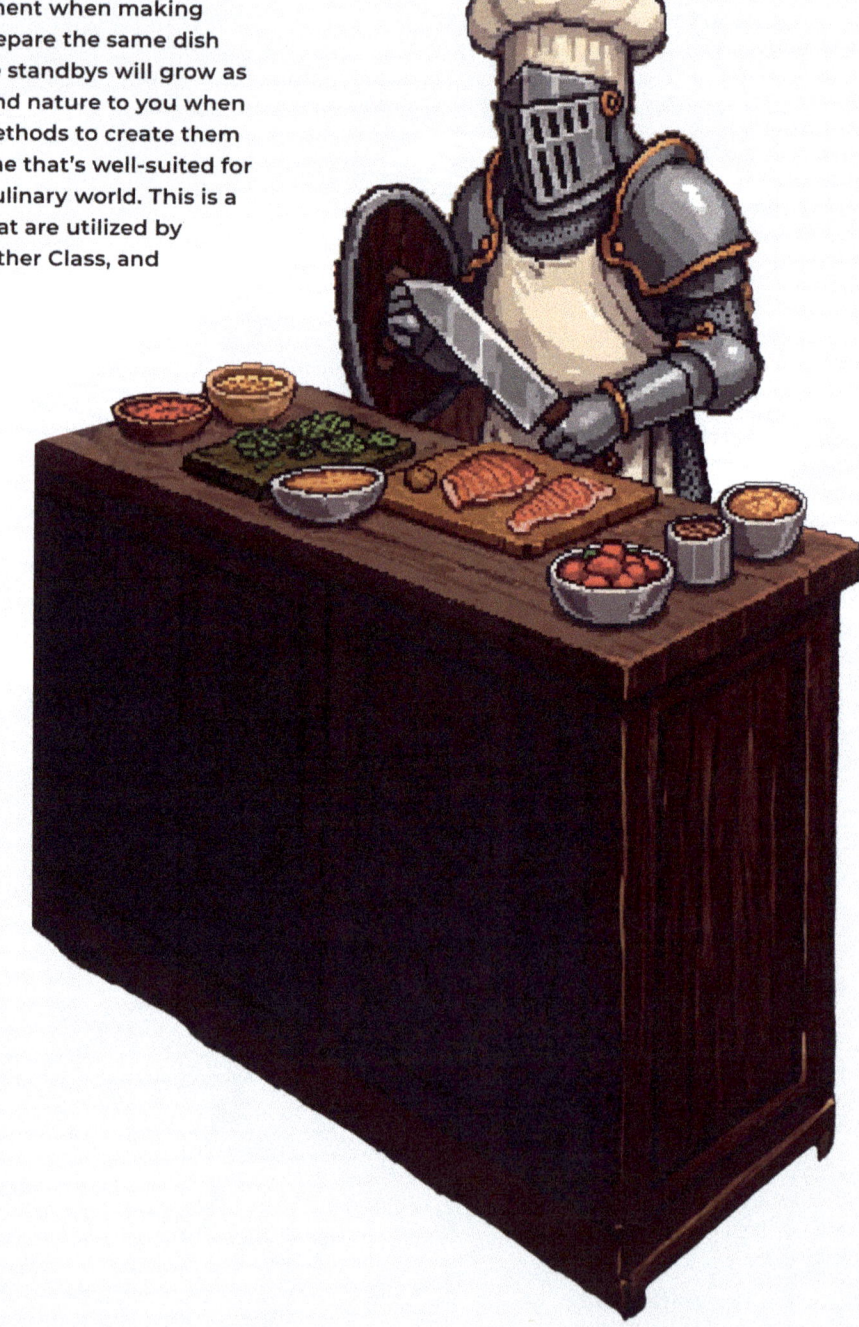

Ranger

The Ranger is used to setting out into the wild, preparing the foods they know, trust, and can gather themselves. You enjoy cooking with whole foods (minimally processed) that you purchase from local farmers when possible and food you've grown yourself when the seasons allow. If this is you, The Ranger is where your heart lies. You'll focus on preparing each of the different components of your meals yourself, and your meals will include unadulterated food that you are in control of. The challenge of making your own pie crust or making large amounts of stock in advance is fun for you because you know the outcome is worth all the effort. And when you go to the market to pick out your ingredients by hand, you feel truly connected to the culinary world and to the food you're going to make. Trying new ingredients that you may have never seen before, or only heard about, is an integral aspect of this Class, so it's suited for those with an intrepid spirit. This Class grows at a quicker rate, and pairs well with The Cleric and The Barbarian, as well as the Knight.

Cooking Style
Resourceful, Adventurous, Hands-On

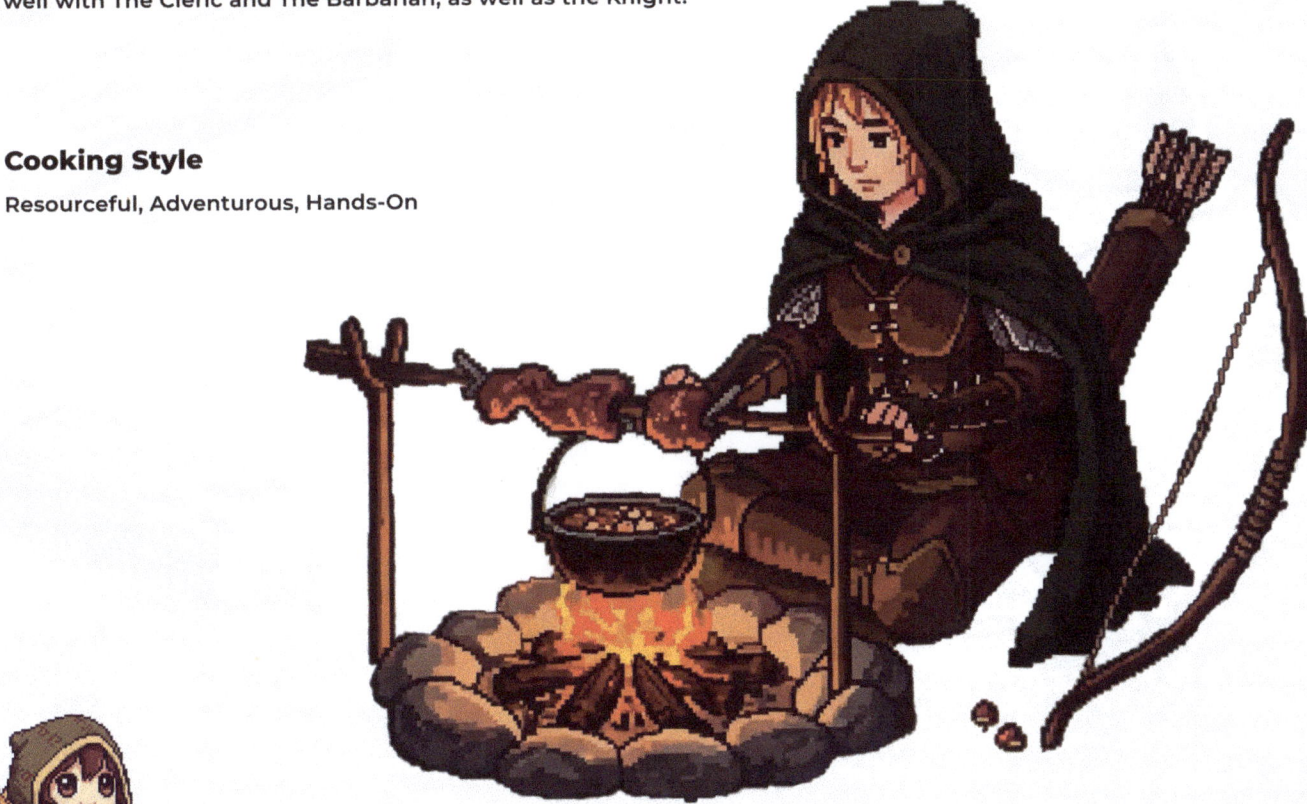

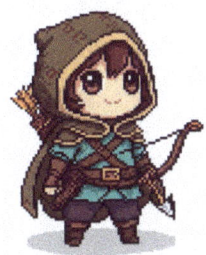

Wizard

The Wizard has taken the time to study, to experiment, to take detailed notes of both their successes and misfortunes, all in the pursuit of creativity and knowledge. If you take delight in experimentation and finding new combinations of flavors and textures that elevate your dishes, then The Wizard is your Class of choice. Taking a recipe, learning it well, then finding ways to augment and change the subtle aspects that can transform the dish is your joy. You love the feeling of coming up with novel ways to prepare and flavor your dishes, and you take pride in sharing your findings with others. This Class requires a fair amount of dedication as understanding a recipe deeply is not something that is done rapidly, and it's guaranteed that you will need to try some things multiple times. Perhaps you'll have an idea that leads you down a road you've never travelled or gives you a new perspective on cooking. These experiences are what you look for, weighing your successes and failures equally. However, this is what draws you to cooking, and the adventures you have in your kitchen is time well spent. This is a moderate growth Class and pairs well with The Cleric and The Ranger.

Cooking Style

Creative, Studious, Multifaceted

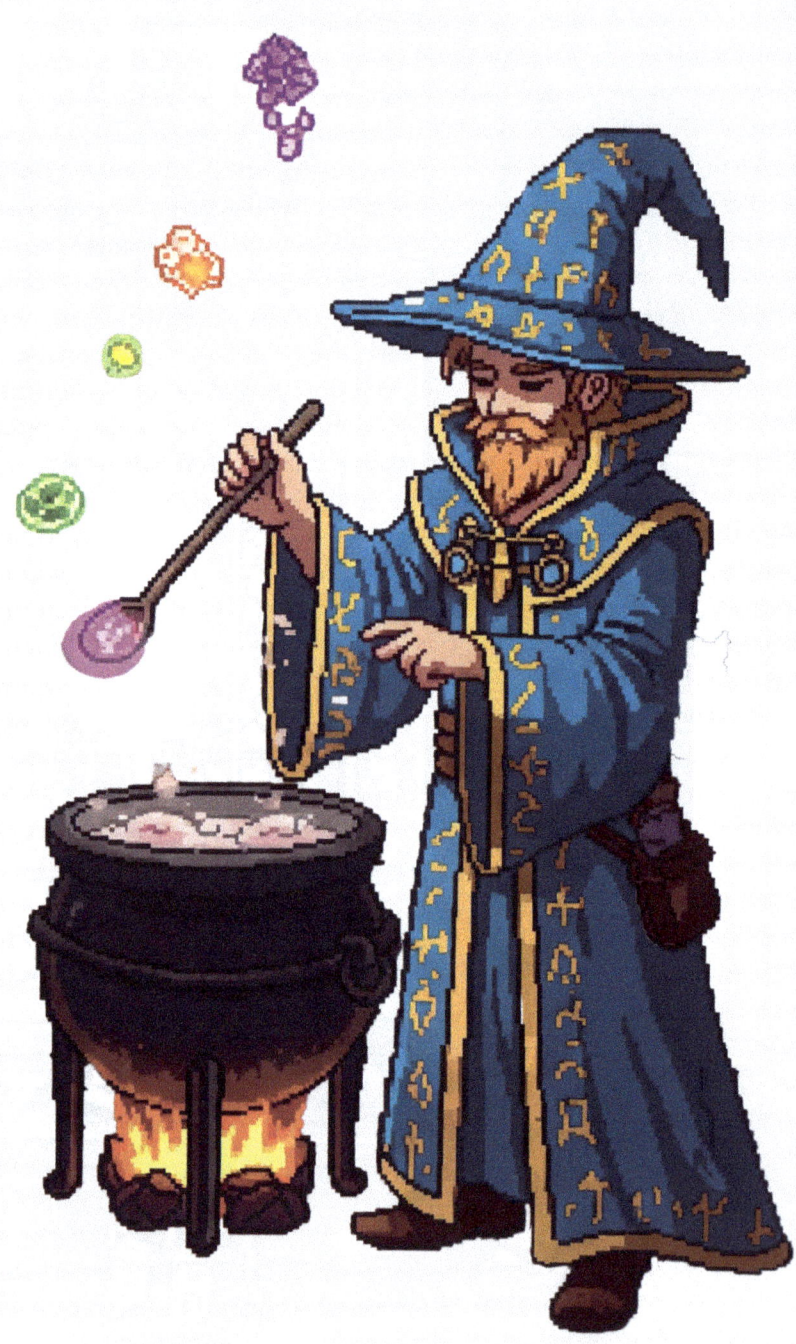

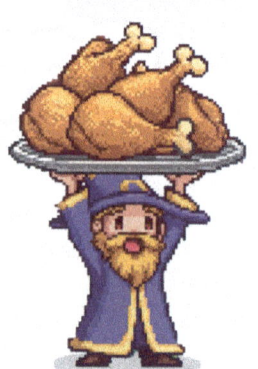

CHOOSE YOUR CLASS

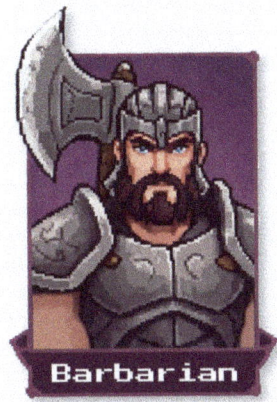

Barbarian

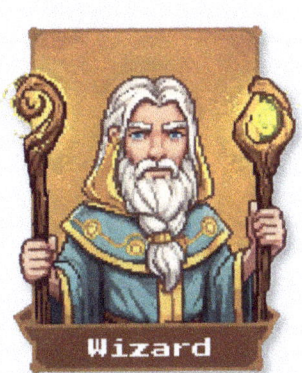

Wizard

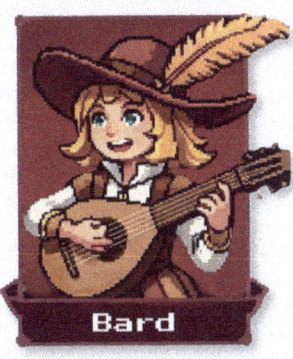

Bard

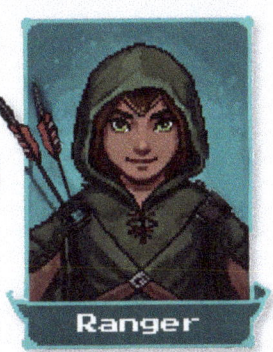

Ranger

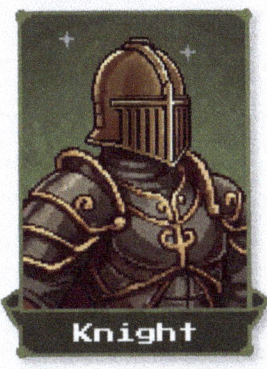

Knight

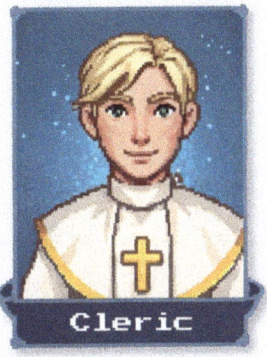

Cleric

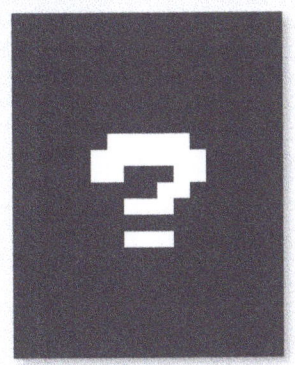

LVLUPCookBook Channel

BEGINNER

A New Day Dawns

Everyone starts out at the Beginning. If this is your first foray into the wide world of cooking, you're right at home. If you've been cooking for a while and are confident in your abilities, take a moment to remember where you started. It never hurts to brush up on techniques and skills that were acquired long ago. And if you're looking to develop these techniques for the first time, pay attention. The Beginner Skill Tree will be the foundation for all the others, as the skills laid out in it are universally used, and work to provide a solid foundation for you to grow into whatever form best suits you.

LEVEL 1

Achievements Unlocked

Good Job, Squire • You know how to properly handle a knife

Chopped • You're familiar with small dice, dice, and large dice, as well as mincing

Well Stocked • You can now make your own Stocks and Broths

A New Day Has Dawned • You've prepared your first full meal with recipes from the book!

Concerning Skill Trees

The Skill Trees in this book are not meant to be weekly meal plans; there are guidelines for that in a previous section. They're a list of actions and goals that should be utilized to challenge yourself and chart your progress as you Level Up in the kitchen. They are not designed to be completed in one or even two weeks but are meant to be referenced as you plan your weekly meal schedules, using recipes you choose from the book to accomplish the challenges set for your chosen Class to help you chart your progress. This means that time, one of the most crucial ingredients in any recipe, is vital to getting the most out of these Skill Trees. Sitting down and powering through the Skill Trees will certainly grant you a lot of Experience Points, but you will be robbing yourself of valuable development time for your skills by not cooking nearly as many recipes.

Think of these Skill Trees as markers to allow yourself to see how far you've come on your journey. The tasks and challenges outlined in them should be attempted as you feel ready. As you climb up the tree, the slower going it'll be but don't feel discouraged, this is the natural course of things when you Level Up. Whether through the necessity of proper planning, or from reviewing your accomplishments and realizing you still need to Level Up a bit before attempting a challenge again, time will pass between your ascension to the next level and new sets of challenges. Some of them may seem like impossible boss battles, but with diligence and varied exploration into the world of cooking, there is no challenge too great for you to overcome.

In short, following a Skill Tree from start to finish in a short time is not the intended way to utilize it. These Trees are meant to be studied and combined; building your character to have multi-class skills is a great way to broaden your knowledge and talent base as a cook, as well as make progress that you can actualize and see in yourself. However, it does take more time. The challenges are meant to be spaced apart from one another, and by doing so, you allow yourself and your skills to grow and power up, unlocking your true potential. Using these Skill Trees as benchmarks will yield much more Experience Points than by trying to grind your way through the levels. Creating meal plans using the recipes in this book will grant you the Experience Points needed to tackle the challenges of the Skill Trees. That being said, it may be a fun challenge for you to build a weekly meal plan using a certain Skill Tree as a guide once you've completed it. This will prove to be a true challenge and will serve as a test that will grant you an awful lot of Experience Points!

Every adventurer should complete the Beginners Skill Tree after choosing their Class. This Skill Tree is the foundation (the trunk) of every other Skill Tree, and will help you become familiar with common terms and knife cuts. There's a section in the Appendices that details these terms and dimensions (see Pg. 379). When following a Skill Tree, it's important to complete each challenge presented at your current rank before ascending to the next one. **Taking shortcuts or skipping steps will leave you unprepared for the challenges that lay ahead and will make it harder for you to Level Up.**

Beginner's Skill Tree

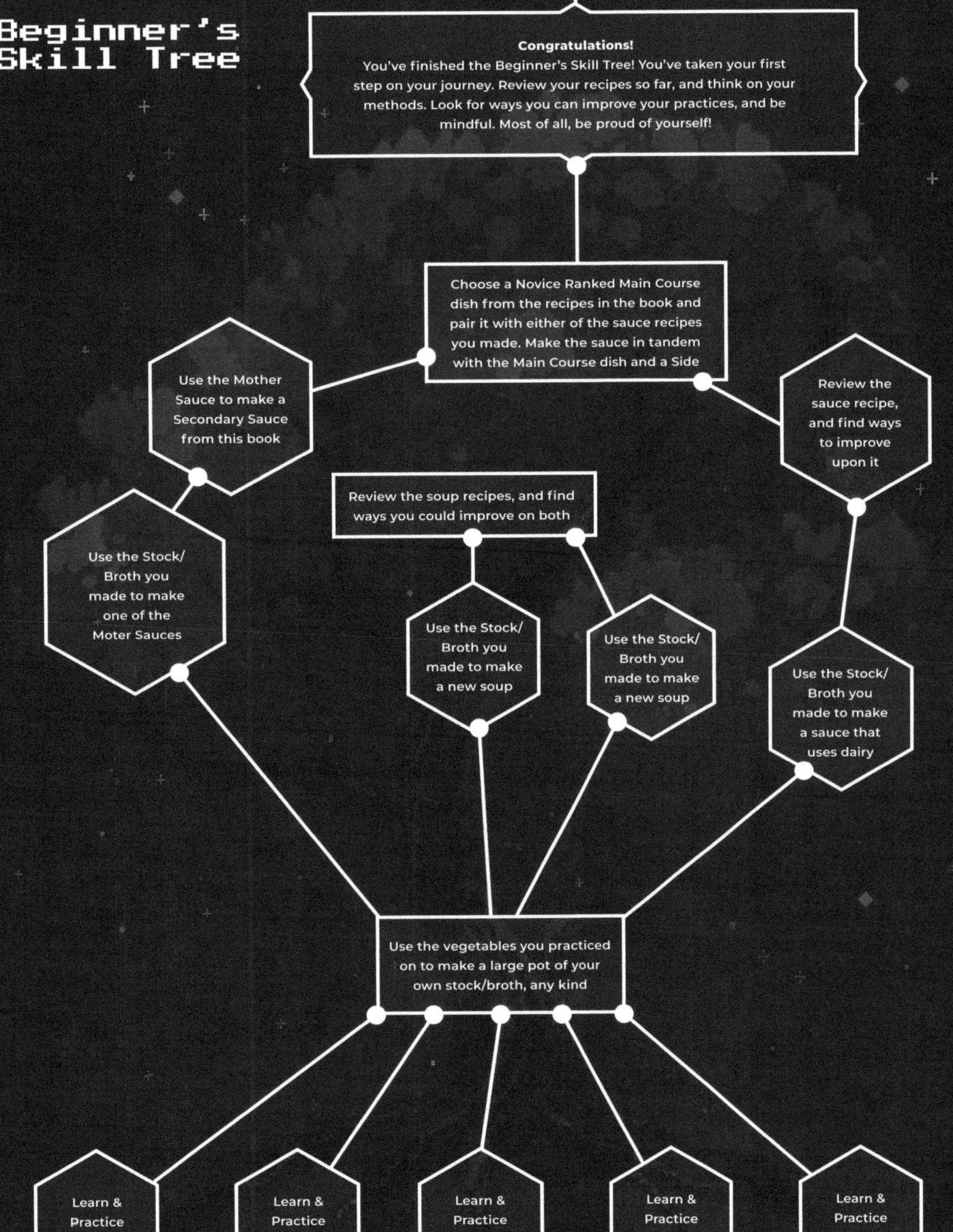

Congratulations!
You've finished the Beginner's Skill Tree! You've taken your first step on your journey. Review your recipes so far, and think on your methods. Look for ways you can improve your practices, and be mindful. Most of all, be proud of yourself!

Choose a Novice Ranked Main Course dish from the recipes in the book and pair it with either of the sauce recipes you made. Make the sauce in tandem with the Main Course dish and a Side

Use the Mother Sauce to make a Secondary Sauce from this book

Review the sauce recipe, and find ways to improve upon it

Review the soup recipes, and find ways you could improve on both

Use the Stock/ Broth you made to make one of the Moter Sauces

Use the Stock/ Broth you made to make a new soup

Use the Stock/ Broth you made to make a new soup

Use the Stock/ Broth you made to make a sauce that uses dairy

Use the vegetables you practiced on to make a large pot of your own stock/broth, any kind

Learn & Practice Brunoise Cut

Learn & Practice Macédoine Cut

Learn & Practice Parmentier Cut

Learn & Practice Julienne Cut

Learn & Practice Chiffonade Cut

START HERE

Barbarian Skill Tree

Prepare yourself a 'feast' by choosing a main dish, Adept level or higher, two sides (Apprentice level or higher) and a dessert. Make the main dish and the sides in tandem, and prepare the dessert so that it's ready to eat when you finish your meal. Review your recipes, and try to plan another 'feast' a few days down the line, with leftovers being utilized from the first one. I advise choosing Expert level recipes that don't seem too intimidating for your first 'feast'. And remember, having friends along makes every adventure more fun.

Review your recipes, and think on what you could do to be more efficient, or what meats would work as substitutes

Purchase the protein in bulk, and get all the meat and broth/stock you need for the recipes from that purchase, and make the recipes, each with a complementing side

Choose 3 different recipes, of Adept level or lower, that utilize the same protein

One piece will be for "Roasted Pork Loin with Cinnamon Apples" the other for "Cha-Siu Pork". Pick 2 apprentice level sides to go with each dish, and make at least 1 in tandem with the Main dish

Purchase a pork loin, cut it into 2 pieces of equal weight

Use the leftover chicken meat to prepare a pot of "Chicken and Dumplin's", save any excess meat for pulled chicken sandwiches

Prepare and make the "Roasted Chicken with 'Pan' Gravy recipe, choose 1 Novice level side to serve with it. Don't eat the whole chicken

Make the "Sweet Heat BBQ Sauce" recipe, and braise the remaining pork to make pulled pork sandwiches and "Nanny's Coleslaw"

Use the meat and the broth/stock to make a pork version of the "Rustic Beef Stew" recipe

Use the bone to make 2 Qt. of Pork Broth or Stock

Purchase a large pork shoulder, and break it down into 2 pieces of equal weight, save the bone if there is one

Bard
Skill Tree

Choose a Main dish recipe (Adept or lower) and think on a way to prepare it to feed a group of people besides just multiplying it (No Soups allowed). Different preparation methods, different portion sizes, different forms of serving, anything goes so long as you serve it in the form of a sharable plate/dish. Pair it with 2 sides/appetizers you know well, and 1 you have not made before. Host a party, and serve all of these to your guests, and revel in the lively and fun atmosphere you created!

Host a party and make all 3 in tandem for the gathering. Take notes on your guests feedback

Choose 3 Soup/Side/Appetizer recipes, with at least 1 being new, and learn them

Pair this multiplied Side with a Novice or Apprentice level Main dish, and serve it to at least 3 other people, making sure to do the proper math so everyone is fed

Make the "French Onion Soup" recipe for at least 3 other people, and pair it with an Apprentice level appetizer

Choose an Adept level side that can be multiplied and made for a group. Learn it, and do the math to multiply it for accuracy

Review the recipes you have chosen so far, and think on how you can be more efficient, and what pairings worked well

Choose two recipes, Apprentice or Novice, that can be made for a group and learn them. Make them for a group, along with a Novice Main dish

Make it, along with a novice level side, for a group. Take notes on their feedback

Choose an Apprentice level soup, learn the recipe so you know the first 4 steps by heart

Make the appetizer for yourself and friends/family and take notes of their feedback

Choose two novice level appetizers, study them, and make them in tandem for a group

Pick a Novice level appetizer recipe and learn it so you know the first 4 steps by heart

Cleric
Skill Tree

Create a full meal (Main Dish, two Sides, and a Sauce) using only vegetarian/healthy ingredients, all cooked in tandem.

Try to cross utilize at least two ingredients, and avoid Gluten as well.

Review the recipe after you've made it, and find ways to make your ingredients list more appropriate for healthy cooking

Choose an Expert level recipe and learn it, replacing only one unhealthy ingredient. Note the difference

Prepare them, and serve one of the curries with something that is neither Rice nor Naan bread

Review the recipes and try to have no overlapping alternatives for ingredients that are unhealthy

Choose two curry recipes and make them both completely vegetarian

Think back on all the recipes you've made so far, and see if there are ways you could make them healthier/less inflammatory

Use that sauce in at least two different meals

Choose an Apprentice level sauce, and research how to best replace the roux with a corn starch slurry

Combine your new recipe and one of the ones you first chose to make a healthy meal

Choose a novice recipe and replace all 'unhealthy' ingredients with healthy alternatives

Review the recipes, and find ways you could improve your method, or the flavor

Research what type of tofu would work best in those recipes, and prepare them

Find at least two Novice recipes in which you can substitute the protein for tofu, and study them

Knight Skill Tree

Prepare a large meal where you make 3 different recipes, Apprentice level or Higher, all in tandem, without reviewing the instructions once. Be sure to study the recipes well, so that you know each step by heart. They can be recipes you've made before, but try to choose at least 1 recipe you haven't made before.

Take that meal plan, and look over the ingredients you need to buy. Find a way to cross-utilize several of them for the next week's meal plan

Utilize the 6 recipes you are most familiar with to form a weekly meal plan

Review all the recipes you've made so far, and choose the recipe that has given you the most trouble. Make that recipe the focus of two different meals

Make that recipe, and make it in tandem with a recipe you made as a Novice

Think back on the meal pairing you just made, and find ways you can improve your method

Take one of the recipes you memorized from the previous skill level and pair it with the new soup recipe

Pick a different knife cut to practice, and choose an Adept recipe that utilizes it

Think about which knife cut you struggle with, and practice it on vegetables to make a stock/broth for the soup recipe you chose

Pick a new recipe, either a Soup or a Sauce, and memorize it

Look over the 4 Recipes you have made so far and find ways you can improve your organization/method, and work to memorize them all

Use those two recipes to make two different meals, with two different Mains/Sides

Choose a novice level "Main Course' and 'Side Dishes' Recipes and memorize them

Ranger Skill Tree

Take everything you've done up to now and make your own Chicken Pot pie from scratch: Chicken you break down yourself, homemade broth/stock to make your own Sauce for the filling, pie crust you made yourself. If you like, replace the Chicken with a more exotic meat; so long as you break it down and use it to craft the necessary ingredients to make the pie, it will fulfill the requirements. Take pride, know that you are fully self-sustaining in your kitchen!

Make your own Basic Butter Crust and use the filling to make a pie from scratch

Go to the local market and pick out fresh fruits to make your own pie filling

Evaluate all the recipes and combinations you've made so far, and pick one to repeat

Use the Mayo you made and the Breasts to make your own chicken salad

Create a sauce from this book and serve it with the Legs

Use the Thighs in a recipe from this book, and serve it with a new sauce recipe

Make a batch of broth/stock with the Carcass & Wings, and use it in at least 2 recipes

Purchase a whole chicken, and break it down into its separate parts (Breasts, Wings, Thighs, Legs, and Carcass)

Make your own Mayo at home

Pick a recipe that uses an ingredient you've never eaten before and make it

Go to your local farmers market and find an ingredient to use in a recipe from this book

Wizard Skill Tree

Choose a Main, a Side, and a Sauce. Find a way to alter the texture and cultural profile of each one, in a way that they all complement one another, without overlapping ingredients and cuisine profiles

Take all that you have learned, and try your hand at making your own herb and spice blend. Use that blend in several recipes.

Choose an adept recipe and replace at least two ingredients with ones you feel will yield the same product

Choose an Adept recipe, and one other of any level, and alter the seasonings so they are distinct, but still complement each other

If confusion, work on finding a good recipe for fusion

Review your choices, and decide if it was fusion, or confusion

Choose an Adept recipe and pair it with a recipe of a different cultural profile that compliments it. Fusion!

Choose an Apprentice level recipe and think of ways to alter the flavor to fit a different cuisine

Choose an Apprentice recipe, and think of ways to alter/enhance the texture of the dish

Take a new recipe and alter not only the texture, but the flavor profile with new ingredients and techniques

Make the recipes, review your changes, and decide what worked well and what didn't

Take those recipes and replace at least two herbs and spices that you feel will yield a good result

Pick two Novice level recipes and learn them well. Research the component herbs and spices.

LVLUPCookBook Channel

NOVICE

Just The Beginning

You've started your journey, and you've probably already made some Novice ranked recipes. You're confident in your abilities, but you're aware of how much farther there is to go.

Remember to take things one step at a time. Keep a steady pace and your journey should be a smooth one.

Now is the time to tackle that Beginner's Skill Tree! A new day has dawned, and you're ready for whatever the road holds for you, with your trusty recipes in one hand and a sharp knife in the other. You can do this!

Soups

Chicken Gnocchi Soup

Decadent
Sweet • Spicy
Savory • Salty

I really enjoy this recipe, and it's become a staple for my meal planning. I probably make this soup once a month, sometimes more often during the colder months of the year. The kale works to create a variety in both texture and appearance, and the excess kale you have from the bunch can be made into some Homestyle Greens (see Pg 83). I use dry herbs for my recipes, but if you like to use fresh ones just remember you need 3 times the volume for the same flavor effect you would get from using dry.

Ingredients

Potato Gnocchi	16oz
Chicken Breast, ½" Cubes	2 C
Roasted Garlic Cloves, Pasted	8 ea
Carrot, Shredded	½ C
Kale, Rough Chop	2 C
White Onion, Diced	¾ C
Butter Or Olive Oil	4 Tbsp
AP Flour	4 Tbsp
Chicken Stock	48 Fl Oz
Heavy Cream, Warmed	12 Fl Oz
Grated Parmesan	¾ C
Thyme, Dry	1 tsp
Oregano, Dry	1 tsp
Basil, Dry	½ tsp
Parsley, Dry	1 tsp
Salt	1 tsp
Black Pepper, Ground	1 tsp
Bay Leaf	1 ea

Prep Time
35 Min

Cook Time
25 Min

Servings
6 - 8 Bowls

6 - 8 Qt Pot
1 ea

Wooden Spoon/Rubber Spatula
1 ea

Wire Whisk
1 ea

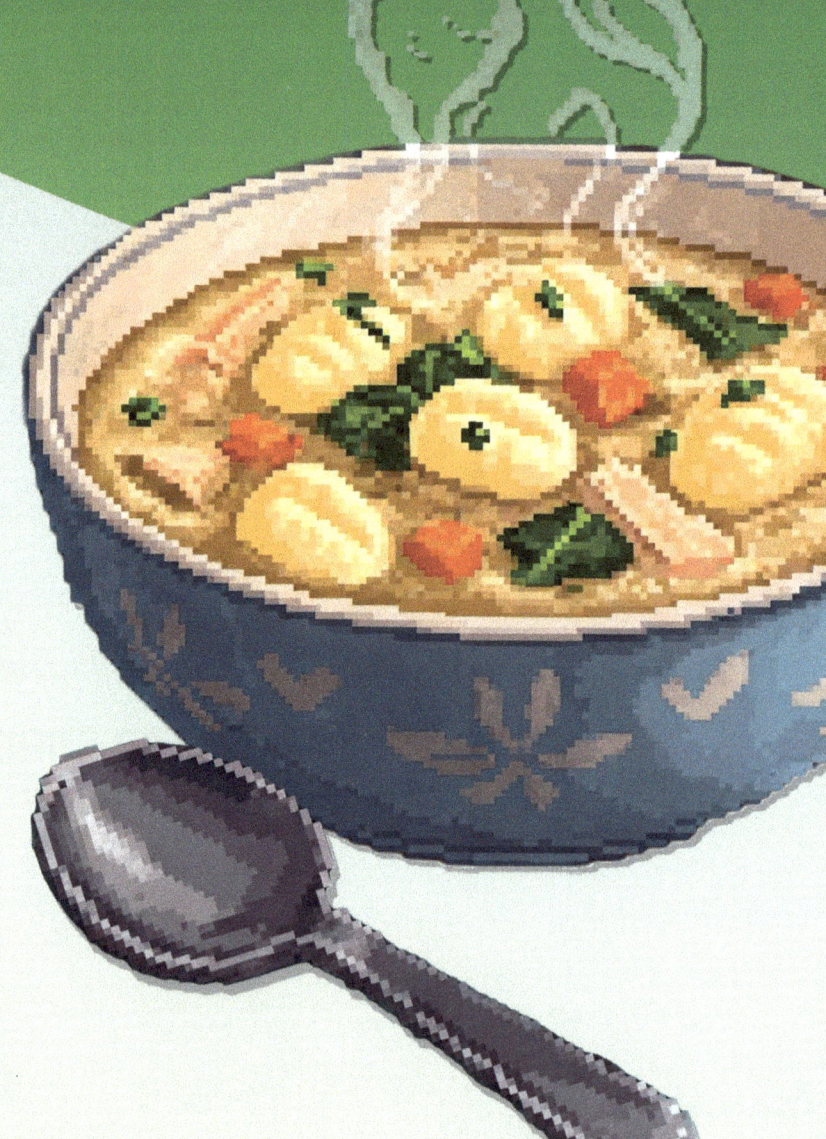

Cooking Directions

1   Place a 6 - 8 Qt. pot over Medium Heat. When hot, add butter/oil.

2   When oil is shimmering, or butter is no longer bubbling, add the onion and cook until translucent, about 5 min.

3   Add the garlic paste and stir well, cooking for 1 minute.

4   Add the flour and seasonings. Stirring often, cook for 3 - 4 minutes.

5   Add 1 cup of the stock to the pot, and stir well, being sure to scrape the bottom of the pot well. When the roux is no longer lumpy add the rest of the stock slowly, stirring constantly. Raise the heat to Medium High.

6   When simmering, add the chicken pieces and cook for 10 minutes.

7   Add the kale and cook for 3 min. more.

8   Add the gnocchi, lower the heat to Medium. Simmer until the gnocchi are floating on the surface, 5 - 7 min.

9   Lower heat to Medium Low, add the carrots and cook for 2 min.

10 Slowly pour in the heavy cream, stirring constantly and gently.

11 Slowly add the parmesan, stirring constantly and gently. Remove pot from heat. Serve Hot, or hold over lowest heat setting for up to 1 hr.

Pumpkin Orange Soup

Decadent
Sweet — Spicy
Savory — Salty

This soup is wonderful for a crisp and clear autumn day or night. It always takes me back to my childhood growing up in New England, and is a very simple way to brighten up a lovely fall afternoon. Try making some smaller side items for placing in the soup once you serve it.

Ingredients

Chicken or Vegetable Stock	32 Fl Oz
Pumpkin Purée, Unsweetened	15 oz
Yellow Onion, Diced	¾ C
Garlic, Minced	1 tsp
Thyme, Dry	1 tsp
Sage, Ground	½ tsp
Black Pepper, Ground	⅛ tsp
Bay Leaf	1 ea
Hot Sauce	½ tsp
Olive Oil	3 Tbsp
AP Flour	3 Tbsp
Juice of 1 Medium Orange	
Zest of ½ A Medium Orange	

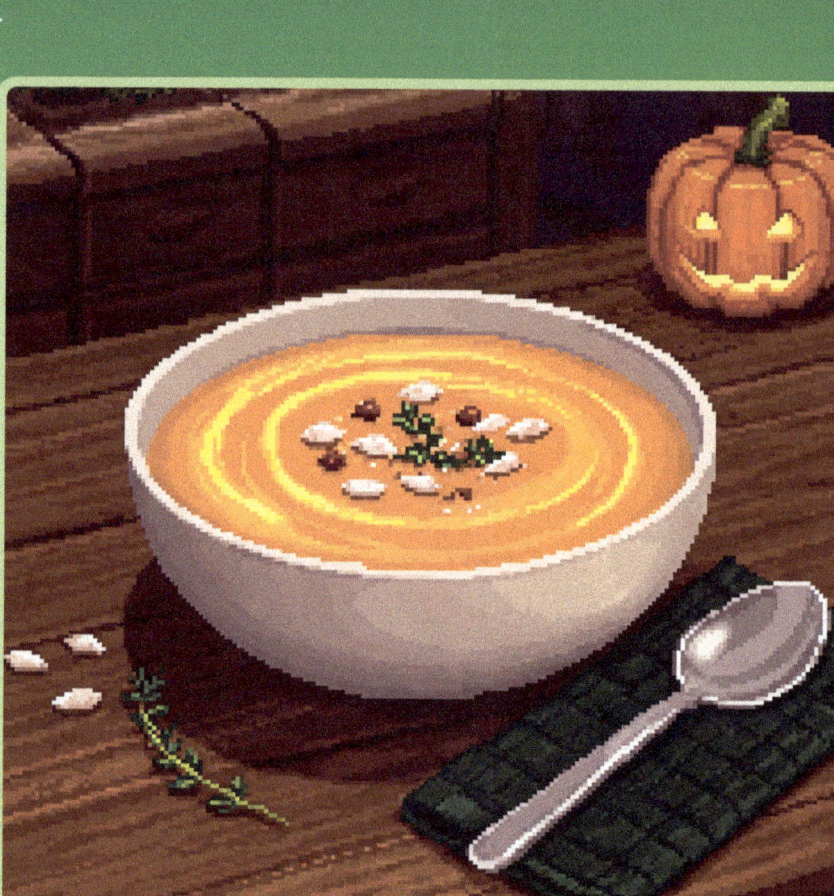

 Prep Time
5 Min

 Cook Time
25 Min

 Servings
4 - 6 Bowls

 Wire Whisk
1 ea

 4 Qt Pot
1 ea

 Wooden Spoon/Rubber Spatula
1 ea

 Zester/ Vegetable Peeler
1 ea

Cooking Directions

1   Place a 4 Qt. pot over Medium heat. When hot, add
    oil. When oil is shimmering, add the onion. Cook until
    slightly browned, about 5 minutes.

2   Add the flour and cook for 2 - 3 min. to bring it to the
    Blond level. Add garlic and cook for 1 minute. Add
    pumpkin purée and dry seasonings, cook for 2 - 3 more
    minutes.

3   Add 1 cup of the stock, and stir well to work out any
    lumps in the roux. Add the remaining stock, the
    orange juice, and the hot sauce. Stir well and raise
    heat to High. Bring to a hard simmer, then lower heat
    to Medium Low. Simmer for 15 minutes, uncovered.

4   Test the flavor and adjust seasoning as desired.
    Remove pot from heat, add orange zest and stir well.
    Serve Hot.

Recipe Tip

Try out different toppings with this recipe! Roasted nuts, roasted
pumpkin seeds (Pepitas), freshly chopped parsley, candied nuts, and
crispy bacon bits are just some of the options that pair well. Get
creative, and make it your own!

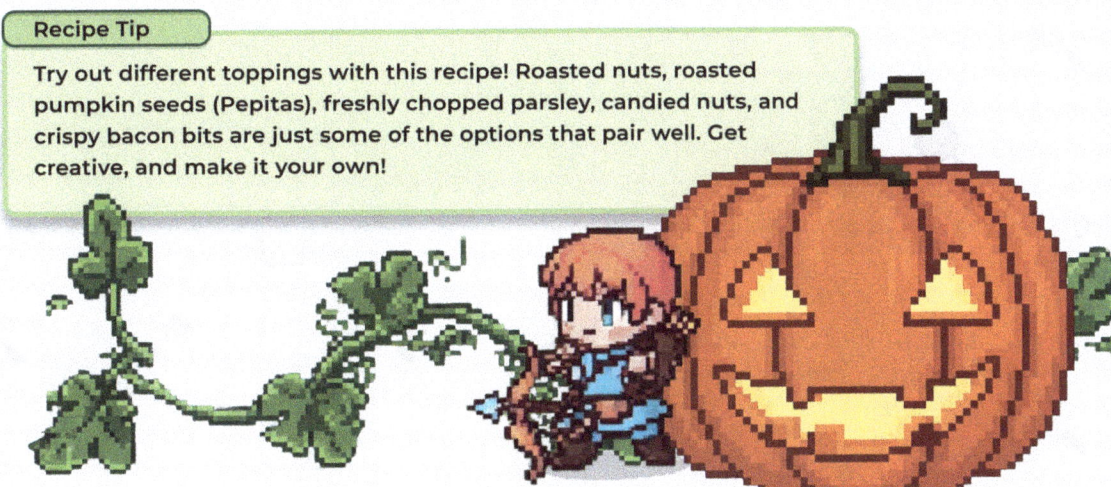

Turmeric Chicken Soup

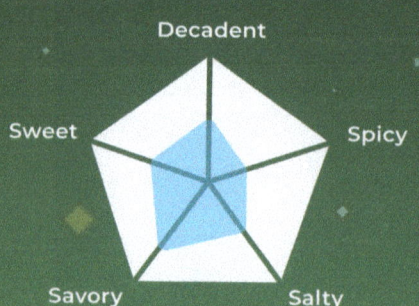

Decadent
Sweet
Spicy
Savory
Salty

This recipe can easily be made vegetarian: Use Vegetable Stock instead of Chicken Stock, and replace the shredded chicken with either extra-firm tofu or extra potatoes. If using extra-firm tofu, be sure to not overcook the tofu, adding it into the pot at the same time as the kale. I personally don't enjoy very spicy food, but ½ tsp. of Cayenne can also be added to the spice mixture to help give this recipe a real kick.

Ingredients

Chicken Breast, 12 oz	1 ea
Water	12 Fl Oz
Carrot, Diced	1 C
Yellow Onion, Diced	¾ C
Celery, Diced	½ C
Cauliflower, Cut Into Florets	1½ C
Gold Potatoes, Diced	½ C
Kale, Washed, Rough Chopped	2 C
Coconut Milk, Unsweetened	14 Fl Oz
Chicken Stock	32 Fl Oz
Garlic, Minced	2 tsp
Ginger, Minced	1 Tbsp
Turmeric	1 Tbsp
Black Pepper, Ground	½ tsp
Garam Masala	½ tsp
Coriander, Ground	½ tsp
Salt	1 tsp
Juice of ½ a Lemon	
Neutral Oil	2 Tbsp

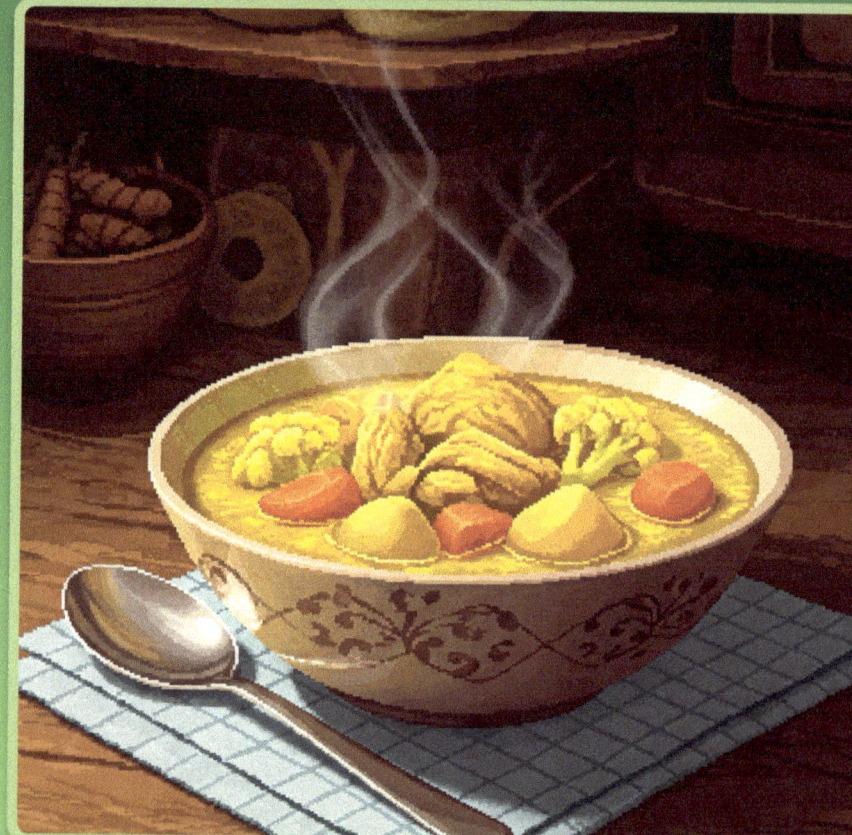

Prep Time
35 Min

Cook Time
45 Min

Servings
6 - 8 Bowls

Small Pot w/Lid
1 ea

Wooden Spoon/Rubber Spatula
1 ea

4 Qt Pot
1 ea

Forks for Shredding
1 ea

Cooking Directions

1   Place the water in a pot just large enough to fit the chicken breast and place over High heat. When simmering, place chicken in the water, reduce the heat to Medium Low and cover with lid. Cook for 30 minutes, until a spoon is easily inserted into the chicken breast.

2   Remove chicken from pot. Set aside. Discard water from pot.

3   While chicken cooks and cools, cut and measure all ingredients. Once cool enough to handle, shred the chicken finely.

4   Place a 4 Qt. pot on Medium High heat. When hot, add the oil. When oil is shimmering add the onions, carrots, and celery, cooking each until soft before adding the next.

5   Add garlic and ginger, cook for 1 - 2 minutes. Add seasonings, potatoes, and cauliflower, stir well.

6   Add coconut milk, lemon juice, chicken and stock. Raise heat to High and bring to a boil.

7   When boiling, reduce heat to Medium Low and simmer for 15 minutes, with the lid on for the first 10 min.

8   Add the kale, stir well and bring back to a simmer. Cook for 5 minutes with lid off.

9   Remove pot from heat, taste test and adjust salt and pepper as needed. Serve Hot.

Sides & Appetizers

Braised Cabbage

NOVICE

Decadent

Sweet — Spicy

Savory — Salty

This classic German side dish pairs well with any kind of protein. The obvious pairing is with Kielbasa or other smoked sausages, but it also pairs with grilled chicken, beef, or seafood. It's a simple recipe that's sure to convince anyone to give cabbage a chance. Since cabbage heads are so large, it's advised to have a second meal in mind that utilizes the cabbage in some way (Vegetable Spring Rolls anyone? see Pg 191) so that you can get the most out of your purchase.

Ingredients

Green Cabbage, Cut into 1 x 1" Pcs	3 C
Scallion Stalks, Chopped	2 ea
Garlic, Minced	2 tsp
Dill, Dry	¼ tsp
Black Pepper, Ground	⅛ tsp
Salt	½ tsp
White Wine (Chardonnay Advised)	½ C
Stock (Chicken Or Vegetable)	½ C
Butter	2 Tbsp

Prep Time
10 Min

Cook Time
45 Min

Servings
2 Cups

4 Qt Pot w/Lid
1 ea

Wooden Spoon/ Rubber Spatula
1 ea

Cooking Directions

1   Place a 4 Qt. pot over Medium High heat. When hot, add the butter.

2   When the butter has stopped bubbling, add the garlic and cook for 1 min.

3   Add the scallions and cook for about 30 sec. then add the cabbage, salt, pepper, and dill. Mix well to incorporate all ingredients.

4   Let cook for 2 - 3 min. before adding the wine. Once the wine is simmering, cook until you can no longer smell the alcohol, about 1 min.

5   Add the stock and stir well. When simmering, cover and reduce heat to Low. Cook for 40 min. not stirring or removing the lid.

6   Taste test and adjust seasoning as desired. Serve Hot.

Buffalo Chicken Dip

Decadent

Sweet

Spicy

Savory

Salty

I was first introduced to this dish during a trip to upstate New York, and I fell in love with it. The tangy heat of the hot sauce and the velvety, almost sweet cream cheese makes for a delicious pairing. Serving with tortilla chips, butter crackers, or vegetable crudité will provide a treat for everyone at your party.

Shredding the chicken ahead of time is the way to go with this recipe, and will cut down on prep time when you go to make the dish. Either cook and shred your chicken at home, or get a rotisserie chicken from the store and get the meat you need from that; both are great options. If you are shredding your own chicken at home, keep in mind that one breast usually yields 1 cup of shredded chicken.

Ingredients

Chicken, Shredded	2 C
Hot Sauce	¾ C
Cream Cheese, Softened	16 oz
Yellow Onion, Minced	¼ C
Colby Cheese, Shredded, Divided	1½ C
Ranch Dressing (Pg 149)	1 C
Paprika	1 tsp
Garlic, Minced	2 tsp
Butter/Oil	½ Tbsp

 Prep Time 15 Min

 Cook Time 40 - 45 Min

 Servings 5 Cups

 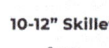 **10-12" Skillet** 1 ea

 Wooden Spoon/Rubber Spatula 1 ea

 8 x 8" Baking Dish 1 ea

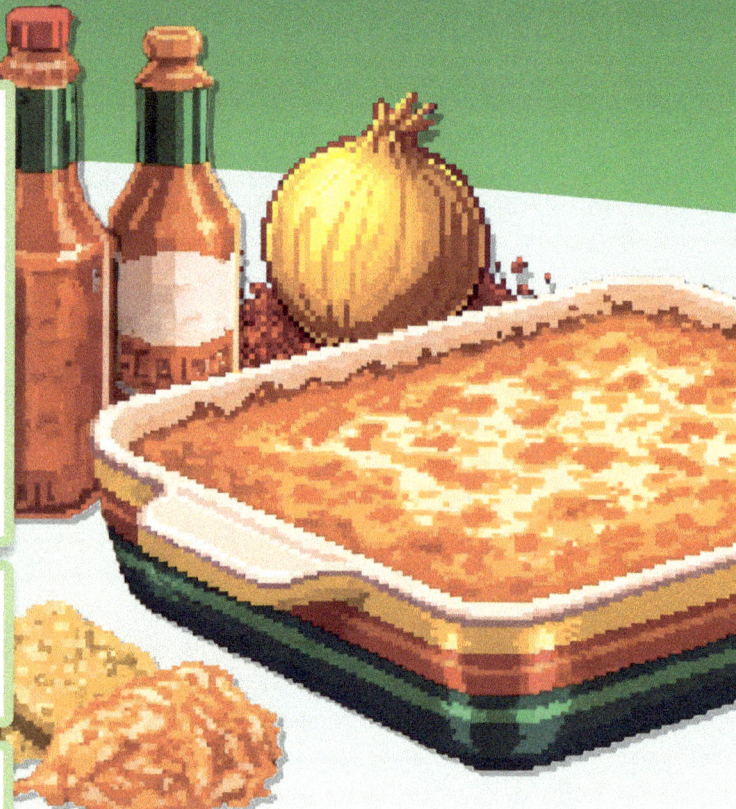

Cooking Directions

1   Preheat oven to 350 with a rack in the center of the oven. Place a 10" - 12" skillet over Medium Heat. Add the butter/oil.

2   When the butter stops bubbling, or the oil is shimmering, add the onion and garlic. Cook for 1 min. until fragrant.

3   Add the hot sauce and shredded chicken, and cook for 3 min.

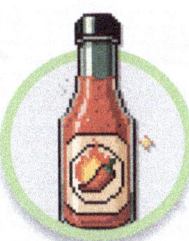

4   Reduce heat to Low and add the ranch and cream cheese. Stirring almost constantly, cook for 3 - 5 min. until completely blended and warm.

5   Remove from heat and stir in ½ of the Colby cheese. It doesn't need to be fully melted. Transfer the mixture to an 8" x 8" baking pan. Evenly distribute the remaining cheese on top. Cover with tin foil.

6   Bake for 30 - 35 min. until the dip is bubbling and hot. Remove from oven, keep covered, and let rest for 10 min. before serving.

NOVICE

Cheese Stuffed Mushrooms

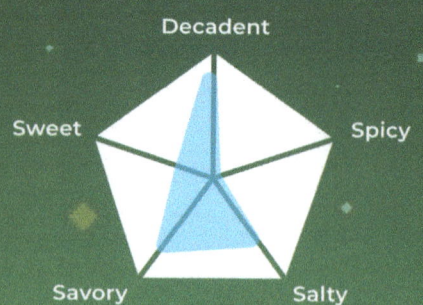

Decadent
Sweet
Spicy
Savory
Salty

I have an affinity for mushrooms of all kinds, but Cremini (Baby Bella) mushrooms are perfect for this recipe. They make for a delightful bite at any gathering, and are simple to make. They can be prepared ahead of time by following all the steps up to actually cooking them. Store the stuffed mushrooms in an airtight container, or covered in plastic, for up to 3 days in the fridge. Simply pull them out when you start preheating your oven, bake as instructed, and they'll be delicious.

Ingredients

Whole Cremini (Baby Bella) Mushrooms	24 ea
Cream Cheese, Softened	16 oz
Parmesan, Grated	½ C
Yellow Onion, Minced	¼ C
Black Pepper, Ground	½ tsp
Garlic, Minced	1 Tbsp
Chili Powder	½ tsp
Butter/Oil	2 Tbsp

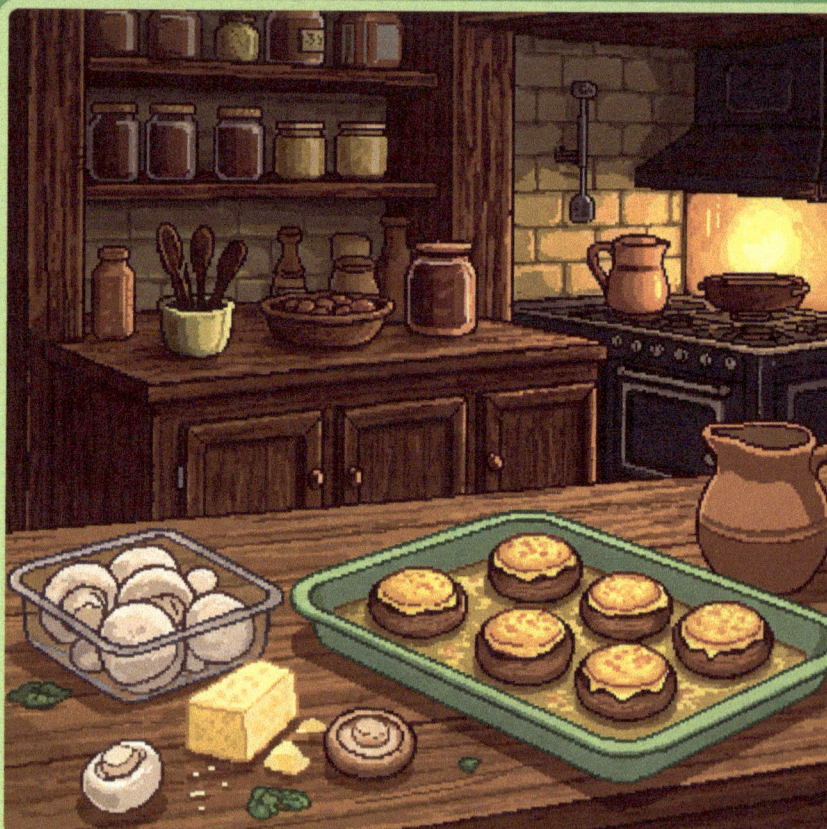

Prep Time
20 Min

Cook Time
25 Min

Servings
24 Mushrooms

8 - 10" Skillet
1 ea

½ Tbsp Scoop/ ½ Tbsp Measuring Spoon
1 ea

8 x 13" Baking Tray
1 ea

Large Mixing Bowl
1 ea

Parchment Paper or Cooking Spray
1 ea

Wooden Spoon/Rubber Spatula
1 ea

Cooking Directions

1   Preheat oven to 350. Make sure there is a rack in the center of the oven.

2   Wash any dirt off your mushrooms and carefully break off stems. Trim any tough parts of the stem off and finely mince them. If you have a food processor, pulse the stems until finely chopped.

3   Place an 8" - 10" skillet over Medium heat. When hot, add the butter/oil.

4   When the butter stops bubbling, or the oil is shimmering, add the minced mushroom, the onion, and garlic to the pan. Cook for 2 - 3 min. until the moisture has evaporated. Remove pan from heat and set aside to cool. Line an 8" x 13" baking tray with parchment paper.

5   In a large bowl, stir together the cream cheese, parmesan, and seasonings. Stir well. Add the mushroom mix from the pan and fully incorporate to the cream cheese mix

6   Use a ½ Tbsp. measuring spoon, or a ½ Tbsp. scoop, to portion the filling into each mushroom cap and transfer each to your prepared baking tray.

7   Bake for 20 min. until the mushrooms are darkened and the cheese is bubbling. Remove from oven, transfer to a serving platter, and let rest for 3 min. before serving.

Creamy Spinach Artichoke Dip

NOVICE

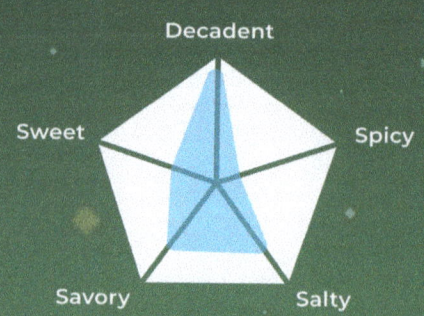

When I was a child, one of things about the holiday season I looked forward to most was making spinach artichoke dip with my mom on Christmas and New Year's Eve. The family would come together, we would play board games and tell stories, all while eating this dip and other delicious appetizers. As an adult, I make this dip whenever I want to bring back those feelings of warmth and comfort. I know you'll enjoy making (and eating) this simple classic as much as I still do.

Ingredients

Cream Cheese, Softened	8 oz
Artichoke Hearts, Drained, Chopped	14 oz
Spinach, Rough Chop	8 oz
Mayo (Pg 145)	¼ C
Garlic, Minced	2 tsp
Parmesan Cheese, Grated	½ C
Mozzarella	¼ C
Basil, Dry	½ tsp
Oregano, Dry	½ tsp
Salt	¼ tsp
Black Pepper, Ground	¼ tsp
Butter/Olive Oil	1 Tbsp

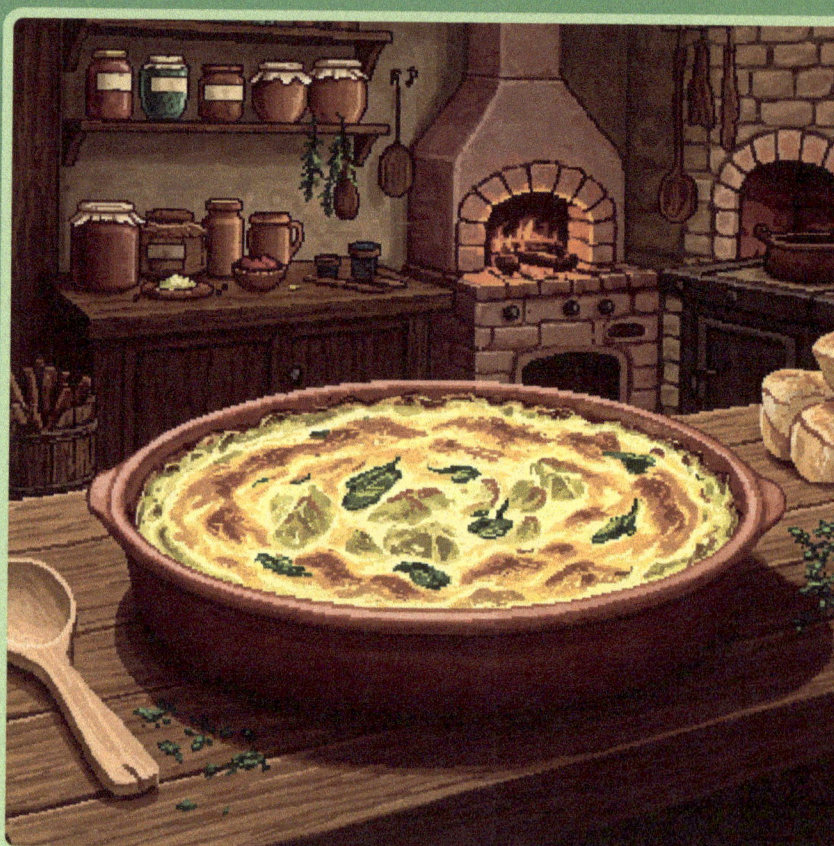

 Prep Time
10 Min

 Cook Time
30 Min

 Servings
1 Pan (8 x 8")

 10 - 12" Skillet
1 ea

Large Mixing Bowl
1 ea

 8 x 8" Baking Dish
1 ea

 Wooden Spoon/Rubber Spatula
1 ea

Cooking Directions

1   Preheat oven to 350, make sure there is a rack in the center of the oven. Place a 10" - 12" skillet over Medium High heat. When hot, add the butter/oil.

2   When the butter stops bubbling, or the oil is shimmering, add the garlic and chopped spinach. Cook until the spinach is wilted and most of the moisture is evaporated, 3 - 4 min. When done cooking, remove pan from heat.

3   In a large bowl, combine the cream cheese, parmesan cheese, herbs, salt, and pepper. Mix well until the cream cheese is spreadable. Add the chopped artichokes and the spinach mix.

4   Stir to combine thoroughly and transfer to an 8" x 8" baking dish. Top evenly with the mozzarella.

5   Bake for 25 min. until the cheese on top is melted and the filling is bubbling. Remove from oven and let rest for 5 min. before serving.

Recipe Tip

Serving this dip with toasted bread rounds, bagel chips, tortilla chips, or crudité will make for a party dish that's sure to please!

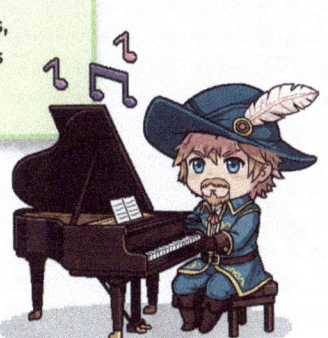

NOVICE

Garlic Mashed Potatoes

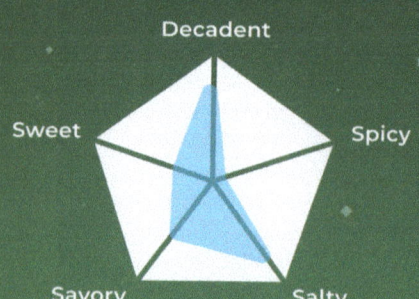

Decadent

Sweet — Spicy

Savory — Salty

Mashed potatoes are a classic staple for any family gathering or an easy week night dinner. Adding the small amount of garlic to the recipe helps provide an unctuous note to the creamy, delicate profile of the potatoes. Of course, feel free to add more or remove it entirely if you prefer.

Ingredients

Russet Potatoes, ½" x ½" x 3" Julienne	1 Lb
Red Potatoes, ½" x ½" x 3" Julienne	1 Lb
Butter, Melted	4 Tbsp
Heavy Cream	6 Fl Oz
Salt	¾ tsp
Black Pepper	¼ tsp
Garlic, Minced	2 tsp

 Prep Time 5 Min

 Cook Time 15 Min

Servings 32 oz

 Potato Masher 1 ea

 6 - 8 Qt Pot 1 ea

 Microwave Safe Bowl 1 ea

 Large Mixing Bowl/Stand Mixer for Mashing 1 ea

 Large Handled Spoon 1 ea

Recipe Tip

Try roasting some garlic bulbs and throwing in about 4-6 cloves per pound of potatoes to give them a sublime undertone that pairs well with almost any dish.

Cooking Directions

1   Place the potatoes into a 6 - 8 Qt. pot and fill with enough cold water so that the water level is about 2" over the potatoes. Place the pot over High heat. Always start your potatoes with cold water to help them retain their starches.

2   While the potatoes begin coming to a boil, place your butter and garlic in a microwave safe bowl/dish. Microwave on High in bursts for 6 - 8 seconds at a time until the butter is melted. I advise covering the bowl/dish with a paper towel during this process. Once the butter is nearly all melted, carefully remove from microwave and set aside.

3   When the potatoes are boiling, your cooking time begins. It should take 9 - 10 min. for the potatoes to cook to the right softness. After 8 min. pull a piece of potato out of the water with a long handled spoon and press it gently against the side of the pot. You'll know the potatoes are ready when they give little resistance and mash easily with gentle pressure. This is a test to see how much more time you need to cook them.

4   When done cooking, strain the potatoes and let them rest for 30 sec. to make sure all the water has sloughed off. Then transfer them to a large mixing bowl. If mashing with a stand mixer, turn it on the lowest setting and work the potatoes for about 30 seconds, then stop and add in your remaining ingredients. Mix for 1 - 2 min. until most of the potatoes have creamed and there are some small chunks left. Be careful not to over-mix, as over-working causes the starches in red potatoes to become gluey.

    If mashing by hand, mash the potatoes together for about 30 sec. then add your remaining ingredients and keep mashing and stirring until your desired consistency is reached.

5   If not eating immediately, transfer to a pot and place on the warming eye of your stove (if available) or on your smallest eye over the Lowest heat setting and cover. The potatoes will hold well for up to 2 hr. this way. Be sure to stir occasionally to prevent the potatoes from sticking to the bottom of the pot.

Homestyle Greens

Personally, I find a combo of Mustard and Collard greens gives the most flavor, but this recipe works well for any of them. Kale can even be used, but it requires less cooking time. Serve with hot sauce, hot pepper vinegar, malt vinegar, or if you are feeling adventurous, try them with a sprinkling of fish sauce to give them a hard hit of salty-savory flavor.

Decadent / Sweet / Spicy / Savory / Salty

Ingredients

Fresh Greens	2 Bunches
(Collard, Mustard, Turnip)	
Butter	4 Tbsp
Yellow Onion, Diced	½ C
Garlic, Minced	1 Tbsp
Salt	¼ tsp
Black Pepper, Ground	¼ tsp
Apple Cider Vinegar	2 Tbsp
Chicken Stock	16 Fl Oz
Smoked Ham Hock Or	
Turkey Neck	1 ea
OR	
Bacon Slices, ¼" Pcs	4 ea

 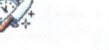

Prep Time
20 - 30 Min

Cook Time
45 - 60 Min

Servings
8 - 10 Portions

Wooden/ Rubber Spatula
1 ea

6 - 8 Qt Pot w/Lid
1 ea

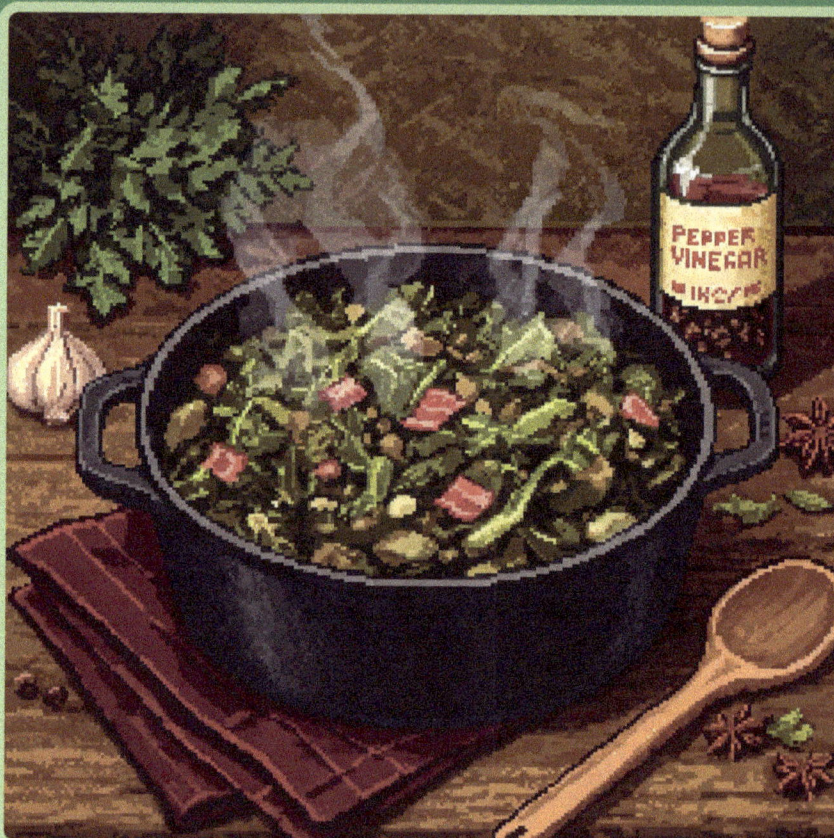

Cooking Directions

1 Remove stems from greens and rough chop leaves into pieces that are 1" - 1½". Wash thoroughly and set aside to drain.

2 Place a 6 - 8 Qt. pot over Medium heat. When hot, add butter and melt until it stops bubbling. Note: if using bacon, omit the butter and cook the bacon pieces until they are crispy. Leave bacon and grease in pot for next step.

3 Add onion to pot. Cook for 5 minutes, until translucent. Add garlic and cook for 1 min. If using a ham hock, turkey neck or turkey wing, place it in the bottom of the pot.

4 Add greens to the pot until it's full. Stir well, keeping the meat on the bottom of the pot. Cover and let the greens cook down for 1 - 2 min. Remove lid, add more greens and repeat the process until all greens are in the pot.

5 Add the vinegar, salt and pepper. Stir well so the meat is evenly distributed, unless using a ham hock/turkey neck. Keep that at the bottom. Cook for 30 seconds, then pour in the stock. Raise heat to Medium High and bring to a simmer. Cover the pot and reduce heat to Medium Low.

6 Cook for 45 - 60 min. until tender. Do not cook for more than 2 hr. Serve Hot, or they can be held on lowest heat setting or up to 2 hr.

Jalapeño Popper Dip

Decadent

Sweet — Spicy

Savory — Salty

I love the flavor of Jalapeño Poppers. But stuffing, battering, and frying is such a time consuming and messy effort for home cooking. So, making this dip is the next best thing. Make it for the next party you are hosting and watch as it quickly disappears onto people's plates.

Ingredients

Colby Cheese, Shredded	1 C
Monterey Jack Cheese, Shredded	1 C
Cream Cheese, Softened	16 oz
Jalapeño Peppers, Seeded, Minced	16 ea
Bacon Slices, Cooked, Finely Chopped	8 ea
Corn Kernels (Fresh Pref.)	1 C
Mayo (Pg 145)	½ C
Black Pepper, Ground	⅛ tsp
Salt	¼ tsp
Chili Powder	½ tsp
Garlic, Minced	2 tsp

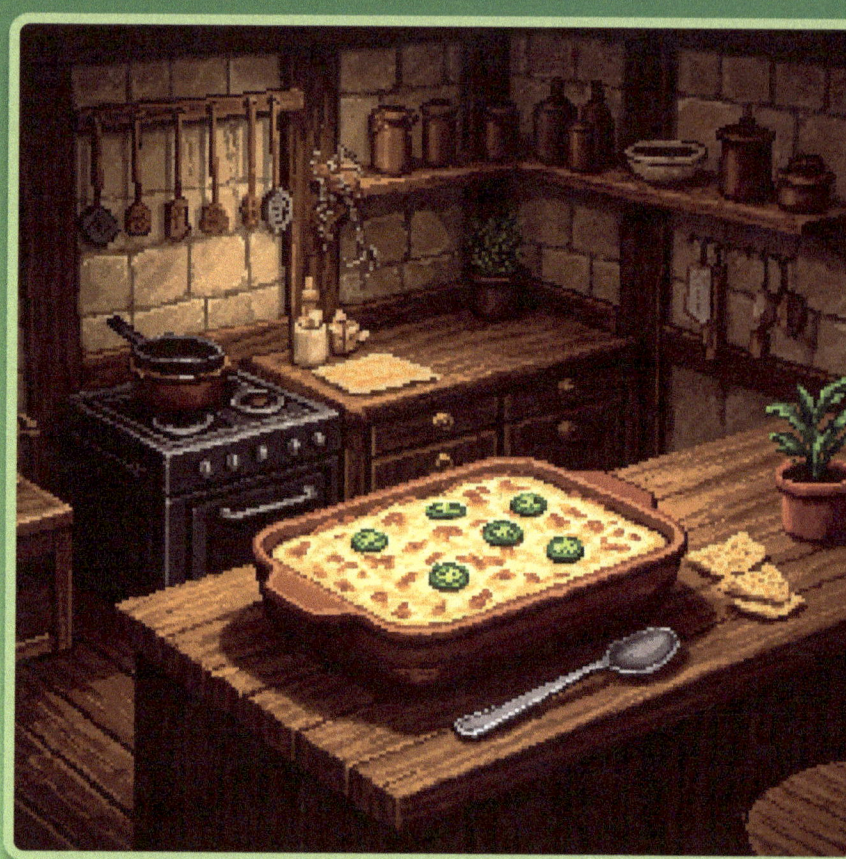

 Prep Time
15 Min

 Cook Time
30 - 35 Min

 Servings
1 Dish (9" x 13")

 9" x 13" Baking Tray
1 ea

 9" x 13" Casserole Dish
1 ea

 Large Mixing Bowl
1 ea

 Wooden/ Rubber Spatula
1 ea

Cooking Directions

1   Preheat your oven to 350. Make sure there is a rack in the center of the oven.

2   Line a baking tray with foil, and place the bacon slices on it. Bake for 12 - 14 min. until bacon is crispy. Remove from oven, and raise heat to 400.

3   Place the cream cheese, mayo, garlic, and seasonings in a large bowl. Mix until the cream cheese is whipped and easily spread.

4   Once the bacon is cool, dice it and add to the bowl.

5   Add the remaining ingredients and mix until well combined.

6   Transfer mixture to a 9" x 13" casserole dish. Place dish in oven and bake until the top is slightly browned and the filling is bubbly, 15 - 20 min.

7   Remove from oven and let rest for 5 min. before serving.

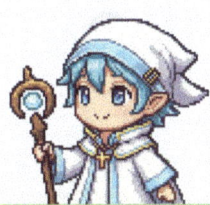

Recipe Tip

Serving with tortilla chips is obvious, but try it also with toasted French bread rounds, vegetable crudité, or pita chips. Anything with a good crunch will complement the creamy texture of this recipe nicely.

NOVICE

Okra & Stewed Tomatoes

Decadent

Sweet

Spicy

Savory

Salty

This recipe is courtesy of my lovely wife, Julia. Her grandfather would make this simple dish often, and she was all too eager to share it with me when I told her that I had never had it before. It quickly became a favorite of ours for nights when we are making old fashioned southern food, or are pinched for time.

Ingredients

Okra, ½" Slices	3 C
Stewed Tomatoes, Canned	14 oz
OR	
Small Tomatoes, Sliced ¼" Thick	6 ea
Yellow Onion, Diced	1 C
Oil Or Butter	1½ Tbsp
Salt & Pepper To Taste	

Prep Time
10 Min

Cook Time
20 Min

Servings
4 - 6 Portions

10" - 12" Skillet
1 ea

Wooden Spoon/Rubber Spatula
1 ea

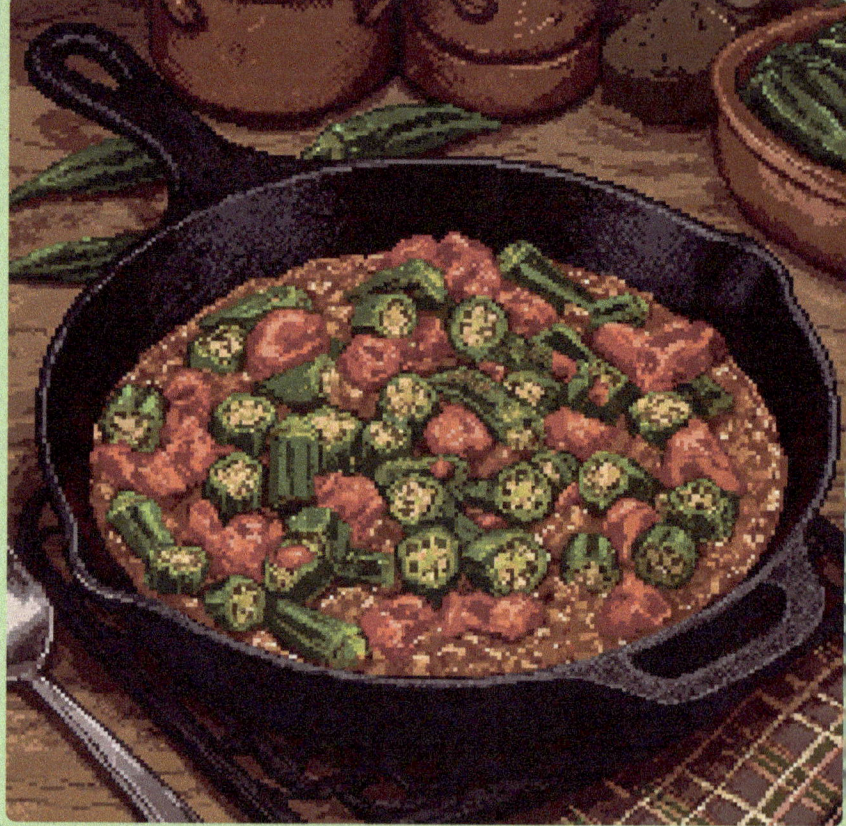

Cooking Directions

1   Place a 10" - 12" skillet over Medium heat. When hot, add oil/butter.

2   When oil is shimmering, or butter stops bubbling, add okra with as many cut sides down as possible.

3   Cook for 5 minutes before stirring, then cook for 5 min. more.

4   Add onion, cook for 5 - 6 minutes, until the onions are slightly browned.

5   Add tomatoes, with their juices, to the pan. Using a wooden spoon or spatula, press the tomatoes and break the large pieces into chunks. Cook for 10 min. stirring often.

6   Add a pinch of salt and pepper, stir and taste test. Adjust seasoning as needed. Hold over Low heat, covered, until needed. Serve Hot.

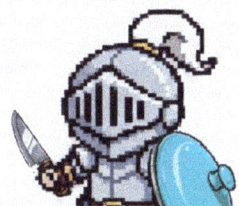

Recipe Tip

This dish tastes just as good cold as it does hot. Try spreading it over buttered crostini as an appetizer, or served cold as a unique addition to a charcuterie board.

Oven Baked Rice

NOVICE

This recipe is great for any dish that requires rice to be served with it. Add 2 Tbsp. of various vegetables to impart unique flavors to the rice when cooking. The options are nearly limitless, so I encourage you to experiment and flex your culinary muscles to pair this rice with all your delicious dishes!

Decadent
Sweet
Spicy
Savory
Salty

Ingredients

Long Grain Rice	2 C
Stock (Any Kind)	32 Fl Oz
Salt	¼ tsp
Yellow Onion, Minced	¼ C
Black Pepper, Ground	¼ tsp
Butter, Small Cubes	2 Tbsp

 Prep Time 5 Min

 Cook Time 1 Hr

 Servings 4 Cups

 9 x 13" Casserole Dish 1 ea

Fork for Fluffing 1 ea

 Large Spoon for Stirring 1 ea

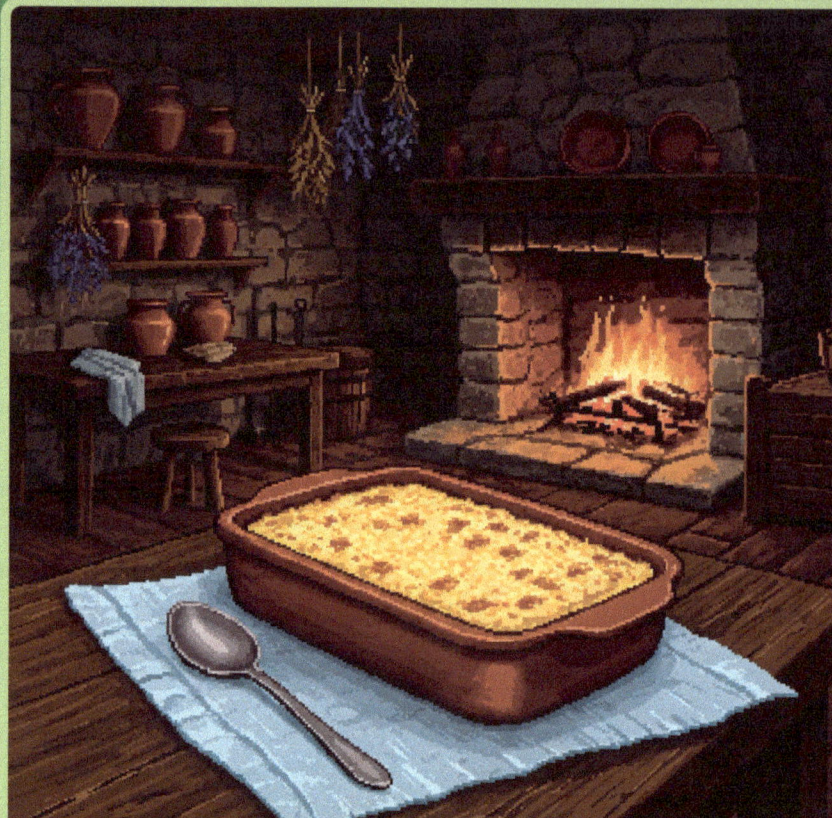

Cooking Directions

1 Preheat oven to 350. Measure and wash rice well, until the water runs clear.

2 Combine all ingredients in a 9" x 13" casserole dish. Stir well to combine.

3 Cover dish tightly with foil. Bake for 1 hour.

4 Remove from oven, uncover, and fluff gently with a fork immediately. Keep covered until ready to use. Will stay hot for up to 1 hour outside of oven.

Recipe Tip

Adding different ingredients to compliment your Main dish is one of the best things you can do with this Side. Green Bell Pepper and White Onion for Cajun food. Curry Powder and Cardamom pods for when making curries. Tomatoes and Scallions when making Central American cuisine, the limit is your sense of adventure!

Rice Pilaf

NOVICE

Using different types of rice, herbs, vegetables, and stocks can produce a wide range of flavors in this dish. This recipe is just a basic, all-purpose Pilaf that goes with just about anything. Experiment, and find out which varieties you enjoy the most with different dishes.

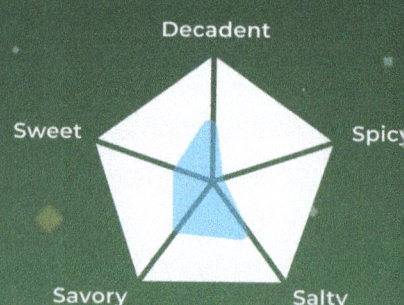

Ingredients

Long Grain Rice, White	1 C
Yellow Onion, Diced	½ C
Carrot, Peeled & Diced	¼ C
Stock (Any Kind)	16 Fl Oz
Oregano, Dry	1 tsp
Black Pepper, Ground	⅛ tsp
Salt	¼ tsp
Olive Oil Or Butter	1 Tbsp

 Prep Time 10 Min

 Cook Time 25 Min

 Servings 2 Cups

 12 - 14" Skillet w/Lid or 2 Qt Pot w/Lid 1 ea

 Wooden Spoon/Rubber Spatula 1 ea

 Fork for Fluffing 1 ea

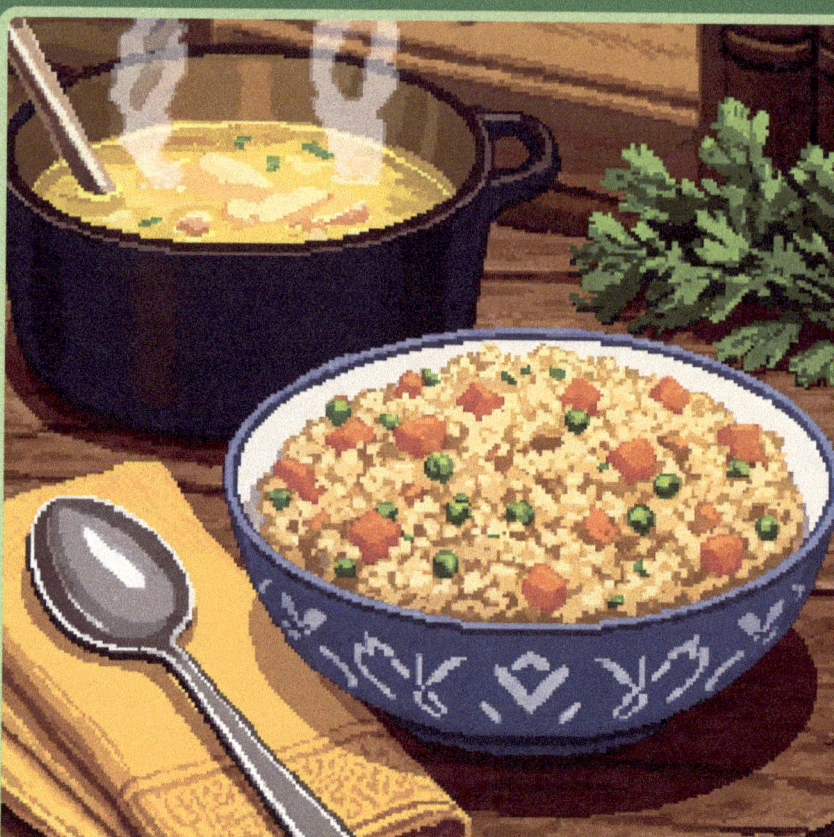

Cooking Directions

1   Place a 12" - 14" skillet (with a lid) or a 2 Qt. pot over Medium heat. When hot, add oil or butter.

2   When oil is shimmering or butter stops bubbling, add rice and stir. Cook for 2 min. until rice begins to brown, and smell nutty and aromatic.

3   Add onion and carrot. Stir well and cook for 1 - 2 minutes.

4   Add seasonings and stock to pan, stirring well. Raise heat to Medium High and bring to a simmer.

5   When simmering, reduce heat to Low and cover. Cook for 15 - 20 min. until all the stock has been absorbed. Remove lid and fluff with a fork immediately. Serve Hot, may be held over lowest heat setting, covered, for up to 1 hr.

Spinach Balls

This recipe is perfect for hosting parties and making quick side options for family gatherings. Dipping in ranch, tzatziki, blue cheese dressing, or just drizzling some hot sauce onto them helps elevate this simple dish into something extra. Stuffing mix can be bought in large bags at the grocery store, if you would prefer to use that over making your own stuffing mix with bread at home.

Decadent — Sweet — Spicy — Savory — Salty

Ingredients

Spinach, Chopped	1½ Lb
Olive Oil, Or Melted Butter	6 Tbsp
Parmesan Cheese, Grated	¼ C
Bread Slices, ¼" Thick Cubes	5 - 6 ea
Eggs, Partially Beaten	3 ea
Yellow Onion, Minced	½ C
Black Pepper, Ground	½ tsp
Garlic Powder	½ tsp
Thyme, Dry	½ tsp
Rosemary, Dry	¼ tsp
Sage, Ground	¼ tsp
Salt	¼ tsp
Olive Oil, For Sautéing	1 Tbsp

 Prep Time 15 Min

 **Cook Time** 20 - 25 Min

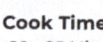 **Servings** 18 - 20 Balls

 11" x 14" Baking Sheet 1 ea

 12" - 14" Skillet 1 ea

 14" x 16" Baking Sheet 1 ea

 Large Mixing Bowl 1 ea

 Wooden/ Rubber Spatula 1 ea

Parchment Paper 1 ea

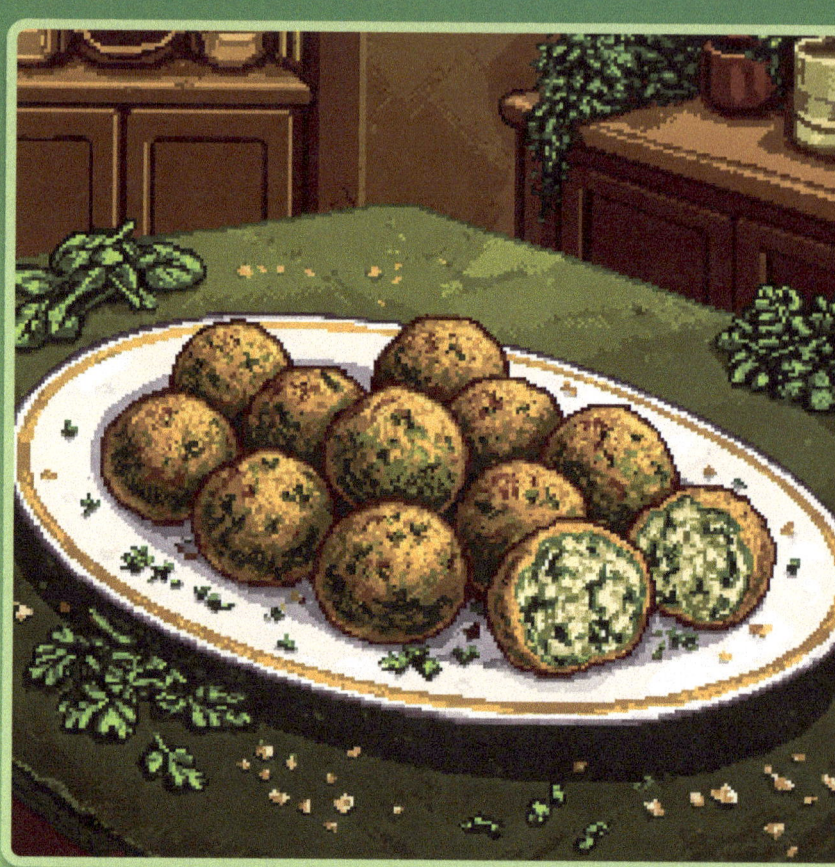

Cooking Directions

1   Preheat your oven to 200. Place the cubed bread pieces on a baking tray and place in oven. Cook until very dry and firm, 10 - 12 min.

2   Place a 12" - 14" skillet over Medium heat and add 1 Tbsp. olive oil. When oil is shimmering, add spinach. Cook until wilted and most of the moisture is evaporated, stirring often. Remove pan from heat. Raise oven temp to 350.

3   Combine all ingredients in a large bowl and mix well to combine.

4   Shape mixture evenly into golf ball sized pieces, pressing them gently to get them spherical.

5   Line a baking sheet with parchment paper and place balls on the sheet evenly spaced. They can be close together, just not touching.

6   Bake for 10-15 min. until slightly firm and browned, with an internal temperature of 145.

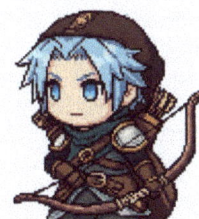

Recipe Tip

If buying stuffing mix at the store, keep in mind: It takes 3 - 4 average sized slices of bread, ½" thick, to make 1 C of stuffing cubes. Use this knowledge to figure out how much stuffing mix you need to buy.

Mains

Beef Chili

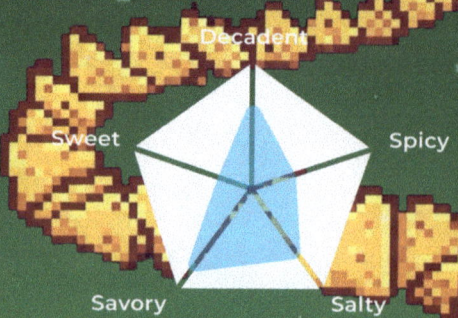

This recipe is a traditional chili recipe, and doesn't utilize some of the more unusual ingredients sometimes used in chili making. This isn't to say you shouldn't feel encouraged to experiment. Try adding peanut butter for a savory-sweetness, or fish sauce to give the tomatoes a distinct meatiness and zip. Or a dash of cinnamon sometimes really helps bring out the earthiness of the beans and meat. If you like heat, add 1 tsp. of cayenne to kick it up a notch.

Ingredients

Ground Beef	2 Lb
Green Bell Pepper, Diced	1 C
White Onion, Diced	1 ½ C
Diced Tomatoes OR	8 C
14 oz. Can Diced Tomatoes	4 ea
Black Beans, Rehydrated OR	3 C
14 oz. Can Black Beans, Rinsed	2 ea
Chili Powder	2 Tbsp
Paprika	2 tsp
Coriander, Ground	1 tsp
Cumin	½ tsp
Black Pepper, Ground	½ tsp
Garlic, Minced	1 Tbsp
Salt	1 tsp
Neutral Oil (Stovetop Cooking)	2 Tbsp
Water or Stock (Stovetop Cooking Only)	8 Fl Oz
Water (Omit if Using Cooked/ Canned Beans)	32 Fl Oz

Prep Time
15 Min

Cook Time
4 - 5 Hr (Stove Top)
3 - 7 Hr (Crock Pot)

Servings
8 - 10 Bowls

12" - 14" Skillet
1 ea

8 - 10 Qt Pot w/Lid (Stovetop Cooking)
1 ea

Wooden Spoon/Spatula
1 ea

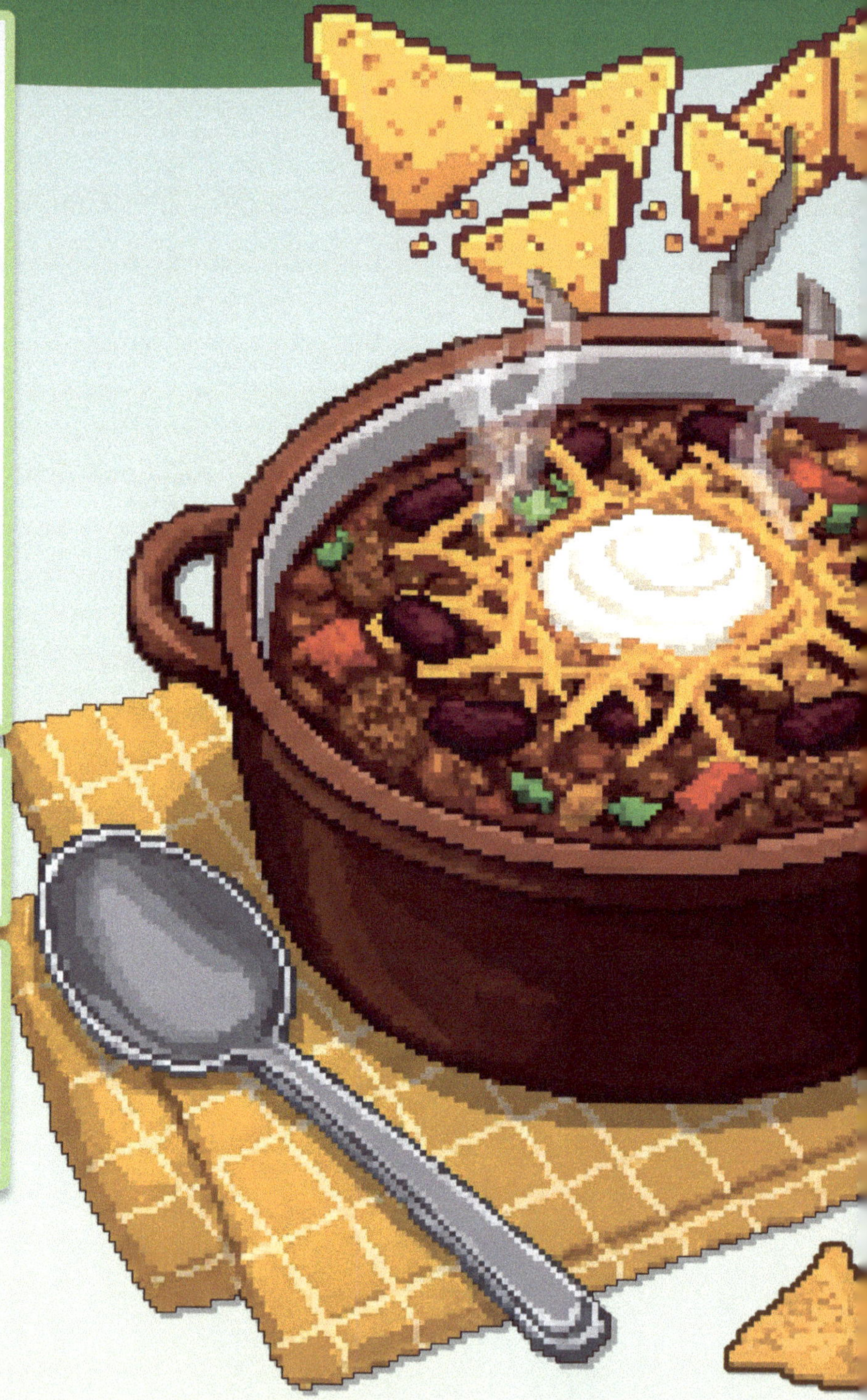

Cooking Directions
(For Crock Pot)

1   Place a 12" - 14" skillet or medium pot on Medium heat. Place ground beef in the pan/pot and cook thoroughly, breaking the meat apart into large chunks.

2   Once fully cooked, drain the fat and water from the beef. Transfer beef to a bowl and set aside. Set your crock pot to the desired cooking temperature (see below).

3   Put the tomatoes, onion, bell pepper and spices in a large (10 Qt. or more) crock pot. Next, add the beans and beef. If using rehydrated, uncooked beans add the extra water as well. Using a ceramic safe spoon or spatula mx ingredients together thoroughly.

4   Place the lid over the crock. If cooking on High setting, cook for 3 - 4 hr. If cooking on Low heat, cook for 6 - 8 hrs.

>>>> STOVE TOP DIRECTIONS >>>>

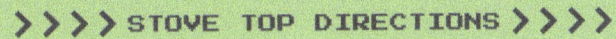

Cooking Directions
(For Stove Top)

1   Follow the directions on the previous page through Step 2.

2   Place an 8 - 10 Qt. pot with a lid over Medium heat. Put the oil in the pot.

3   When oil is shimmering, add the onion, bell pepper, and seasonings to the pot and cook for 5 - 7 min.

4   Add tomatoes, beans, and beef. Stir and incorporate all ingredients thoroughly. Add the water/stock. Bring to a hard simmer, then reduce heat to Medium Low. Cover pot with aluminum foil, then place the lid. Cook for 4 - 5 hr. checking on the chili every 90 min. or so. Make sure not to let too much moisture evaporate, and add more liquid if needed.

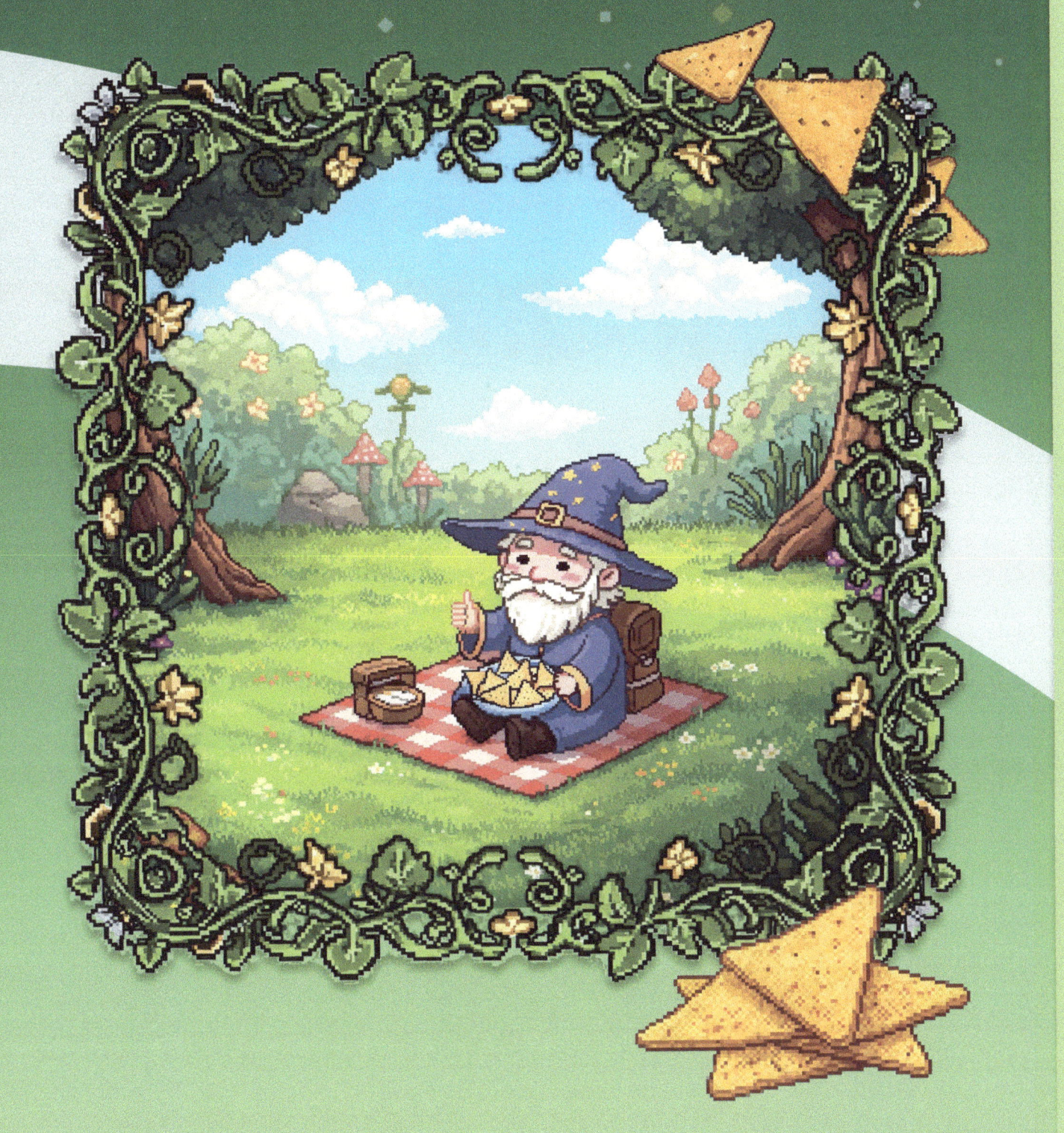

Chicken Salad

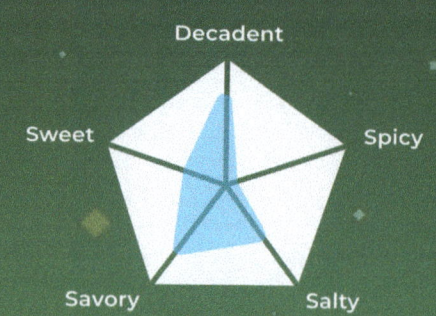

This all-purpose chicken salad recipe makes for a great sandwich or addition to a bed of greens. It works well as a base for your own experimentation, as it's neutral flavor lends itself to being manipulated and altered with a wide variety of herbs and spices. Flex your culinary muscles and get creative!

Ingredients

Chicken Breasts	2 ea
Water (If Shredding Chicken)	12 Fl Oz
Celery, Minced	⅓ C
White Onion, Minced	⅓ C
Mayo (Pg 145)	⅔ C
Salt	½ tsp
Black Pepper, Ground	¼ tsp
Mustard Powder	½ tsp
Garlic Powder	¼ tsp
Parsley, Dry	¼ tsp

Prep Time
35 Min

Cook Time
30 Min

Servings
6 - 8 Sandwiches

   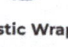 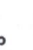 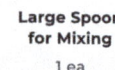

4 Qt Pot w/Lid
1 ea

Plastic Wrap
1 ea

Large Spoon for Mixing
1 ea

Forks for Shredding
2 ea

Wire Whisk
1 ea

Large Bowl for Shredding
1 ea

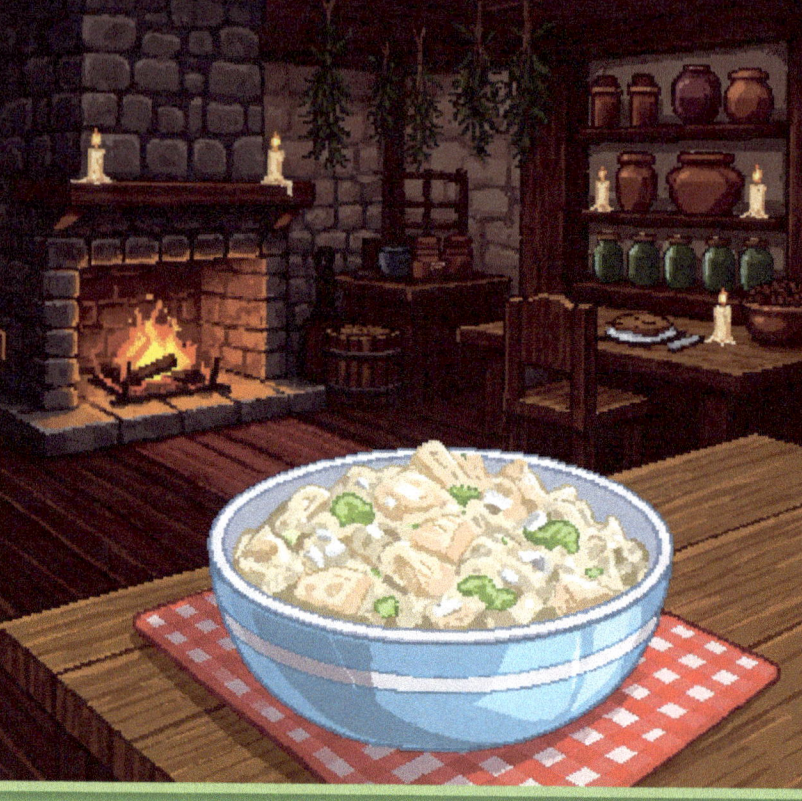

Cooking Directions

1   Place the water in a pot just big enough to hold the chicken breasts. Put the pot over High heat and bring to a simmer. When simmering, place the chicken in the pot, cover, and reduce heat to Medium Low. Cook for 30 min. until a spoon can be easily inserted into the chicken.

2   Remove the chicken from the pot and place in a large bowl. Discard water. Using two forks shred the chicken into fine pieces. Place shredded chicken in fridge to cool down.

3   Combine all ingredients except the celery and onion in a large bowl and whisk until combined. Add the onion, celery and shredded chicken. Fold gently with a rubber spatula until well combined. If the mixture looks too dry, add more mayo 1 Tbsp. at a time.

4   Cover with plastic wrap or transfer to an airtight container. Refrigerate for 2 hr. minimum or overnight before serving. Holds in refrigerator for 3 - 4 days.

> **Recipe Tip**
>
> If you want to save time, you can always purchase a rotisserie chicken from the store and shred the meat needed off of that. The leftovers can be saved for other dishes to make throughout the week, so you can get multiple meals out of one purchase. Cross-Utilization for the win!

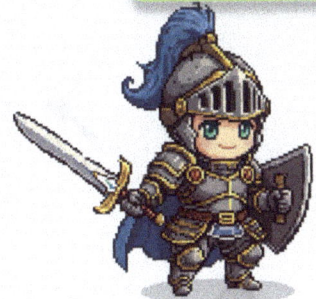

Duck Leg Confit

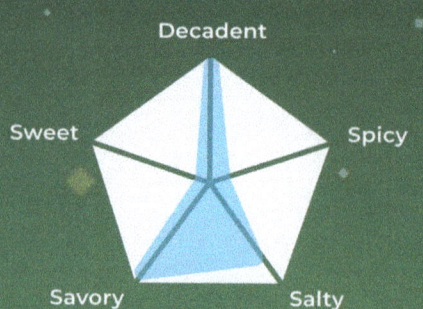

Decadent

Sweet · Spicy

Savory · Salty

This classic recipe is deceptively simple to make, even if it does take a lot of time. Don't be discouraged, this haute cuisine dish is within everyone's grasp, and won't disappoint those who take the plunge and give it a go.

The gravy recipe I gave with this dish is a simple and basic one. I encourage you to get creative and try adding various ingredients to it yourself. I highly recommend trying it with various sauces in this book; don't be afraid to experiment! However, there's a reason pan gravies are the classic companions of dishes like Duck Leg Confit: they're delicious.

Ingredients

Duck Leg Quarters	4 ea
Stock (Chicken or Duck)	12 fl oz
White Wine	6 fl oz
Garlic, Minced	1 tsp
Oregano, Dry	⅛ tsp
Rosemary, Dry	⅛ tsp
Black Pepper, Ground	⅛ tsp
Salt	¼ tsp
Duck Fat From Pan	2 Tbsp
AP Flour	2 Tbsp
Butter or Lard for Greasing the Pan	

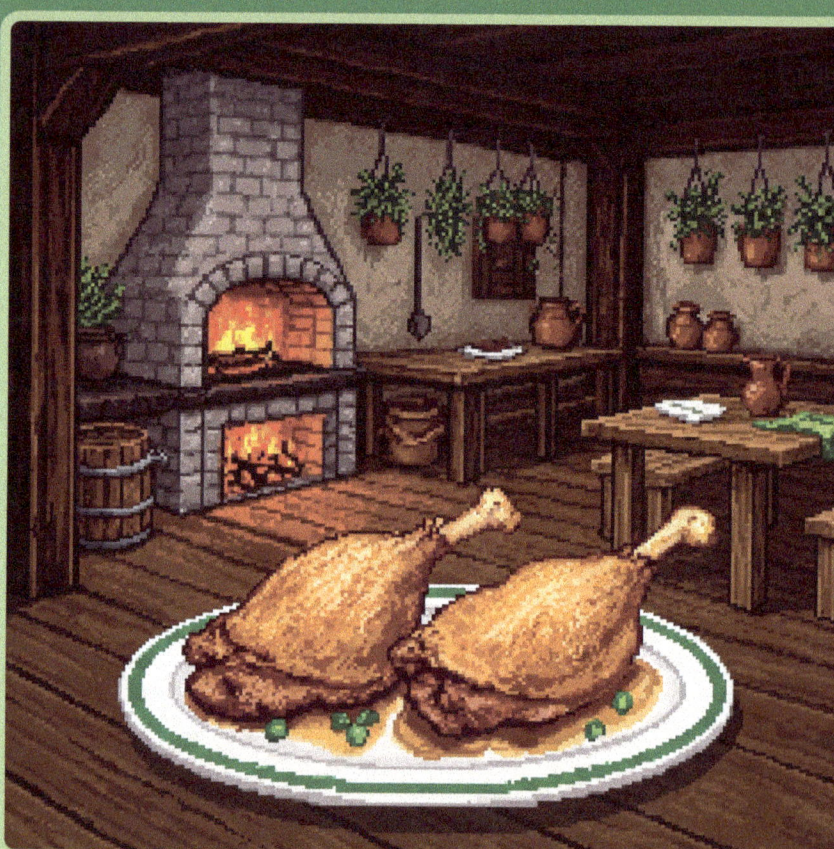

Prep Time
30 - 40 Min

Cook Time
2 - 2¼ Hr

Servings
4 Whole Legs

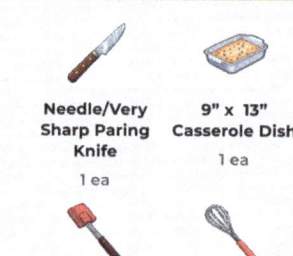

Needle/Very Sharp Paring Knife
1 ea

9" x 13" Casserole Dish
1 ea

3 Qt Pot or 8 - 10" Skillet
1 ea

Rubber Spatula
2 ea

Wire Whisk
1 ea

Large Spoon
1 ea

Cooking Directions

1   Pat the legs dry with paper towels.

2   Using a needle or a very sharp knife, prick the skin all over as much as possible. Focus on the skin that covers fat the most. Do your best to avoid piercing the skin through to the meat. This step is vital as it helps produce a crispy skin.

3   Turn the duck legs over, meat side up, and salt them generously. Let them rest on the counter for 25 - 30 min. Don't worry, they won't spoil.

4   Place the duck legs in a 9" x 13" casserole dish, skin side up, in such a way that they are close but not overlapping and touching as little as possible. Find the best way to arrange them, remove them from the dish and grease the bottom of the dish well, then replace them skin side up still.

5   Place the dish into a cold oven, on a rack that's in the middle. Set the heat to 285 (300 if not a digital oven). It cannot be stressed enough: DO NOT preheat the oven.

6   Let the duck cook for 2 hr. and check on it after 1½ hr. The fat should be well melted with the legs partially submerged in it, the skin getting crispy.

7   After 2 hrs. turn the oven up to 375 and cook for 10 min. then check the duck and continue cooking until the skin is very crispy. There may be some spots that aren't as crispy as others. This is a sign that those parts weren't pierced as well as others. But that's ok, it's better to have some patches that aren't too crispy, rather than some burnt ones.

> > > > CONTINUED > > > >

8   Remove from the oven and let cool for 10 min. before removing from the pan.

9   While the duck is cooling, place a small sauce pot or medium sized skillet over Medium heat. When hot, spoon 2 Tbsp. of the duck fat into the pan then add 1½ Tbsp. of flour to the pan. Stir constantly and cook for 3 - 4 minutes to bring to the Blond Level. Add the wine and stir constantly, making sure to work out any lumps in the roux. Next, add the seasonings and cook for 1 minute more. Then, add the stock and stir until the roux is completely dissolved and mixed into the liquid. Bring to a simmer and cook for 4 - 5 minutes until desired thickness is reached. If too thick, add stock 1 Tbsp. at a time until the right consistency.

10 Remove duck legs from the pan and place on paper towels to absorb excess grease before serving.

11 Place the duck leg on a plate and spoon 3 - 4 oz. of the gravy around the leg. Avoid putting it directly on the leg to retain the crispiness of the skin.

Recipe Tip

If keeping the grease for later use (which I highly recommend) be sure to strain it through a fine sieve or cheesecloth while still liquid. It will keep in the fridge for about 6 - 8 weeks.

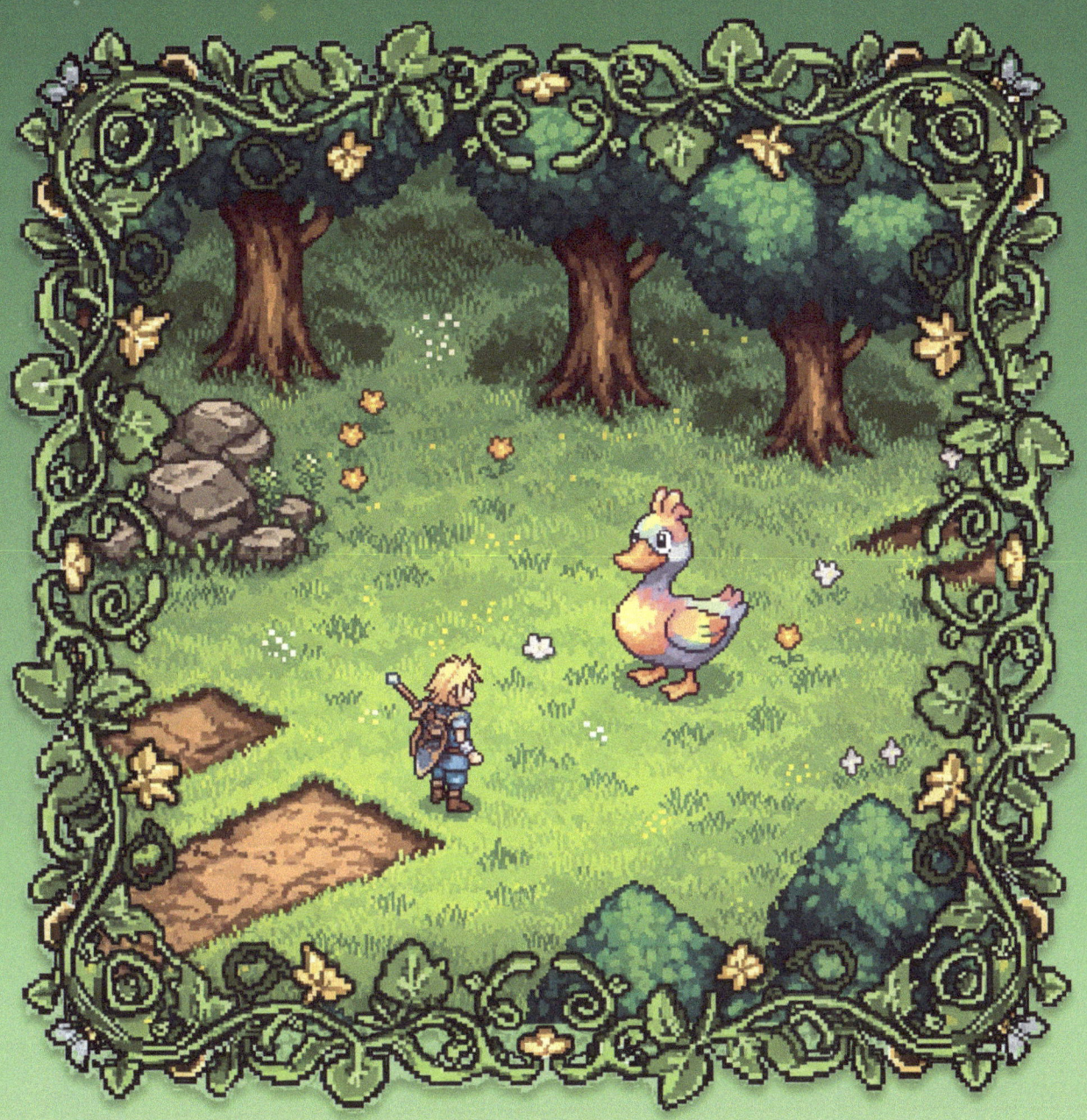

Fluffy Ground Beef

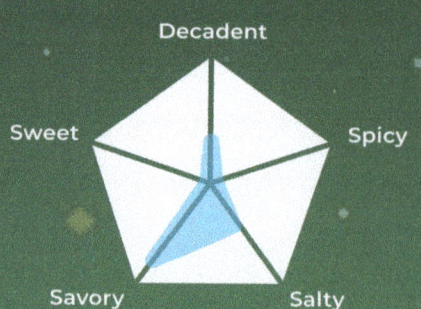

This recipe is a great base for all sorts of dishes. Need meat for lasagna, a meat sauce, or stuffed shells? Need fluffy beef for your Shepherd's Pie, or maybe a meaty mac and cheese casserole? This recipe works for a wide variety of options. The sky's the limit, so flex those culinary muscles and get creative!

Ingredients

Ground Beef, 85/15 preferred	2 Lb
Salt	1 tsp
Black Pepper, Ground	½ tsp
Garlic Powder	1 tsp
Carrot, Minced	¼ C
Yellow Onion, Minced	¼ C
Water/Stock	16 fl oz

Prep Time	Cook Time	Servings
5 Min	1 Hr	2 Lb

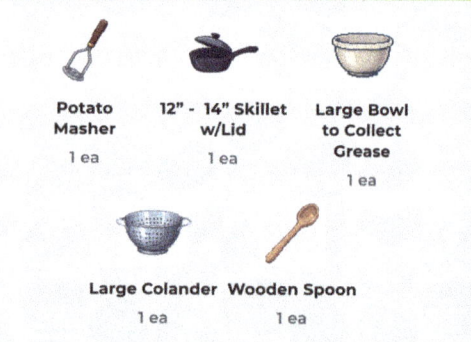

Potato Masher	12" - 14" Skillet w/Lid	Large Bowl to Collect Grease
1 ea	1 ea	1 ea

Large Colander	Wooden Spoon
1 ea	1 ea

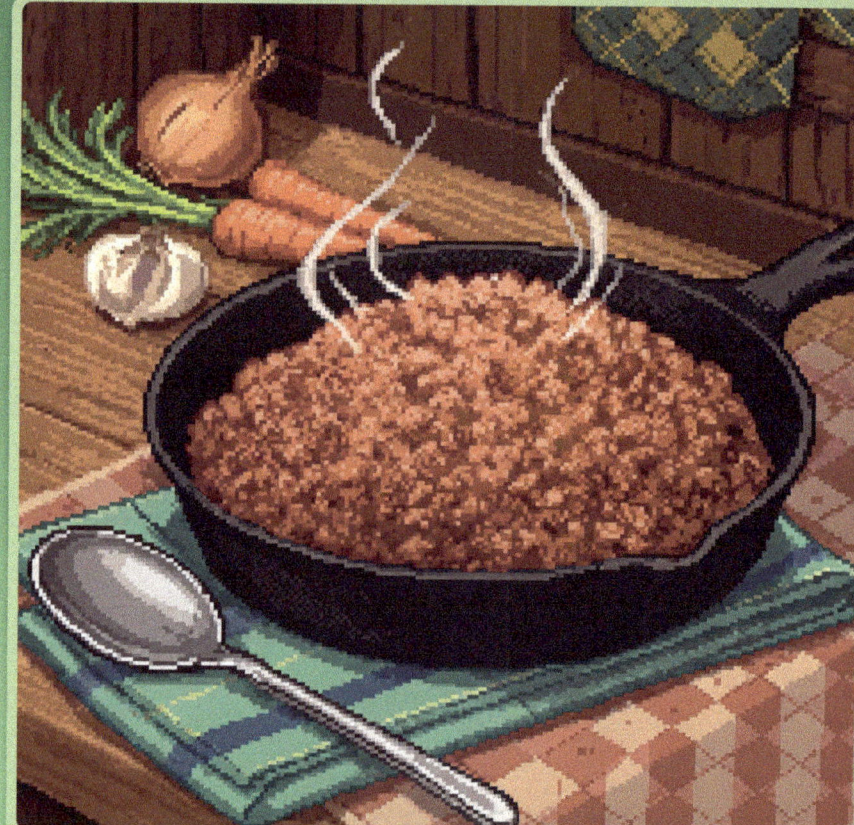

Cooking Directions

1   Place a 12" - 14" skillet (with lid) or a large pot over High heat.

2   Put all ingredients into the skillet/pot and break the meat into large chunks using a wooden or metal spatula.

3   Bring the liquid to a hard simmer. Lower heat to Medium Low and cover.

4   Cook for 1 hr.

5   Remove the lid and use a potato masher to break apart the beef until completely mashed and broken into tiny pieces.

6   Strain the mixture in a colander over a large bowl. Discard the liquid, but not in the sink because the beef fat will clog your drains.

7   Transfer to a heat safe container and cool for 45 min. out of fridge, stirring often, before placing in fridge. If using immediately, no need to worry about cooling. Be sure the meat is completely cooled before covering. Can be stored for up to 5 days.

Old School Pot Roast

This dish can be very easy to make. The searing isn't necessary, just recommended. If you aren't looking for a thickened gravy, you can also skip making the roux and simply place all ingredients in a crock pot before lunch, set it to Low, and walk away until dinner time.

I recommend serving this dish with biscuits, or some good quality bread for soppin' up all that gravy. Once you've Leveled Up, try it out with some homemade French Bread (see Pg 371).

Radar chart: Decadent, Sweet, Spicy, Savory, Salty

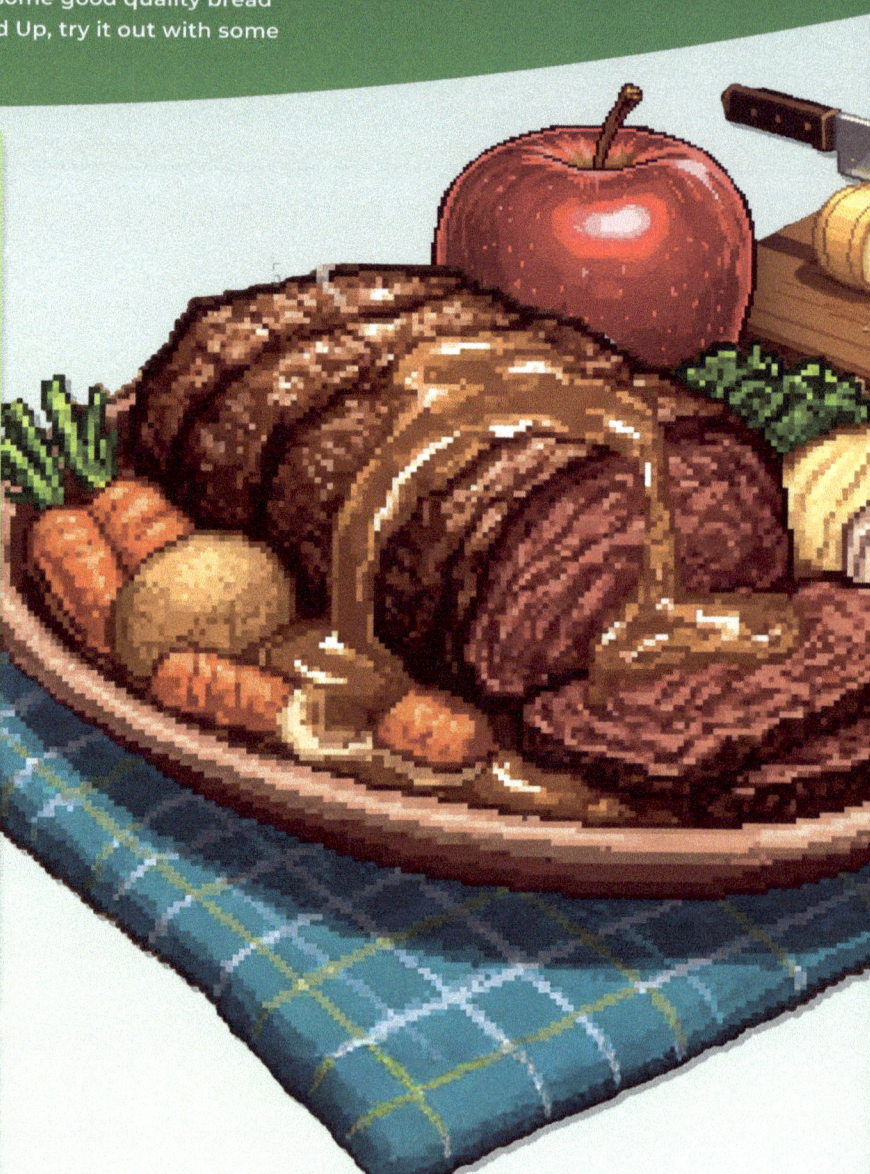

Ingredients

Chuck Roast	3 - 4 Lb
Carrots, Cut Into Rounds	1 C
Yellow Onion, Large Dice	1 ½ C
Mushrooms, Quartered	½ C
Celery Stalks, ½" Slices	2 ea
Large Red Apple, Diced	1 ea
Beef Stock	16 Fl Oz
Bay Leaf	2 ea
Salt	2 tsp
Black Pepper, Ground	½ tsp
Rosemary, Dry	1 tsp
Thyme, Dry	1 tsp
Garlic, Minced	2 tsp
AP Flour	10 Tbsp
Oil (For Roux)	9 Tbsp
Oil (For Searing)	1 Tbsp

 Prep Time 20 Min

 Cook Time 3 Hr (Oven) 4 - 8 Hr (Crockpot)

 Servings 6 - 8

 6 - 8 Qt. Pot w/Lid or Dutch Oven 1 ea

Wire Whisk 1 ea

 Pair of Tongs 1 ea

 Wooden Spoon/Rubber Spatula 1 ea

Cooking Directions
(For Crock Pot)

1   Place a 6 - 8 Qt. pot over Medium High heat. When hot, add 1 Tbsp. of oil. When shimmering, place the roast in the pot and sear for 2 - 3 min. per side. Meanwhile, cut the apple and place the pieces at the bottom of the crock. Remove meat from the pot and place in crock. Set the crock to Low if you are cooking it for 6 - 8 hrs. and on High if you are cooking it for 4 - 5 hr.

2   Add the remaining oil. When shimmering, add the carrots, celery, onion and mushrooms. Cook for 5 min. stirring often. Add the flour and cook for 3 - 4 min. stirring constantly to bring it to the Blond Level.

3   Add the garlic and cook for 1 min. more. Add a small amount of the stock and scrape the bottom of the pan well. Add the rest of the stock, stirring well to make sure there are no lumps. It'll thicken intensely, but that's good. The water from the vegetables and meat will thin it out to the right consistency.

4   Remove the pot from the heat. Add the salt, pepper, rosemary, bay leaves and thyme and stir. Carefully transfer the vegetables to the crock, pouring them over the roast. Be sure to scrape as much of the thickened stock out of the pot as possible.

5   Cover the crock and cook according to your time schedule. Serve Hot.

> > > > OVEN DIRECTIONS > > > >

Cooking Directions
(For Oven)

1   Preheat oven to 300.

2   Place a 6 - 8 Qt. pot over Medium High heat. When hot, add 1 Tbsp. of oil. When shimmering place the roast in the pot. Sear for 2 - 3 min. per side. Remove from pot and set aside.

3   Add remaining oil, then the vegetables. Cook for 5 min. stirring often. Then add the flour. Cook for 3 - 4 min, stirring constantly to bring it to the Blond level.

4   Add the garlic, cook for 1 min. Add a small amount of the stock and scrape all the browned bits from the bottom of the pan. Then add the remaining stock and whisk well. It'll thicken intensely, but that's good.

5   Add the seasonings and the apple pieces to the pot and stir well. Place the roast back in the pot and agitate so the roast is near the bottom and mostly submerged in the gravy.

6   If not using a Dutch oven, cover the pot tightly with foil before placing the lid on. Once covered, move to the oven and cook for 3 hours. Check on the roast halfway through to make sure there is always enough liquid in the pot so the roast is half submerged. Cook until a spoon can be inserted into the roast easily, and can be torn apart easily. Serve Hot.

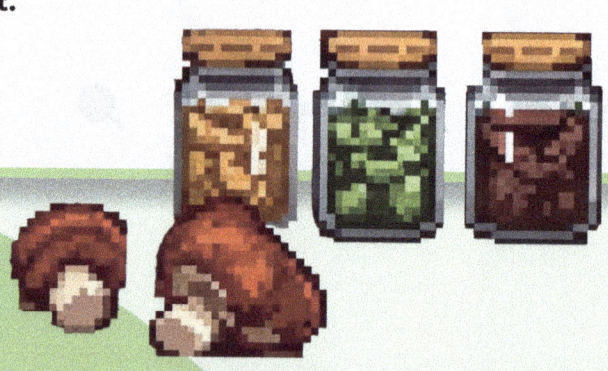

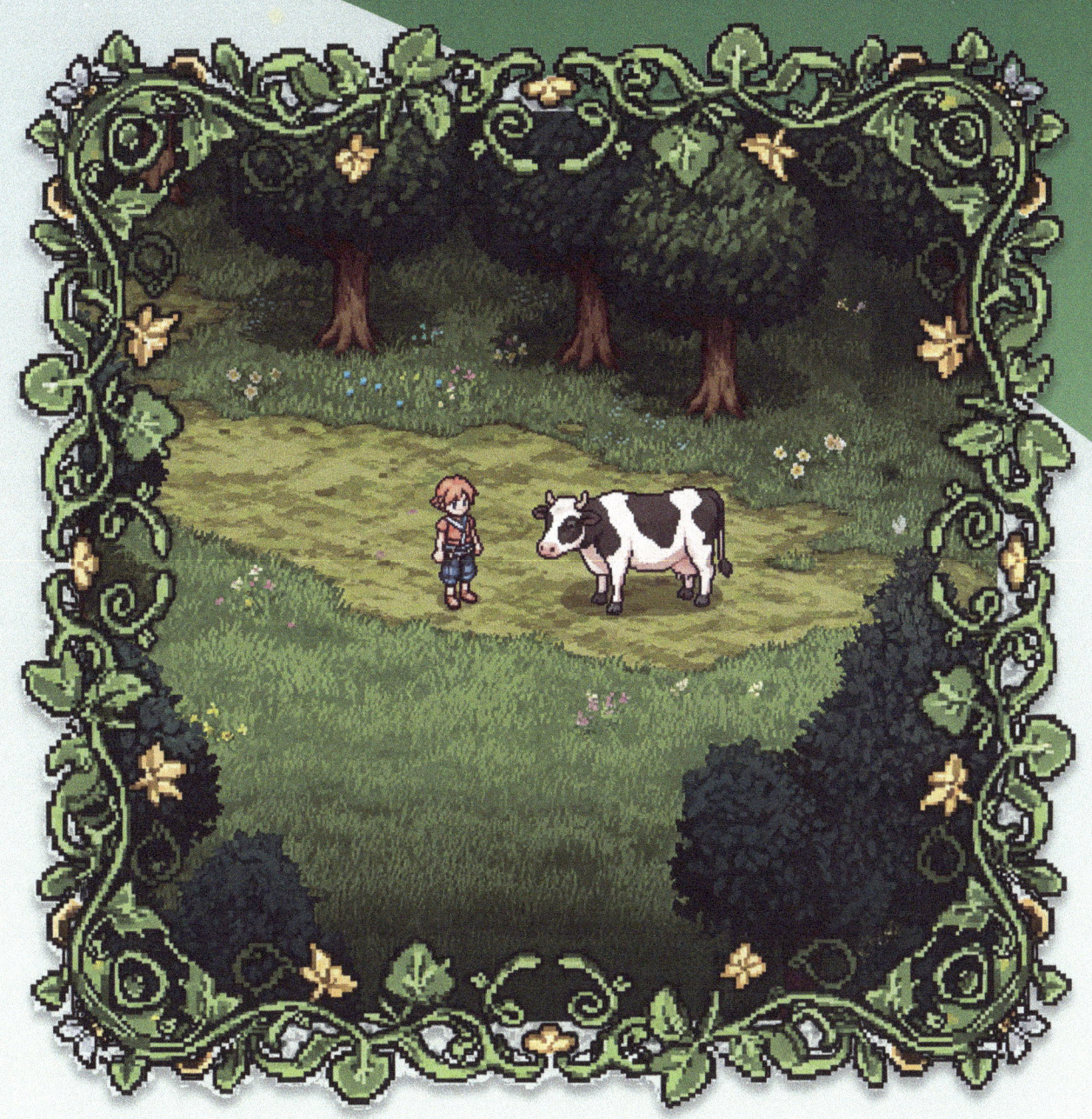

Osso Bucco (Braised Beef Shanks)

This recipe is another example of a classic dish that's beyond easy to make. I recommend serving the shanks over mashed potatoes, roasted vegetables, or large pearl couscous. When transferring the shanks, be careful. The meat will very easily come apart. Since the braising liquid will be full of a large amount of liquid fat, it's not very useful to use as a garnish. That being said, preparing a separate sauce on the stove top is the recommended course of action. I suggest the Cherry Bordelaise (Pg 321) or the Classic Stock Gravy (Pg 241). Any kind of flavorful, rich sauce will pair very well with this dish.

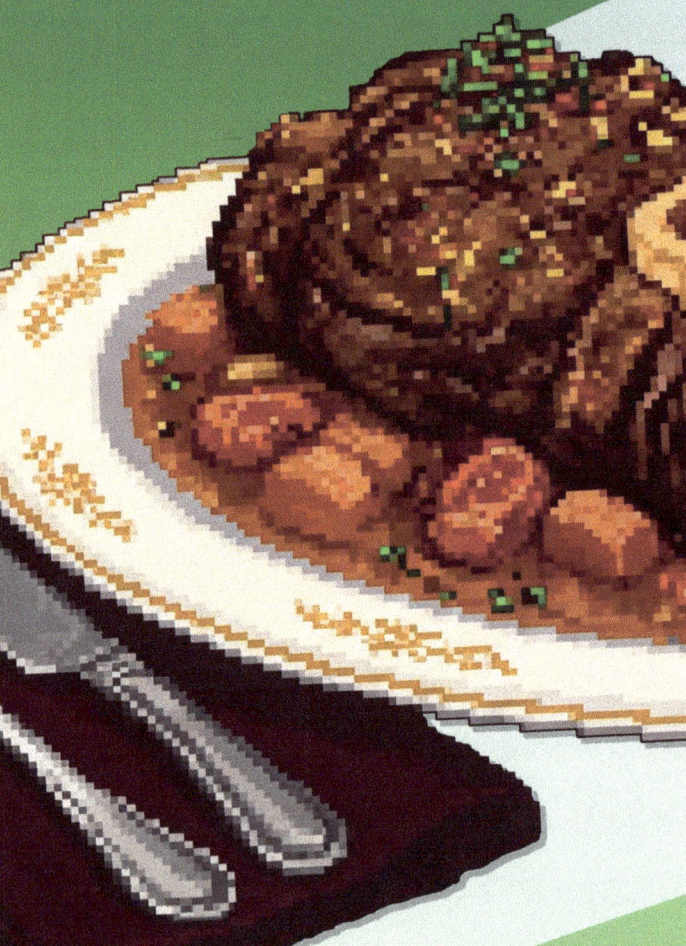

Ingredients

Beef Shanks (3 - 4" Thick)	2 - 3 Lb
Oil or Butter	2 Tbsp
Garlic, Minced	2 Tbsp
White Onion, Sliced	½ ea
Carrot, Diced	¾ C
White Wine	½ C
Tomato, Diced	2 C
Beef Stock	8 Fl Oz

 Prep Time 10 Min

 Cook Time 15 Min + 4 - 6 Hr

 Servings 4 ea

 6 - 8 Qt. Pot w/Lid 1 ea

 Wooden Spoon 1 ea

 Pair of Tongs 1 ea

Decadent
Sweet
Spicy
Savory
Salty

Cooking Directions
(For Oven)

1. Preheat oven to 300. Place a 4 - 6 Qt. pot (with lid) or a Dutch oven over Medium High heat. When hot add the oil or butter.

2. When the oil is shimmering, or the butter stops bubbling, sear the beef shanks for 2 - 3 min. per side. Remove from pot and set aside.

3. Add onion slices to pot, cook for 5 - 7 min. stirring often, until the onion is soft.

4. Add the carrot and garlic. Cook until fragrant, 1 - 2 min.

5. Add the wine and stir, make sure to scrape the browned bits (the fond) off the bottom of the pan. Then add the stock and tomatoes.

6. Return the shanks to the pan, moving them around so that they are as submerged as possible. Cover the pot. If not using a Dutch oven, cover with foil before putting the lid on.

7. Place the pot in the oven and cook for 4 - 5 hr. Cook until a spoon can be inserted easily into the meat, and the meat can be easily torn. Serve Hot.

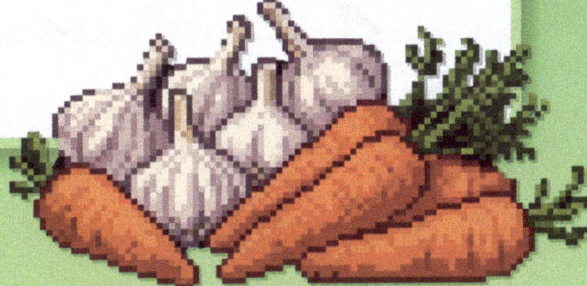

〉〉〉〉 CROCK POT DIRECTIONS 〉〉〉〉

Cooking Directions
(For Crock Pot)

1   Follow steps 1 - 5 from previous page.

2   Set your crock pot to Low. Place your seared shanks in the crock.

3   Carefully transfer the vegetables and liquid to the crock, pouring it evenly over the shanks.

4   Cover with the lid and cook for 5 - 6 hr. Serve Hot.

Recipe Tip

You may also use veal or lamb shanks with this dish. Beef shanks are usually the easiest to obtain in stores, but if you find either of the other options, pick them up and make this delicious offering the next time you feel like treating yourself and your family and friends to a real treat!

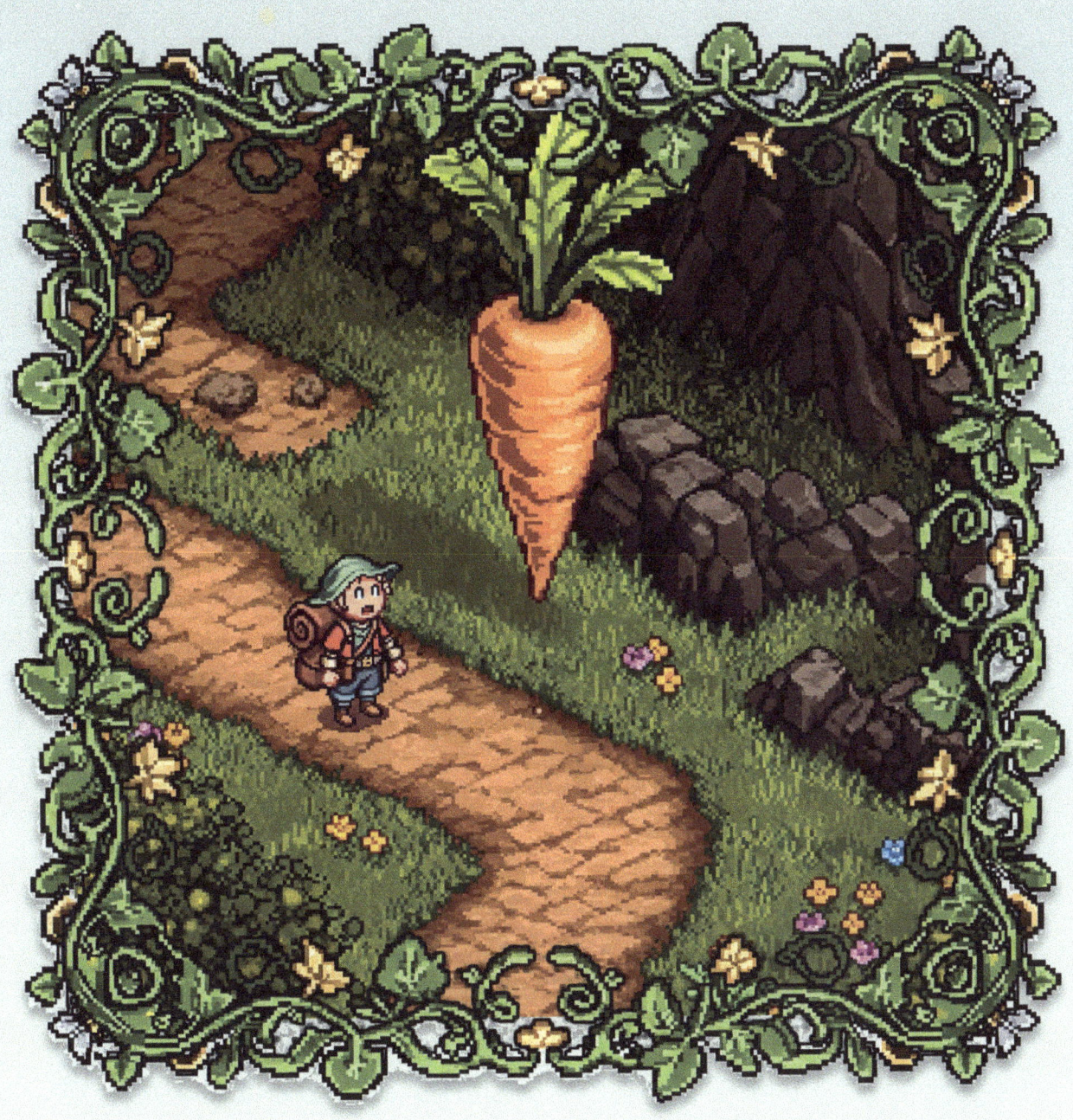

Restaurant Style Taco Beef

Decadent

Sweet — Spicy

Savory — Salty

This meat will have a mild flavor without any extra seasoning, and the lack of excess fat makes it the go-to choice for making tacos, enchiladas, quesadillas, and more. Adding extra seasonings and cooking in a pan with a little water can really ramp up the flavor in your recipes, and help the meat stick together a little better. Don't worry, it won't ruin the texture of your fluffy ground beef.

Ingredients

Ground Beef, 85/15	2 Lb
Salt	1 tsp
Chili Powder	1 tsp
Cumin	2 tsp
Garlic Powder	1 tsp
Black Pepper, Ground	½ tsp
White Onion, Small Dice	½ C
Water/Stock	16 fl oz

 Prep Time
5 Min

 Cook Time
1 Hr

 **Servings**
2 Lb

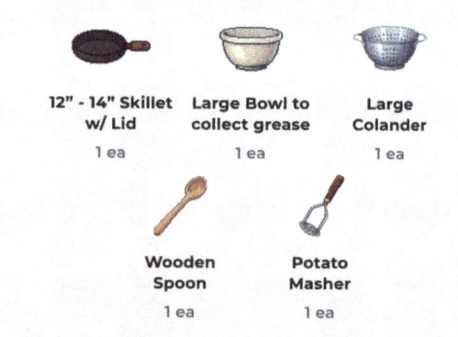

12" - 14" Skillet w/ Lid
1 ea

Large Bowl to collect grease
1 ea

Large Colander
1 ea

Wooden Spoon
1 ea

Potato Masher
1 ea

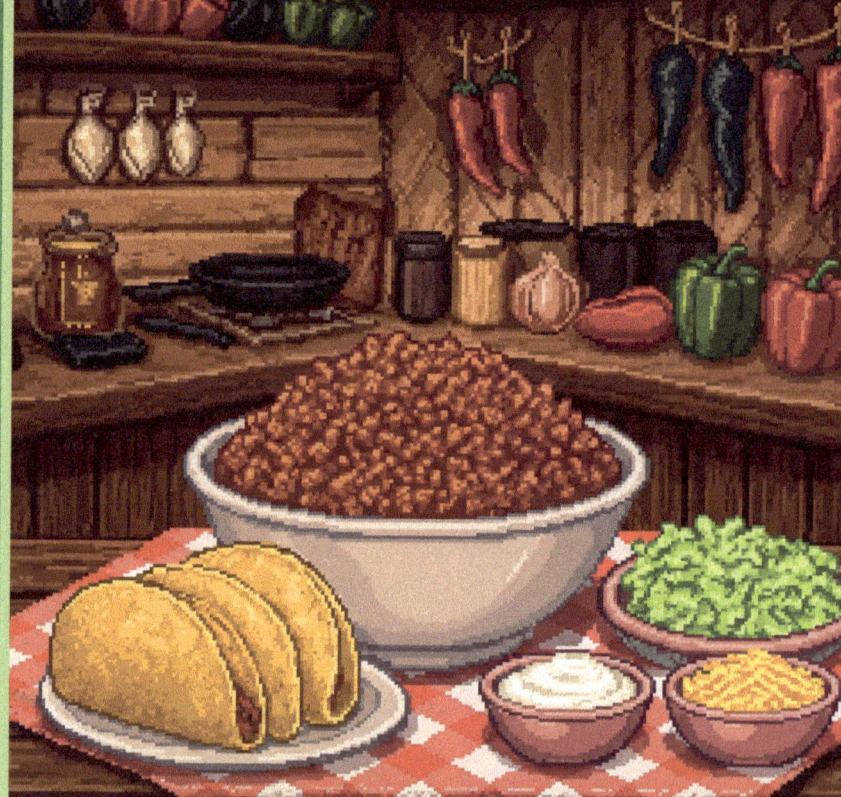

Cooking Directions

1   Place a 12" - 14" skillet (with lid) or a medium pot over High heat.

2   Put all ingredients in the pan, using a wooden spoon to break the meat into large chunks. Bring to a hard simmer.

3   Reduce the heat to Medium Low and cover. Cook for 1 hr.

4   Remove lid and use a potato masher to break apart the meat until completely mashed into fine, small pieces.

5   Strain the beef in a colander over a large bowl. Discard the liquid, but not in the sink because the beef fat will clog your drain.

6   Cool in a container on the counter for 45 min. stirring often before placing it in the fridge if not using immediately. Be sure the meat is completely cool in the fridge before covering. Can be held for up to 3 days before use.

Rustic Beef Stew

This beef stew is a delicious dish that requires no additional sides. Of course, you can always make them if you desire, but the dish itself has vegetables, starches, and protein, making it a complete meal in a bowl. The one thing I would recommend is having some French Bread (see Pg 371) to sop up any gravy left in your bowl. Another way to do it would be to omit the potatoes and serve this stew over a bed of egg noodles or long grain rice to give it a variety of texture.

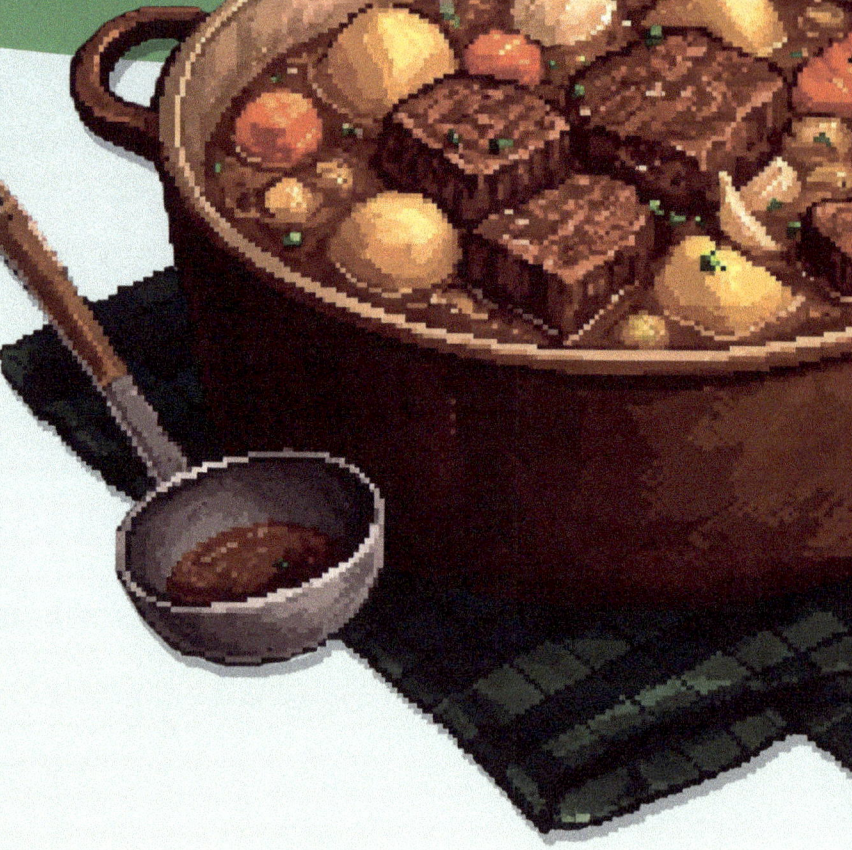

Decadent
Sweet — Spicy
Savory — Salty

Ingredients

Chuck Roast, 1½" Pcs	2 Lb
Carrot, Cut Into Rounds	1 C
Yellow Onion, Large Dice	1 ½ C
Mushrooms, Quartered	½ C
Celery Stalks, ½" Slices	2 ea
Garlic, Minced	2 tsp
Small Red Potatoes, Cut in Half	½ Lb
Salt	2 tsp
Bay Leaf	2 ea
Black Pepper, Ground	1 tsp
Rosemary, Dry	½ tsp
Thyme, Dry	¾ tsp
Parsley, Dry	1 tsp
Sage, Ground	½ tsp
Beef Stock	24 Fl Oz
AP Flour	6 Tbsp
Oil (For Roux)	5 Tbsp
Oil (For Searing)	1 Tbsp

 Prep Time
15 Min

 Cook Time
3½ - 4 Hr (Stovetop)
6 - 8 Hr (Crockpot)

 Servings
6 - 8 Bowls

 Wire Whisk
1 ea

 Pair of Tongs
1 ea

 Wooden Spoon/Rubber Spatula
1 ea

  6 - 8 Qt. Pot w/Lid
1 ea

Cooking Directions
(For Stove Top)

1. Place a 6 - 8 Qt. pot over Medium High heat. When hot, add 1 Tbsp. of oil. Once it's shimmering, place the meat in the pan, making sure not to overcrowd the pan. Sear the pieces for 1 - 2 min. per side, browning 2 sides of each cube. Work in batches if needed.

2. Once done searing, transfer the meat to a bowl and set aside. When all the meat is seared, add the rest of the oil (if making roux during cooking).

3. Add the onion, carrot, celery, and mushrooms. Cook for 3 - 4 min. until they begin to get soft. Add the garlic and cook for 1 min. If using premade roux, now is the time to place it in the pot and stir well. If not, add the flour and cook for 4 - 5 min. stirring constantly to bring it the the Blond Level.

4. Add 8 oz. of the stock to the pot and stir well, scraping up all the browned bits (the fond) from the bottom of the pan and working out any lumps in the roux.

5. Add the remaining stock slowly, stirring as you do. Bring to a simmer and thicken. It'll thicken intensely, but that's good. The liquid from the vegetables and meet will thin it to the right consistency.

6. Return the meat to the pot, add your seasonings.

7. Bring to a boil and cover the pot with foil before placing the lid on it. Reduce the heat to Low or Medium Low (whichever maintains a light simmer on your stove better).

8. Cook for 3 - 3½ hr. Be sure to check on the stew every hour or so, adding more liquid if necessary. It's done when the meat can be easily torn apart. Serve Hot.

Cooking Directions
(For Crock Pot)

1   Follow steps 1 - 5 from the previous page.

2   Set your crock pot to the Low heat setting. Place your seared meat in the crock.

3   Once the gravy has been thickened, carefully transfer it from the pot into the crock. Be sure to scrape up any extra gravy that is on the sides and bottom of the pot with a rubber spatula.

4   Cover and cook for 5 - 6 hr. until the meat is soft and easily torn apart. Serve Hot.

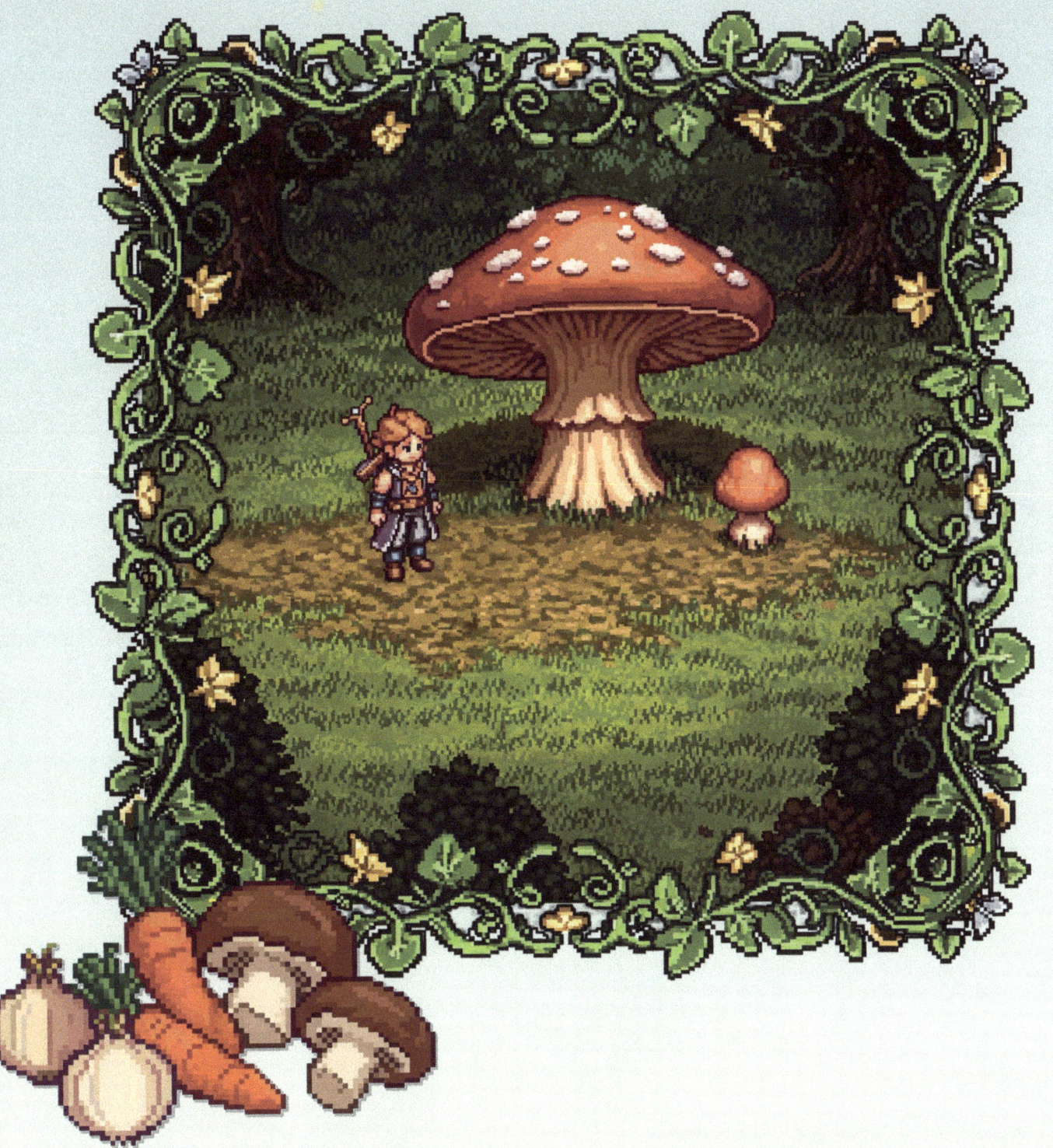

Simple Chicken Pot Pie

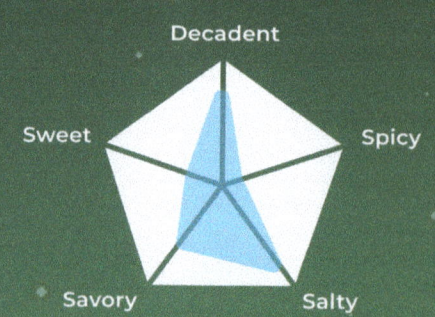

Decadent

Sweet   Spicy

Savory   Salty

This recipe is a bit of a standout in this book, as it contains mostly prepared items from the store. While we all love cooking at home and using whole foods for our recipes, there isn't always time to do that. This recipe is a great way to give yourself a home cooked meal that is warming and satisfying without a lot of preparation and work. Turn this recipe into an Expert level recipe by making every component from scratch for a real challenge! Just replace the cream of mushroom soup with homemade Chicken Veloute.

Ingredients

9" Deep Dish Pie Crusts	2 ea
Pie Dough Rolls (from Store)	2 ea
Chicken Breasts, ½" Pcs	2 ea
Yellow Onion, Diced	1 C
Garlic, Minced	1 Tbsp
12 oz Bag of Frozen Veg Medley	1 ea
Soy Sauce	2 Tbsp
Large Egg, Beaten, for Brushing	1 ea
Cream of Mushroom Soup, Condensed	22 oz
Neutral Oil	1 Tbsp
Salt & Pepper for Chicken	
Bowl of Cold Water for Shocking	

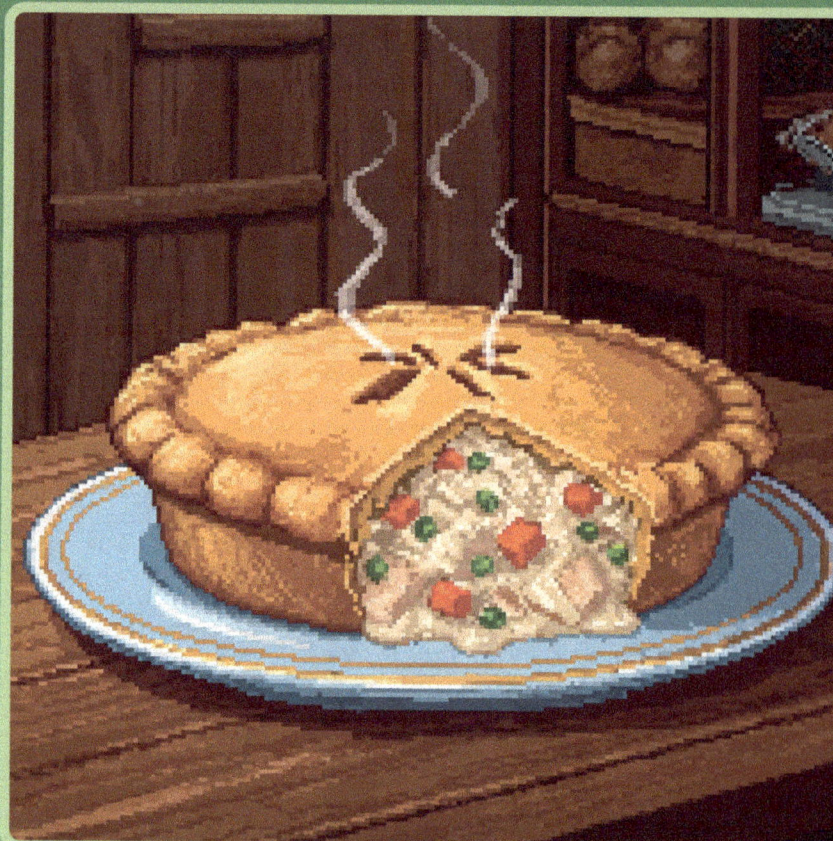

Prep Time
15 Min

Cook Time
40 - 45 Min

Servings
2 Pies

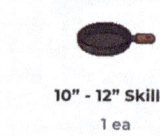

10" - 12" Skillet
1 ea

Large Mixing Bowl
1 ea

Small Pot for Thawing Frozen Veg Medley
1 ea

Large Spoon
1 ea

Large Colander
1 ea

Cooking Directions

1   Thaw the frozen pie crusts in fridge overnight. Place
    both them and the dough rolls on the counter for about
    20 min. before starting. Preheat the oven to 350.

2   Toss the chicken pieces in a generous amount of salt
    and pepper.

3   Place a 10"- 12" skillet on Medium High heat. Also place
    a small pot, filled ⅔ of the way with water, on
    High heat.

4   Add ½ Tbsp. of oil. When the oil is shimmering, place
    the chicken in the pan. Cook for 5 - 8 min, stirring
    halfway through. Remove chicken from pan and set
    aside. Take pan off of heat and turn off stove eye.

5   When the water is boiling, add the vegetables and
    immediately remove the pot from heat. Strain the
    vegetables right away and place in the bowl of
    cold water to stop them from cooking. Strain
    again and set aside.

6   Place the pan you cooked the chicken in over Medium
    heat, add the rest of the oil. When it's shimmering add
    the onion. Cook for 3 min. Then add a ¼ cup of water to
    the pan and scrape up the browned bits from the bottom
    of the pan (the fond) and cook until the water has
    evaporated. Remove from heat and set aside.

7   In a large bowl, combine the chicken, onion, and
    other remaining ingredients (except the egg) and
    stir well to combine.

8   **Transfer ½ of the mixture into each pie dish. Unroll the pie dough and place one over each dish. Trim the excess from the edges then press together to seal.**

9   **Cut 3 slits in the top crust to vent, brush with the egg, and sprinkle a little salt on top.**

10   **Bake for 40 - 45 min. until golden brown. Let rest for 10 min. before cutting into the pie.**

Recipe Tip

This recipe makes 2 pies, so it's perfect for making dinner and then freezing another pie for a later meal. Just wrap the pie in plastic wrap and tin foil before placing in the freezer. When ready to bake the frozen pie, simply remove the wrapping and bake at 350 for 1 hr. 15 min.

Recipe Tip

The excess dough can be used to make ornamentation for the pie crust. Try getting creative with various designs. Leaves and spirals are fairly simple decorations and really elevate the look of this simple dish.

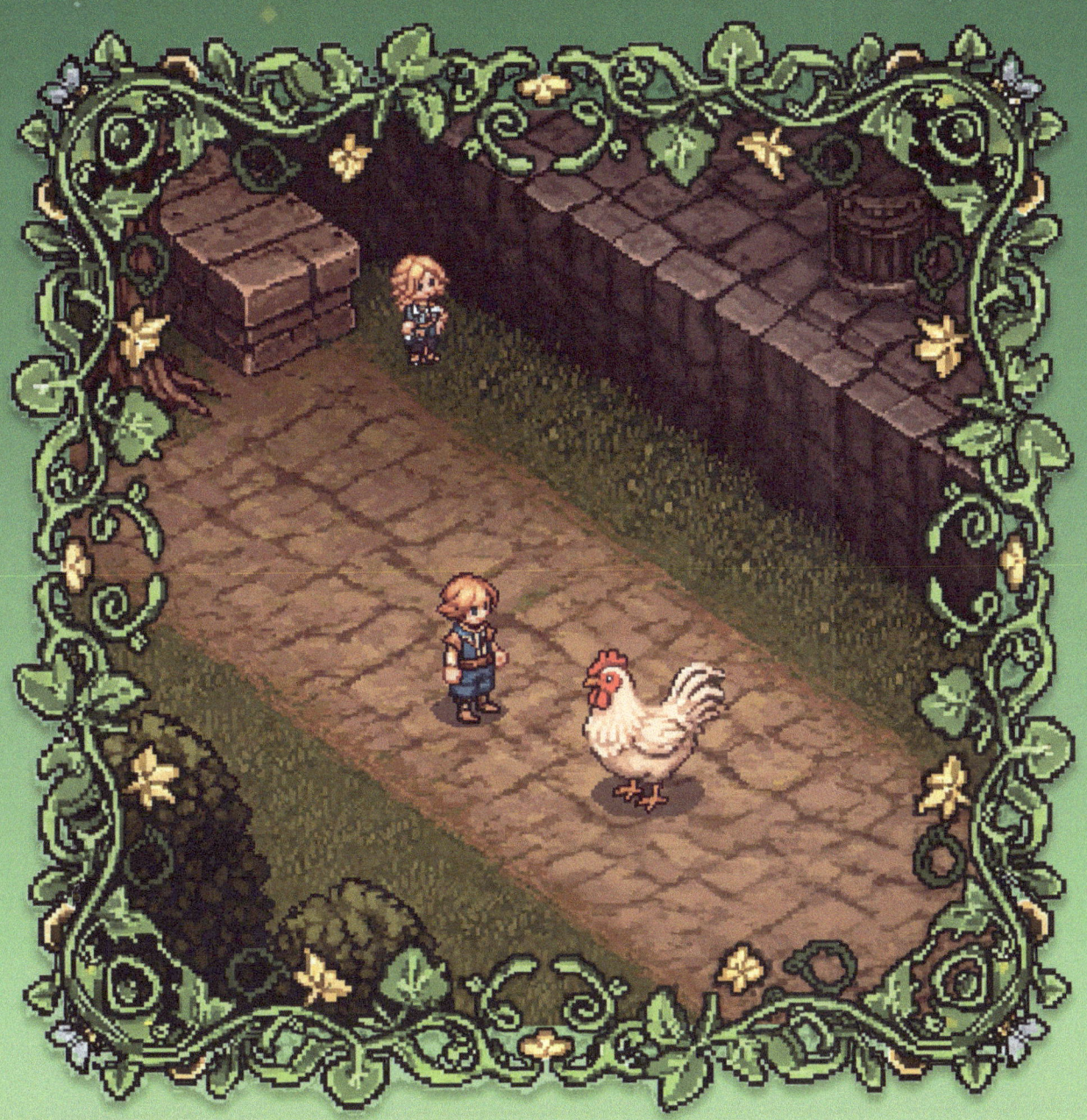

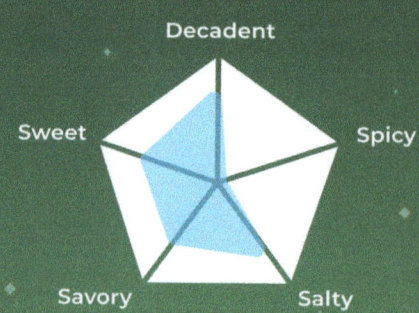

Summer Chicken Salad

This is a refreshing chicken salad recipe for the hot days of summer. The grapes and walnuts add a crunch and body to it that helps elevate the average chicken salad sandwich. Serve on whole wheat bread for a subtle sweetness that pairs well with the savory elements of the nuts and chicken.

Ingredients

Chicken Breast	2 ea
Water	12 Fl Oz
Walnuts Or Pecans	¾ C
White Grapes, Cut In Half	1 C
Mayo (Pg 145)	⅔ C
Dijon Mustard	1 Tbsp
Salt	½ tsp
Garlic Powder	¼ tsp
Dill, Dry	¼ tsp
Black Pepper, Ground	¼ tsp

Prep Time
35 Min

Cook Time
30 Min

Servings
4 - 6 Sandwiches

3 - 4 Qt Pot w/Lid
1 ea

Large Spoon for Mixing
1 ea

Forks for Shredding
2 ea

Large Bowl for Shredding
1 ea

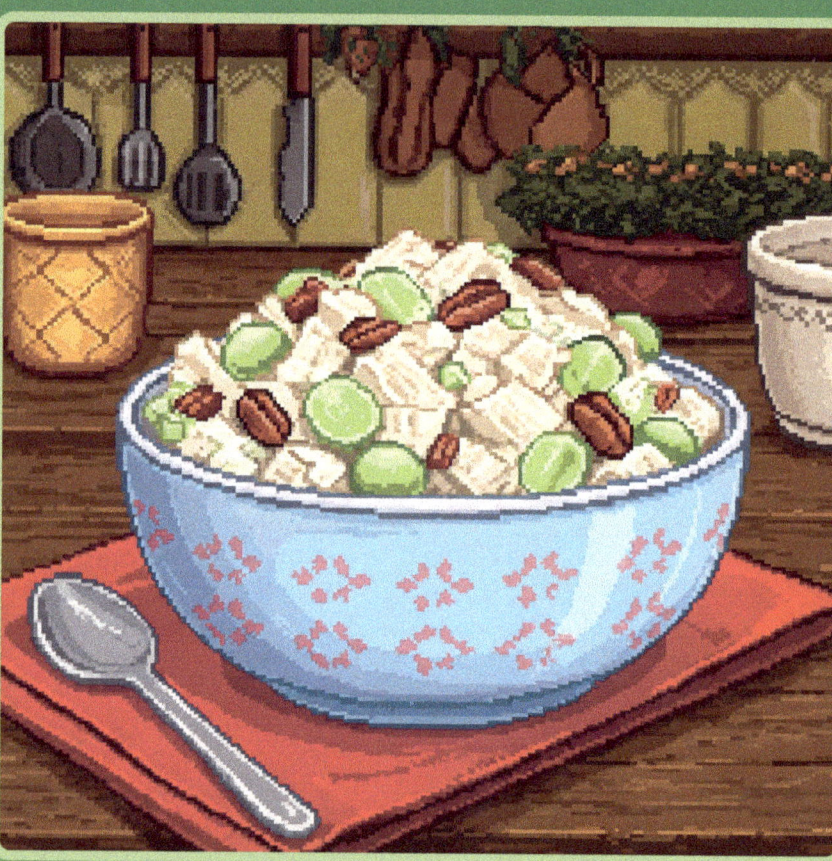

Recipe Tip

Try toasting the nuts to add a depth of flavor. Or, instead of grapes, try out different kinds of fruit! Any kind of fruit with an edible skin would work well, or a kind that has a lower water content. Experiment and have fun!

Cooking Directions

1   Put the water in a pot just big enough to hold the chicken and place over High heat. When simmering, place chicken in pot. Lower heat to Medium Low, cover and cook chicken for 30 min. until a spoon is easily inserted.

2   Remove chicken from pot and place in large bowl. Using two forks, shred the chicken into fine pieces. Place in the fridge to cool.

3   Prepare the remaining ingredients and combine everything except the grapes and nuts in a large bowl. Whisk until smooth.

4   Add the grapes, nuts and cooled chicken into the bowl and fold gently with a rubber spatula to combine. When well mixed, cover in plastic wrap or transfer to an airtight container. Place in fridge and let rest for 2 hr. minimum, or overnight before serving. Holds in fridge for 3 - 4 days in an airtight container.

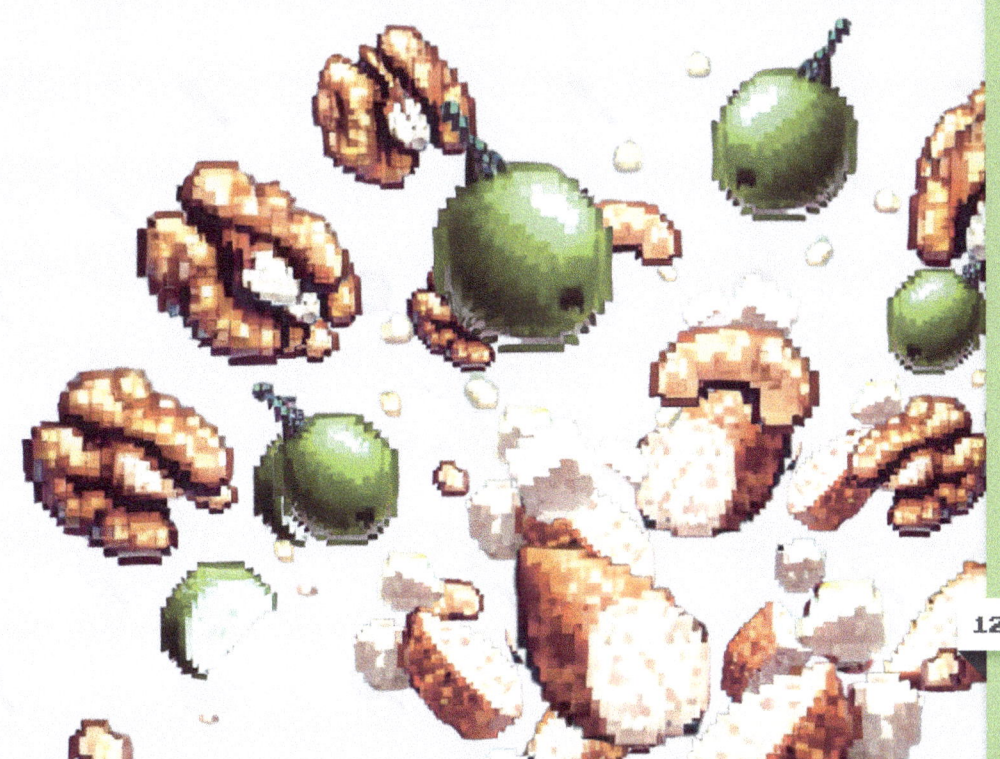

Dressings & Sauces

Bleu Cheese Dressing

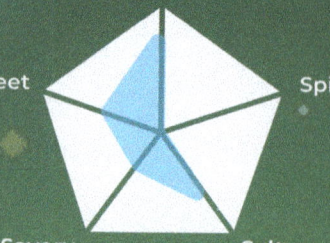

Decadent

Sweet

Spicy

Savory

Salty

Making your own bleu cheese dressing is the perfect way to highlight salads or wing night. Once you start, it'll be hard to go back to store bought. Try it on wedge salads, add some of your favorite hot sauce or chipotle sauce to give it a kick before putting it on sandwiches, and of course use it as a dip for your crudité and Buffalo wings! It's just delicious.

Mother Sauce: Mayonnaise

Ingredients

Bleu Cheese Crumbles (by weight)	6 oz
Mayonnaise (Pg 145)	½ C
Heavy Cream	6 Fl Oz
Lemon Juice	1 Tbsp
White Sugar	½ tsp
Garlic, minced	½ tsp
Salt	⅛ tsp
Black Pepper, ground	¼ tsp

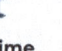
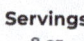
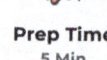
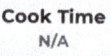

Prep Time
5 Min

Cook Time
N/A

Servings
8 oz

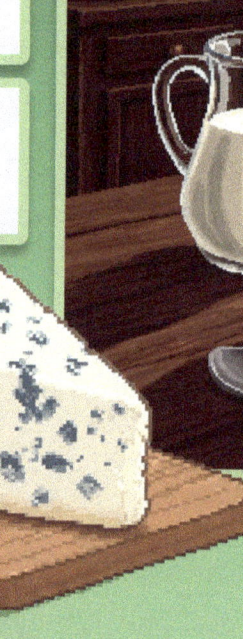

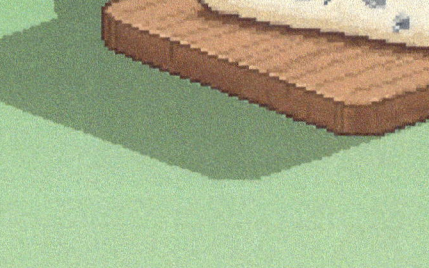

Cooking Directions

1   Place the bleu cheese in a medium bowl and add the
    heavy cream. Using a rubber spatula, mix together
    until well combined. It should look slightly clumpy
    and creamed together.

2   Add the remaining ingredients and gently fold them
    into the bleu cheese mix, becoming more vigorous
    as you stir to fully incorporate the ingredients.

3   If it seems too thick to you, add more heavy cream
    1 tsp. at a time.

4   Taste test and adjust salt and pepper levels to your
    taste. Store in an airtight container and refrigerate
    for at least 2 hr. before use. Holds in fridge for 7 days.

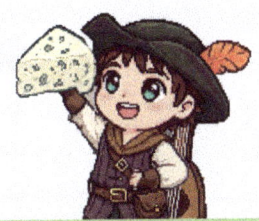

Recipe Tip

The type of Bleu Cheese used to make the dressing makes a
difference! Double Creme will yield a softer and sweeter
flavor, while a variety like Roquefort will be stronger and
sharper. Experiment and enjoy!

Enchilada/Taco Sauce

NOVICE

This sauce is a wonderful addition to taco night, and is the go-to for making a pan of enchiladas or when frying chile rellenos. It's hard to find a Central American dish that this sauce doesn't compliment well. I find that white vinegar adds a tang to the profile of this recipe that makes it really pop, but apple cider vinegar works well too.

Decadent
Sweet
Spicy
Savory
Salty

Mother Sauce: Veloute

Ingredients

Chile powder (Guajillo or similar)	1 Tbsp
Cumin	1 tsp
Garlic powder	½ tsp
Oregano, dry	¼ tsp
Salt	¼ tsp
Cinnamon (optional)	⅛ tsp
Tomato Paste	2 Tbsp
Stock (Chicken or Veg)	16 fl oz
Vinegar (White or Cider)	1 tsp
Lard/Butter/Olive Oil	3 Tbsp
AP Flour	3 Tbsp
Black Pepper to taste	

Prep Time
5 - 10 Min

Cook Time
12 - 15 Min

Servings
16 oz

Wooden Spoon/Rubber Spatula
1 ea

Pot w/Lid
1 ea

Wire Whisk
1 ea

Spoon for tasting
1 ea

Cooking Directions

1   Place a 2 Qt. pot over Medium heat. Add the oil/butter/lard. When melted, add the flour.

2   Stir constantly and cook for 4 - 5 min. to bring it to the Blond level. Then add the tomato paste and cook for 1 min. more.

3   Add all dry ingredients and cook for 1 min. Then add ½ of the stock and whisk well, making sure to work out any lumps in the roux. Add the rest of the stock and whisk until smooth.

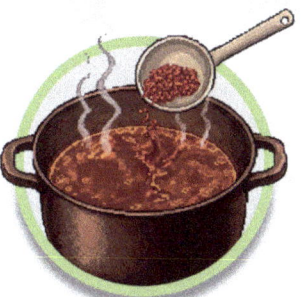

4   Raise heat and bring to a boil, then reduce the heat to Medium Low and simmer for 5 - 7 min. whisking often, until it thickens to coat the back of a spoon (nappe).

5   Remove pot from heat, add the vinegar and whisk to combine, then taste. Add extra salt and pepper to taste.

6   Let rest for 30 min. before transferring to an airtight container and placing in the fridge. Stir occasionally and make sure that it is completely cooled before covering. Holds for 5 days in the fridge, 3 months frozen.

Garlic Aioli

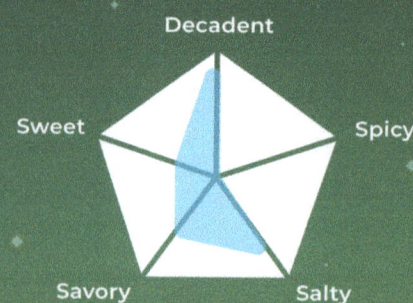

Decadent

Sweet · Spicy

Savory · Salty

This condiment is a simple and tasty addition to anything that goes well with mayo. Put on burgers, sandwiches, french fries; the options are many and varied.

This recipe is for an Italian style aioli, but really you can make any type. An aioli is simply a mayonnaise based condiment, with acidic components and various herbs and spices added to it. Try out different combos and discover your favorites.

Mother Sauce: Mayonnaise

Ingredients

Roasted Garlic Cloves, pasted	8 ea
Oregano, dry	½ tsp
Basil, dry	½ tsp
Parsley, dry	½ tsp
Lemon Juice	1½ Tbsp
Salt	¼ tsp
Balsamic Vinegar	2 tsp
Black Pepper	¼ tsp
Mayo (Pg 145)	1 C

Prep Time
5 Min

Cook Time
N/A

Servings
8 oz

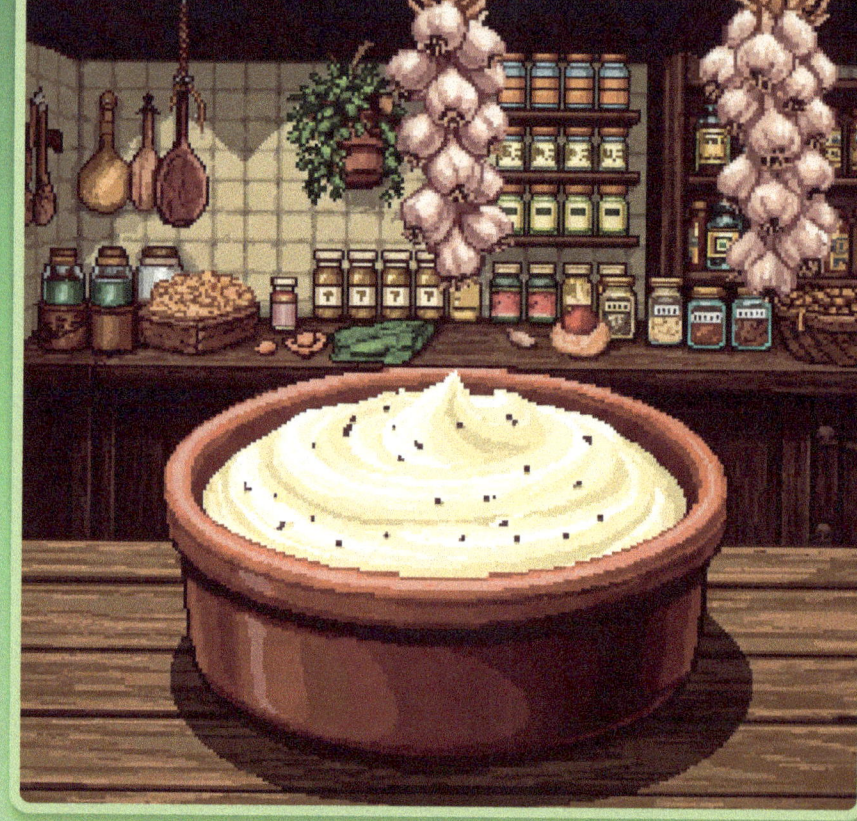

Cooking Directions

1   Combine all ingredients in a bowl. Whisk well,
    fully incorporating them, for about 2 min.

2   Place in an airtight container and refrigerate
    for 1 hr. before use. Holds for 10 - 14 days.

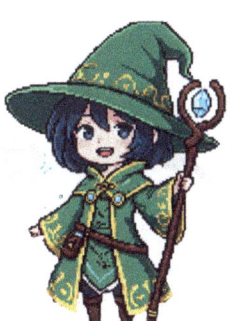

Recipe Tip

Lime juice can be used instead of lemon juice to give it a
brighter and slightly lighter feel on the palate. Try out
different acids and see what you enjoy.

Garlic Alfredo Sauce

Decadent

Sweet

Spicy

Savory

Salty

This is a basic Alfredo recipe, but it's fantastic. It's my go-to when I need to make a quick meal for my wife and I. Eat it with chicken, broccoli, caramelized onion, practically anything that goes into a pasta dish. Beef is the only protein you should be careful of pairing with this sauce. The intense flavor of beef tends to overpower the delicate sweetness of the cream. Try using roasted garlic in place of raw; it changes the profile of the dish in a lovely way.

Mother Sauce: Bechamel

Ingredients

Milk	16 Fl Oz
Garlic, minced	2 tsp
White (or Black) Pepper, ground	¼ tsp
Parsley, dry	½ tsp
Parmesan Cheese, grated	¼ C
Olive Oil	1½ Tbsp
AP Flour	1½ Tbsp

Prep Time
5 Min

Cook Time
N/A

Servings
16 oz

10" - 12" Skillet/ Saucepan
1 ea

Spoon for tasting
1 ea

Wire Whisk
1 ea

Wooden Spoon/Rubber Spatula
1 ea

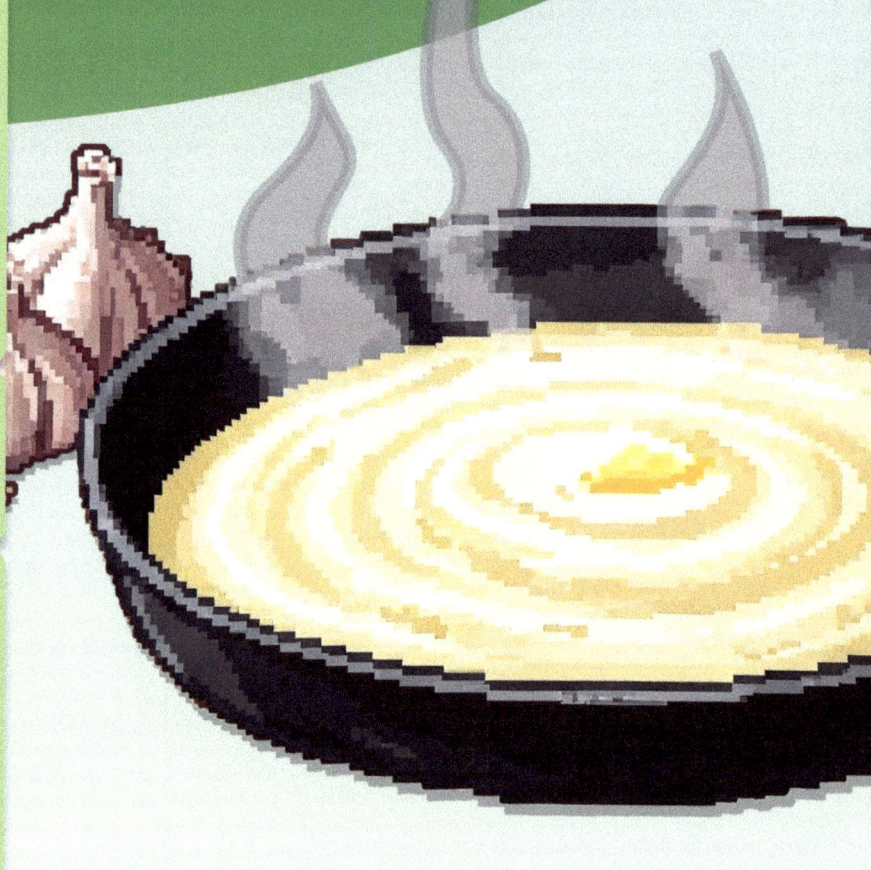

Cooking Directions

1   Place a 10" - 12" sauce pan over Medium heat.
    When hot, add the olive oil.

2   When shimmering, add the garlic and cook for 1 min.

3   Add the flour and cook for 2 - 3 min. This will
    bring it to the Blanc stage.

4   Pour in 4 oz. of the milk, whisking well to
    break up any lumps in the roux.

5   When smooth, add the rest of the milk slowly
    and whisk to combine the roux fully.

6   Bring to a simmer and reduce the heat to Medium
    Low. Whisking often, cook and reduce until it
    coats the back of a spoon (nappe).

7   While whisking, add in the parmesan gradually,
    making sure it doesn't clump up. This should
    give the sauce a thicker, slightly stringy quality.

8   Whisk in the salt and pepper, serve Hot. Make sure to
    cool completely before storing in an airtight
    container. Will hold in fridge for 4 days.

> **Recipe Tip**
>
> Make your roux ahead of time! Or combine all the
> ingredients, except the oil, flour, and parmesan, and store
> that in the fridge or up to 7 days. When cooking time comes,
> you'll be ready!

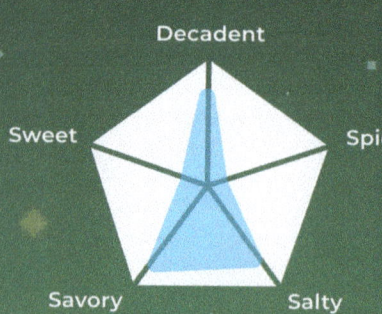

NOVICE

Ginger Dressing

This recipe holds a special place in my heart. Ever since I was a child, I have always enjoyed going to Hibachi restaurants, where the chefs cook the food in front of you on a large grill. In the best ones I have been to, there is always a ginger dressing for the salad that they also as a dipping sauce. The flavor of that condiment enticed me from the first time I tried it as a child. When I became interested in learning how to cook seriously, I began my journey with this recipe. I spent many years (almost 17, on and off) working on recipes trying to recreate the specific flavor that I've come to know and love so well. And finally, my perseverence paid off. Now, you too can enjoy the savory, salty, unctuous flavor that replicates those delicious dressings perfectly.

Temporary Emulsion

Ingredients

Green Bell Pepper, minced	2 Tbsp
White Onion, minced	1½ Tbsp
Carrot, minced	2 Tbsp
Ginger, 2" pc. minced	1 ea
Soy Sauce	2½ Tbsp
Rice Vinegar	1 Tbsp
Peanut Oil	3 Tbsp
Mirin/Shaoxing wine	½ Tbsp
Black Pepper, ground	¼ tsp
Sesame Seeds (optional)	1 tsp

Prep Time
5 Min

Cook Time
N/A

Servings
8 oz

Small or Medium
Sized Food Processor
(Not Required)
1 ea

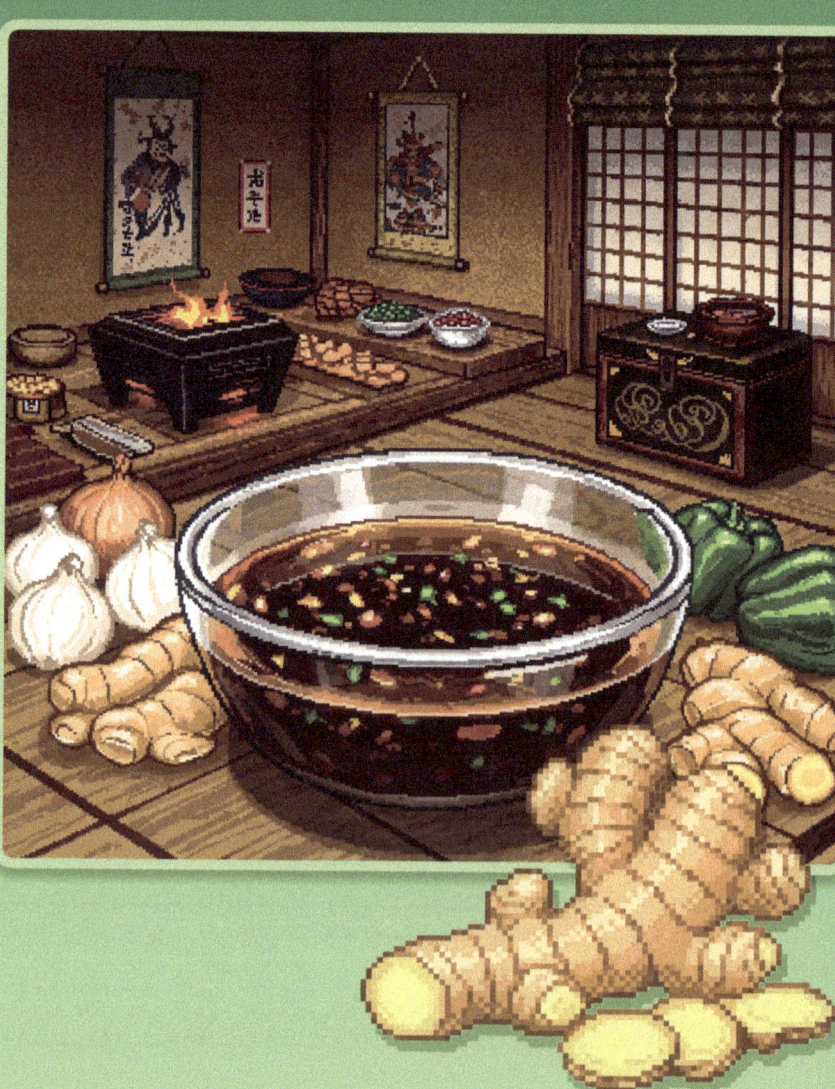

Cooking Directions

1   Place all ingredients in a food processor and blend
    until smooth. If you don't have a food processor
    make sure to mince the vegetables as finely as you
    can. Transfer ingredients to a bowl and whisk
    vigorously for 1 - 2 min. to fully incorporate the
    vinegar with the oil.

2   Store in an airtight container and let rest in fridge
    for 2 hours before use. Holds in the refrigerator
    for 7 days.

Recipe Tip

The tangy, unctuous profile of this dressing lends itself to
salads made using lighter greens and more delicate
vegetables. Inversely, it's perfect for pairing with pieces of
grilled beef or chicken. Experiment and have fun!

Italian Vinaigrette

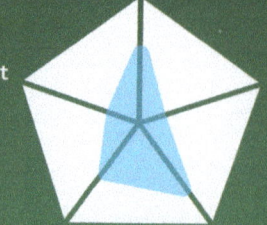

This basic recipe lends itself to experimentation. Try adding minced bell pepper and onion to give it a twist, or red pepper flakes for some heat. Fresh herbs can be used instead of dry, just remember that you need 3 times the amount of fresh herbs to dry ones. Also, this increase in volume will necessitate the use of more liquids. So long as you keep a ratio of 3:1 for Oil to Vinegar, you'll be able to adjust this recipe adequately for fresh herbs.

Temporary Emulsion

Ingredients

Olive Oil	6 Tbsp
Red Wine Vinegar	1 Tbsp
Balsamic Vinegar	1 Tbsp
Basil, Dry	½ tsp
Black Pepper, Ground	⅛ tsp
Parmesan Cheese	2 tsp
Oregano, Dry	¼ tsp
Garlic, Minced	½ tsp
Salt	¼ tsp

Prep Time	Cook Time	Servings
5 Min	N/A	4 oz.

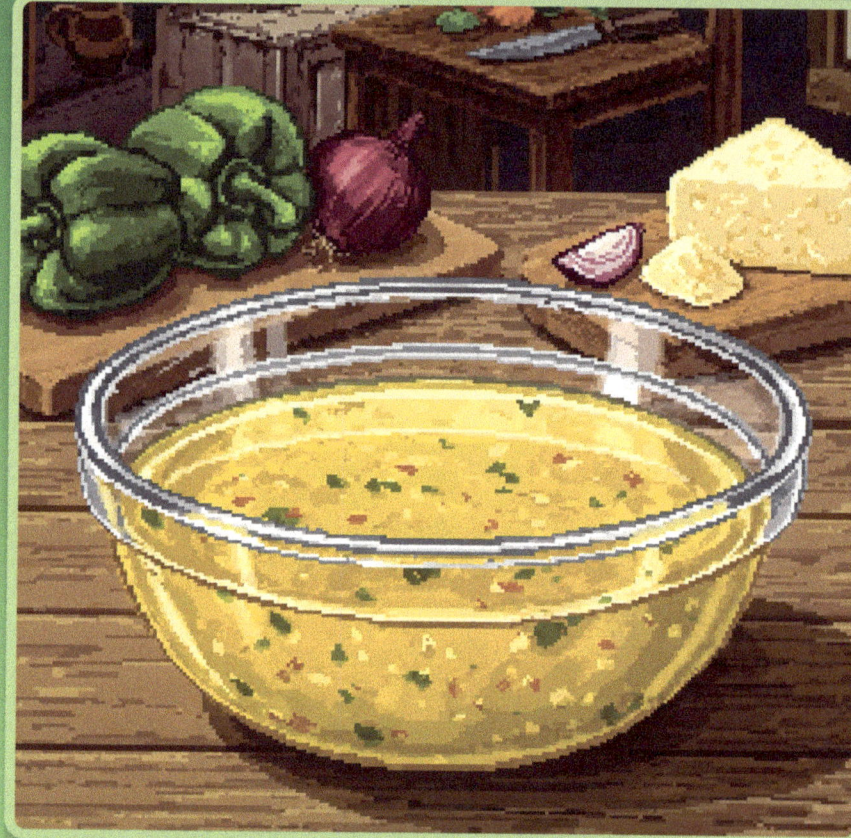

Cooking Directions

1   Place all ingredients in a large mixing bowl.
    Whisk vigorously for 3 - 5 minutes.

2   Transfer to an airtight container and refrigerate.
    Holds in fridge for 7 - 10 days.

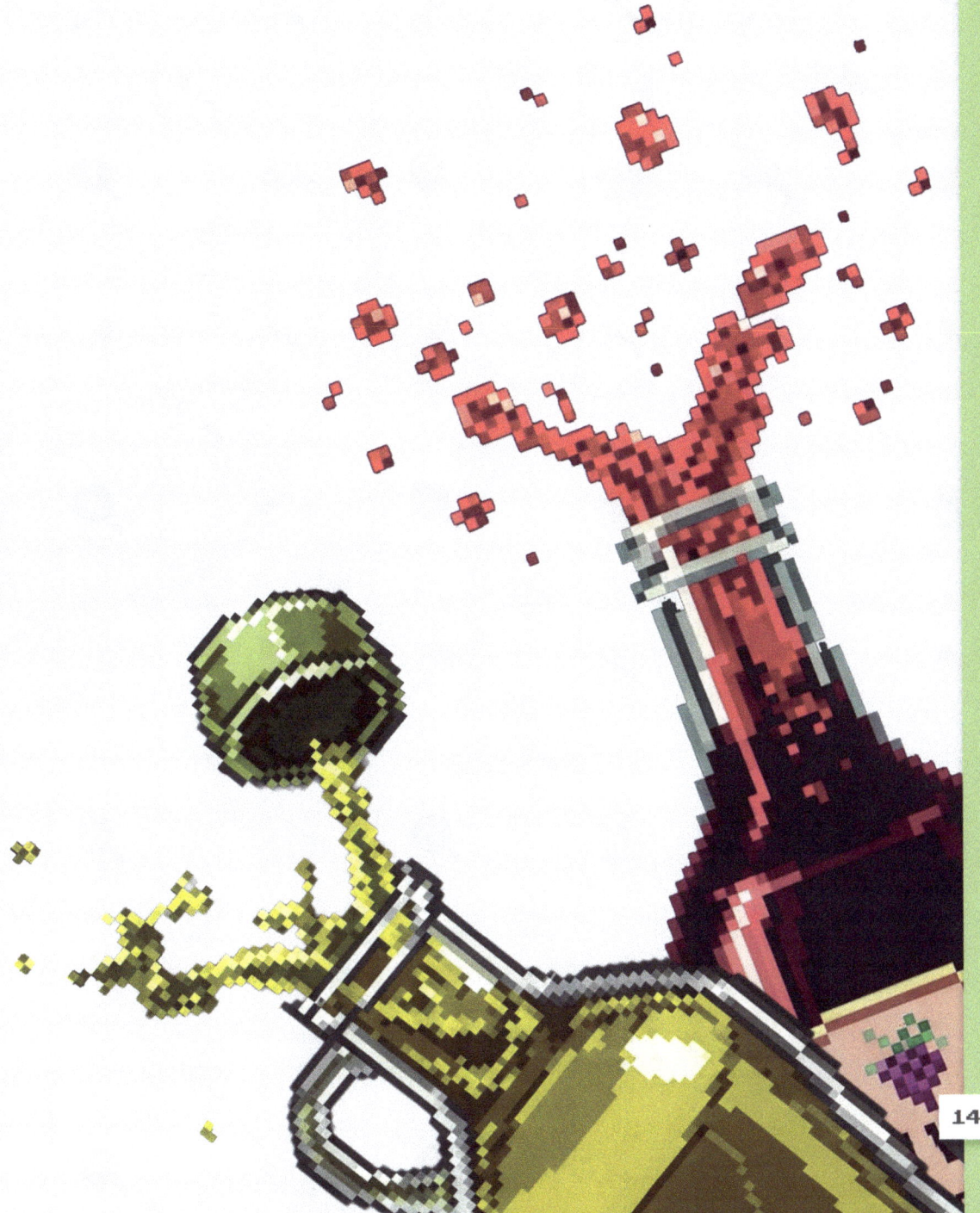

Lo Mein Sauce

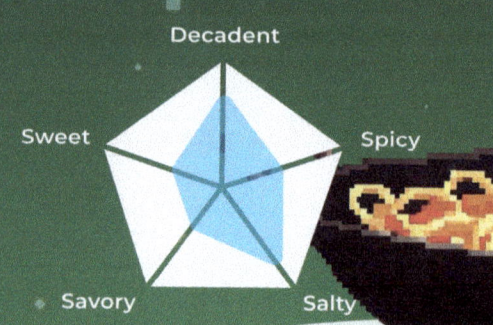

Decadent

Sweet

Spicy

Savory

Salty

This recipe is the secret to making your own delicious lo mein stir fry at home. The MSG isn't a necessary ingredient, but it is the secret to so many of the beloved dishes ordered from Chinese restaurants across the country. Feel free to kick up the amount of sriracha in the recipe to accommodate your preference for heat.

Ingredients

Soy Sauce	¼ C
White Sugar	1 Tbsp
Sesame oil	2 tsp
Ginger, ground	½ tsp
Sriracha	1 tsp
Garlic, minced	2 tsp
Cornstarch	1½ tsp
Water for Cornstarch Slurry	1½ tsp
MSG	⅛ tsp

Prep Time 5 Min   **Cook Time** 3 Min   **Servings** ¼ Cup

Wire Whisk & Bowl for Cornstarch Slurry 1 ea   **Small Pot** 1 ea

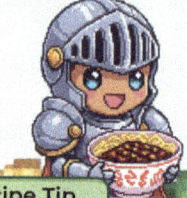

Recipe Tip

Don't be afraid of playing around with this recipe to make it your own! It works well as both Lo Mein and Fried Rice seasoning, so get creative!

Cooking Directions

1 Place the cornstarch in a small bowl and add the water. Whisk together so it's fully incorporated.

2 Combine all ingredients, except cornstarch slurry, in a small pot and stir well.

3 Place over High heat and bring to a simmer. Mix the slurry to reincorporate it fully, then add it to the pot, whisking constantly to thicken.

4 Once thickened, remove from heat and transfer to a heat safe bowl. Cool in fridge.

5 Holds for 7 days in the refrigerator.

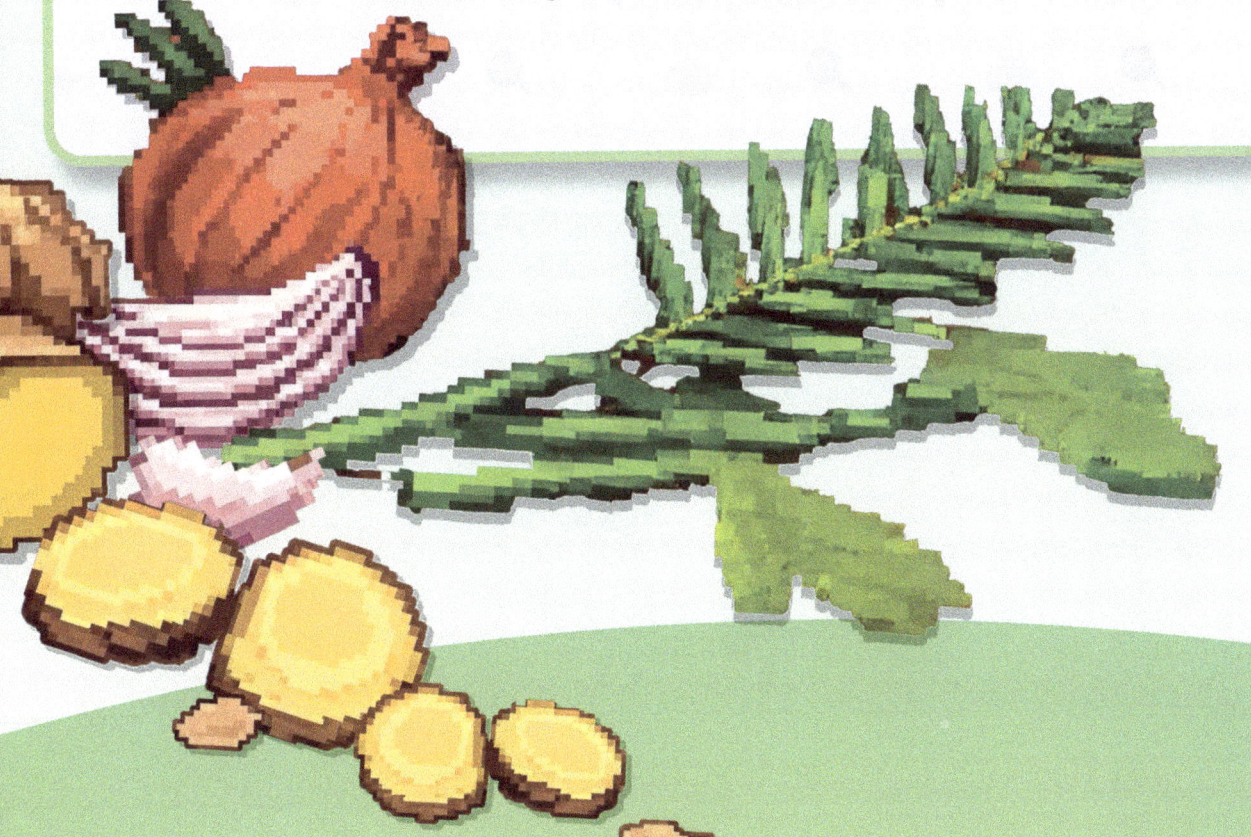

Mayonnaise

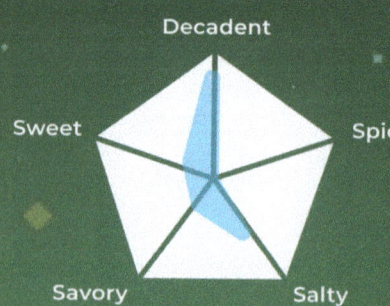

Decadent
Sweet
Spic
Savory
Salty

I love dipping my fries in this mayonnaise, and the flavor it adds to sandwiches is superb. Making your own aioli with this mayo as a base is fantastic, and it's not so difficult that you can't make a large batch for your own coleslaw, or potato/chicken/tuna salad. When mixing it make sure to not add the oil too quickly. 1 Tbsp. at a time might seem tedious, but it guarantees that your mayo binds properly and doesn't turn into a soupy mess.

Ingredients

Large Egg, Room Temperature	1 ea
White Vinegar	1 Tbsp
Mustard Powder	1 tsp
Neutral Oil	1 C
Salt	¼ tsp

Prep Time
5 Min

Cook Time
N/A

Servings
12 oz

Small or Medium Food Processor or Stand mixer (Not Required)
1 ea

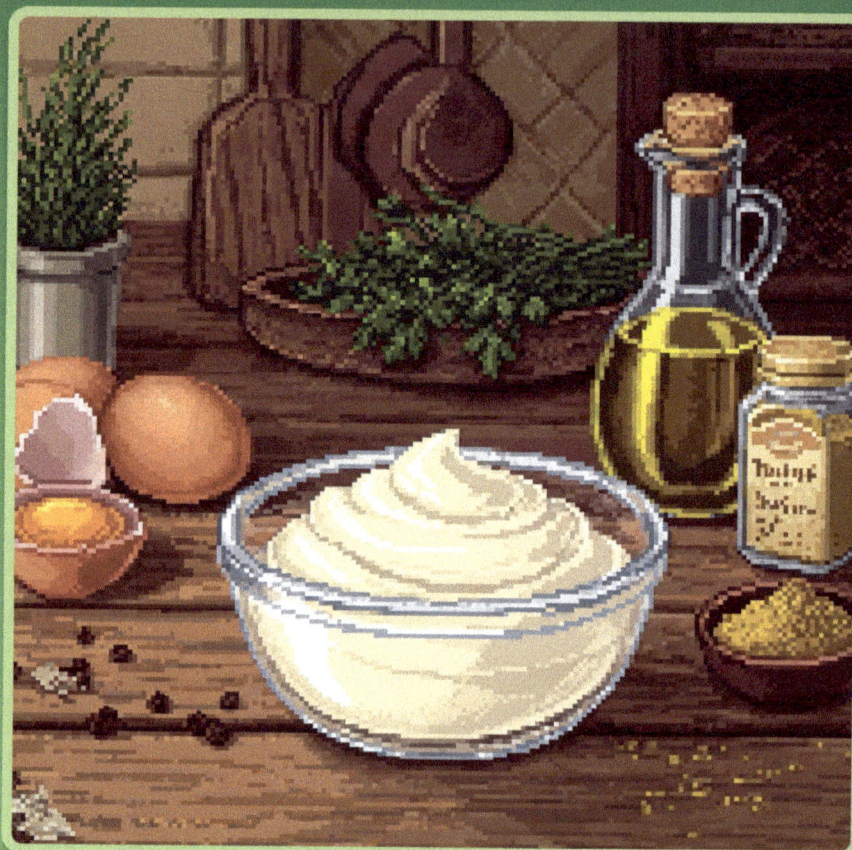

Cooking Directions

1 Crack the egg into a food processor and pulse 8 - 10 times. If using a stand mixer, use the whisk attachment and mix on the 3rd speed setting for about 10 sec. If mixing by hand, whisk for about 15 sec.

2 Add the vinegar and pulse 5 more times. Add the mustard powder and salt, pulse 5 more times. If using a stand mixer, lower the mixing speed to the 2nd setting and add the vinegar, mustard powder, and salt. Mix for about 10 more sec. If mixing by hand, add those same ingredients and whisk for about 20 seconds.

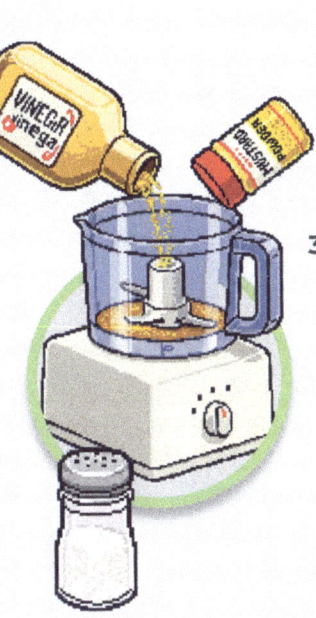

3 1 Tbsp. at a time, add the oil and blend for 4 - 5 seconds between each Tbsp. This step is very important; if you add the oil too quickly the mix won't emulsify and will become irreversibly runny. If using a stand mixer, raise the speed to the 4th or 5th setting and add the oil 1 Tbsp. at a time, while the machine is running, with 4 - 5 sec. between each Tbsp. If mixing by hand, add the oil 1 Tbsp. at a time, whisking vigorously for 30 - 40 seconds between each one.

4 Once all the oil has been added blend for 10 seconds more to fully incorporate the mixture. If using a stand mixer, mix on the 2nd or 3rd speed setting for about 15 seconds to fully incorporate. If mixing by hand, once all the oil has been added whisk vigorously for 1 more min. Taste test and adjust the salt level to your liking.

5 Place in an airtight container and refrigerate. Holds for 14 days.

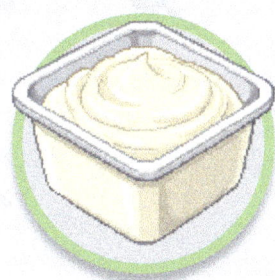

Mustard Vinaigrette

NOVICE

This dressing is a nice change of pace from your basic vinaigrettes. The mustard gives it a tang that compliments the darker and healthier greens that are good for a heartier salad. It also works great as a topping for sandwiches of all kinds.

Decadent

Sweet · S

Savory · Salty

Temporary Emulsion

Ingredients

Olive Oil	3 Tbsp
Red Wine Vinegar	2 Tbsp
Green Bell Pepper, Minced	2 Tbsp
Dijon Mustard	1 Tbsp
Salt	¼ tsp
Parmesan Cheese	1 tsp
Neutral Oil	3 Tbsp
White Onion, Minced	1 tsp
Garlic, Minced	½ tsp
Basil, Dry	¼ tsp
Black Pepper, Ground	⅛ tsp

Prep Time
10 Min

Cook Time
N/A

Servings
4 oz

Small or Medium Sized Food Processor (Not Required)
1 ea

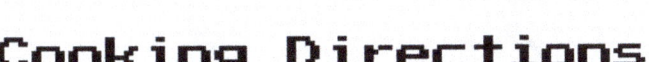

Cooking Directions

1   Combine all ingredients in a food processor and blend until smooth. If you don't have a food processor make sure to mince the vegetables as finely as you can. Transfer all ingredients to a bowl and whisk vigorously for about 1 min. to fully incorporate the oil and vinegar.

2   Transfer to an airtight container and refrigerate for 2 hr. before using. Holds for 7 days.

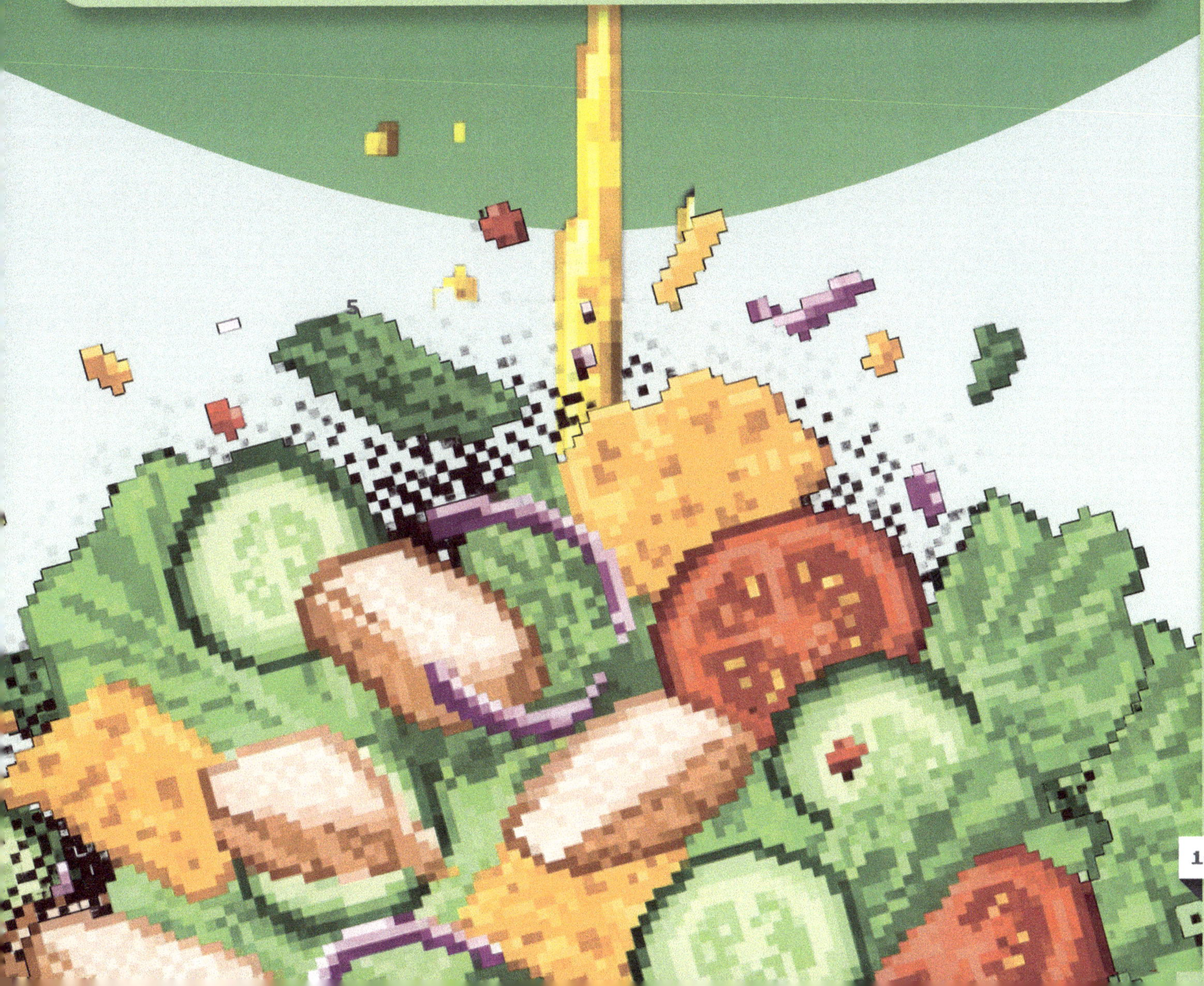

Ranch Dressing

Decadent

Sweet   Spic

Savory   Salty

Making your own Ranch is, in my opinion, like making your own Mayonnaise at home. Once you start doing it, it'll be difficult to go back to store bought. Putting it on salads, dipping fried foods, drizzling on sandwiches, are all great options for this recipe.

Buttermilk Ranch is a common favorite, but since buttermilk can only be bought in large containers, I have found that using Heavy Cream and Lemon Juice will produce a similar flavor profile, without making the ranch as heavy as Buttermilk. However, Buttermilk is excellent for making pancakes, waffles and baked goods with, so it's not too hard to justify buying a large container. Consider your budget and weekly meal plan, and pick which option works best for you.

Mother Sauce: Mayonnaise

Ingredients

Mayo (Pg 145)	1 C
Buttermilk (or Heavy Cream)	8 Fl Oz
Onion Powder	½ tsp
Black Pepper, Ground	⅛ tsp
Lemon Juice (if using Heavy Cream)	1 Tbsp
Parsley, Dry	1 Tbsp
Garlic, Minced	2 tsp
Dill, Dry	¼ tsp
Salt	1 tsp

Prep Time
5 Min

Cook Time
N/A

Servings
16 oz

Cooking Directions

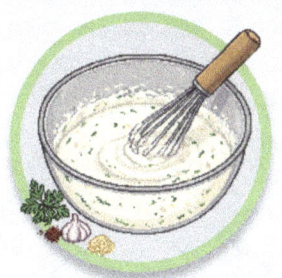

1   Combine all ingredients in a large bowl. Whisk vigorously for about 1 min. until fully combined.

2   Store in an airtight container and refrigerate for 2 hr. before use. Holds in the fridge for 7 - 10 days.

NOVICE

Rustic Pomodoro Sauce

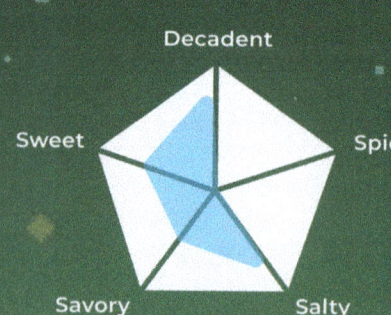

Decadent
Sweet
Spic[y]
Savory
Salty

This sauce is delicious on its own for use with spaghetti, lasagna, making stuffed shells or manicotti; the list goes on. It's also the base for more complex sauces, such as Puttanesca, Fra Diavolo, and Campagnolo. Fortunately for you, these sauces are also in my book so you too can make them at home. (See Pgs 323, 247, 245)

Mother Sauce: Tomato

Ingredients

28 oz. Can of Whole Tomatoes	1 ea
Basil, Fresh, Finely Chopped	¾ oz
Oregano, Dry	¼ tsp
Garlic, Minced	1½ tsp
Carrot, 3" pc. Peeled	1 ea
Olive Oil	½ Tbsp
Salt	½ tsp
Black Pepper, Ground	⅛ tsp

Prep Time
10 - 15 Min

Cook Time
2½ Hr

Servings
28 oz

Can Opener
1 ea

Large Mixing Bowl
1 ea

Wooden Spoon/Rubber Spatula
1 ea

3 - 4 Qt Pot w/Lid
1 ea

Cooking Directions

1   Open the can and transfer the tomatoes to a large bowl. Using a potato masher, or your hands (preferred), mash and break apart the tomatoes into small pieces. Remove any basil leaves that may be packed with the tomatoes.

2   Place a 3 - 4 Qt. pot over Medium heat. When hot, add the oil.

3   When shimmering, add the garlic and cook for 30 sec. until fragrant.

4   Add the tomatoes, making sure to get all the excess juice into the pot. Then add the remaining ingredients (except the carrot) and stir well.

5   Cover and bring to a simmer. When simmering, drop the heat to Medium Low or Low to maintain a gentle simmer.

6   Cook, covered, for 2 hr. stirring every 30 min.

7   Uncover and add the carrot piece to the pot. Stir it in, cover again, and cook for 30 more minutes.

8   Remove from heat, uncover, and remove the carrot. If not using immediately, transfer to a heat safe container and cool on the counter for 30 minutes before placing in refrigerator. Be sure to stir occasionally and make sure it is completely cool before sealing. Holds for 5 - 7 days.

Sizzling Sauce for Fajitas

Ever wonder how restaurants get their fajitas to sizzle so loudly when they come out of the kitchen? This sauce, along with those crazy hot pans, is the secret. The soy sauce adds a savory element to the dish, and the oil and lime juice crackle and pop loudly, producing a delightful aroma. Now, when you make fajitas at home, you can have that sound and smell too. Make sure the sauce is room temperature when you go to use it, and be careful when handling the pan, as it needs to be very, very hot for the sauce to work it's magic.

Decadent · Spicy · Salty · Savory · Sweet

Ingredients

Soy Sauce	¼ C
Lime Juice	¼ C
	(2 Limes)
Neutral Oil	3 Tbsp

 Prep Time 5 Min

 Cook Time N/A

 **Servings** 6 oz

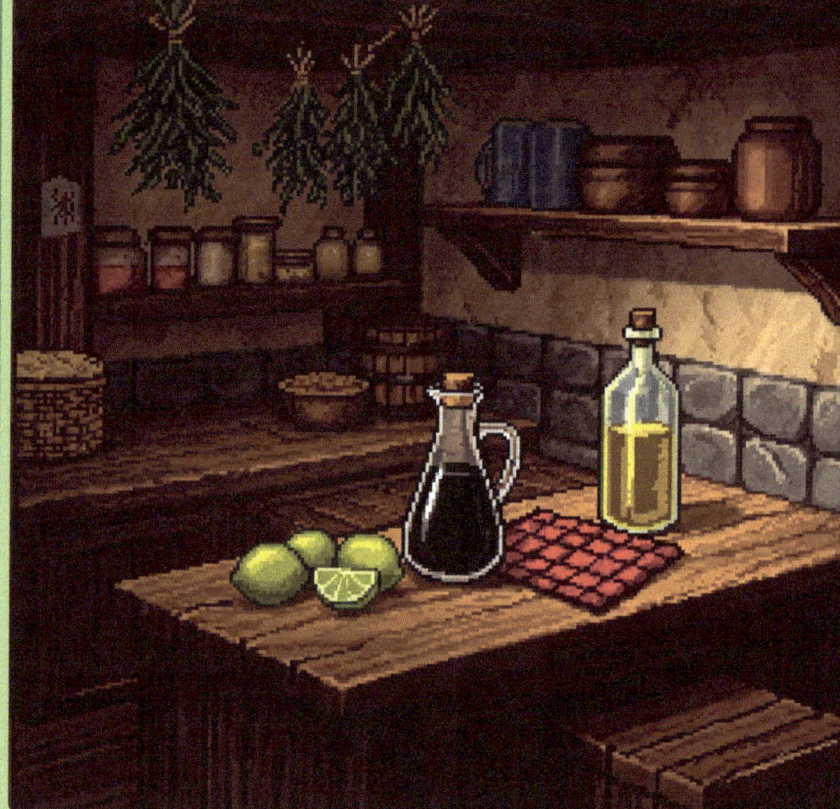

Cooking Directions

1 Combine all ingredients in a bowl and whisk well to combine. Transfer to an airtight container, or even better, a squirt bottle to store in the fridge. Will hold for 7 - 10 days.

Recipe Tip

Making fajitas at home can be intimidating, so try this sauce out with some vegetable stir fries first, to both practice your knife cuts and get a feel for how to best use this simple sauce. Be adventurous, try adding other flavorings to it! You might be surprised how versatile this recipe can be!

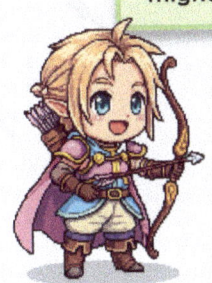

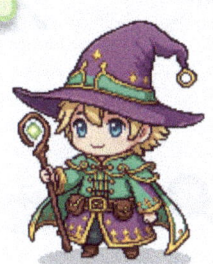

NOVICE

Sweet Chili Sauce

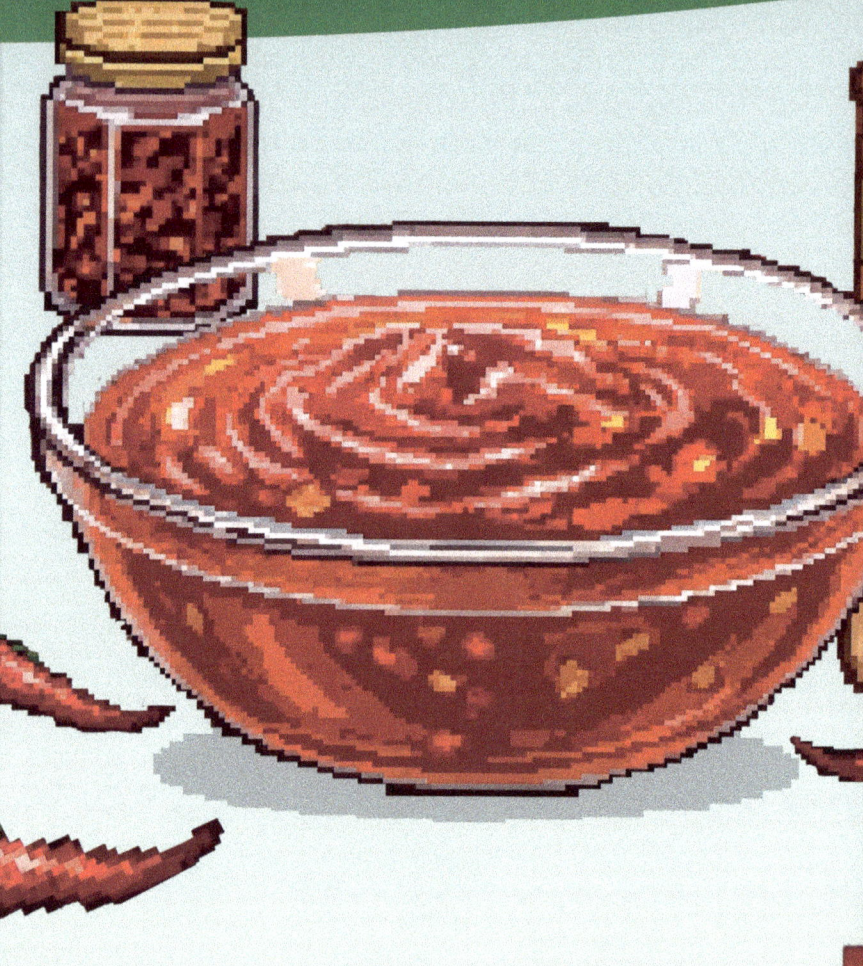

This sauce is great for dipping egg rolls, cheese sticks, chicken fingers and dumplings. It also makes for a great glaze on grilled chicken or pork, and drizzling it on sandwiches is a way to make them really pop. Experiment with it, and you'll be surprised at the combinations you come up with.

Decadent · Sweet · Spic[y] · Savory · Salty

Ingredients

Rice Vinegar	8 Fl Oz
White Sugar/ Honey	¾ C
Water	½ C
Ginger, Minced	1 Tbsp
Garlic, Minced	1½ Tbsp
Hot Chili Peppers, Minced	3 Tbsp
OR	
Red Pepper Flakes	1½ Tbsp
Soy Sauce	2 tsp

 Prep Time 10 Min

 Cook Time 30 - 35 Min

 Servings 8 oz

 Small Pot 1 ea

 Wire Whisk 1 ea

 Medium Bowl for Mixing 1 ea

 Wooden Spoon/Rubber Spatula 1 ea

Cooking Directions

1 Combine all ingredients in a bowl and whisk
   vigorously for 1 - 2 min. until fully combined.

2 Transfer to a 1 Qt. pot, making sure to scrape the
   bowl clean, and place over Medium/Medium High
   heat. Bring to a boil slowly, whisking often.

3 When boiling, lower the heat so it's gently
   simmering and cook for 20 - 25 min. until it
   reaches a syrup like consistency.

4 Remove from heat and let cool on counter
   for 1 hr. before transferring to an airtight
   container. Reheat gently before use. Will
   hold in refrigerator for 3 weeks.

Desserts & Baking

Basic Butter Crust

Decadent

Sweet

Spicy

Savory

Salty

I've never been much of a baker, so I have to give credit to my wife Julia for this basic, never-fail pie crust recipe. Whether you're making a savory entrée pie, or a dessert pie, this crust won't let you down. This recipe makes enough dough for the top and bottom crusts of a pie, but if you're making a pie that doesn't require a top (pecan, chocolate cream, lemon meringue) just cut the recipe in half. And if your recipe calls for a deep dish pie crust, simply multiply the recipe by 1.25 to get the extra dough necessary to cover the base of your dish.

Ingredients

AP Flour	2½ C
Butter, Cold, Cubed	½ tsp
Salt	1 C
Very Cold Water	½ C

Prep Time
10 Min

Cook Time
N/A

Servings
9" Pie

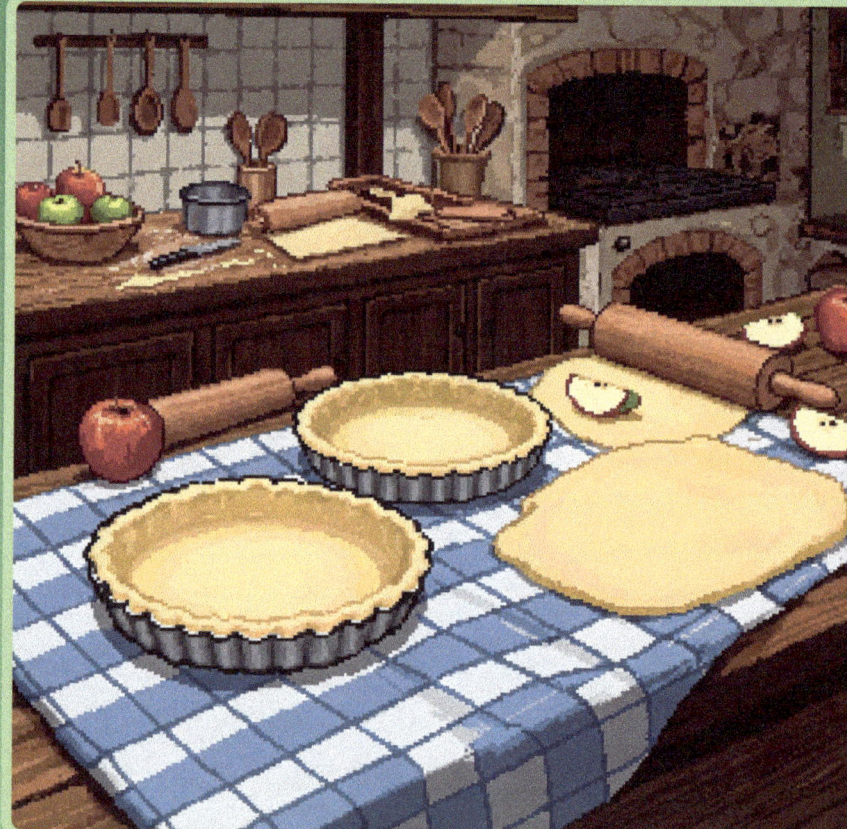

Cooking Directions

1   Sift the flour and salt into a large bowl.

2   Add the cubes of butter to the bowl; using a dough cutter or your hands incorporate the butter into the dough thoroughly. It should become thick and mealy.

3   Add the water to the mixture and knead together using a rubber spatula, or hands, until the dough becomes shaggy.

4   Remove from the bowl and place on a floured surface. Continue kneading for about 1 min. until the dough is smooth.

5   Form into a disc and wrap tightly in plastic wrap. Rest in the refrigerator for at least 1 hour. Then let rest on the counter for 15 min. before use.

6   Will hold in fridge for 2 days before use.

Beer Bread

This is a very basic recipe that makes a hearty loaf of slightly sweet bread that's great for a side with soups, chili, or anything you take off the grill. Try buttering up a piece on both sides and griddling it to give it some crunch. Maybe even make some French toast with it and serving it up with some vanilla ice cream. The options are varied and many!

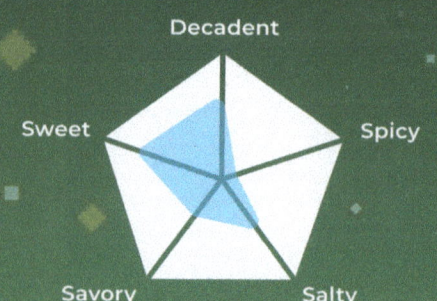

Ingredients

Self-Rising Flour	3 C
Sugar	2 Tbsp
Lager or Other Golden Ale	12 Fl Oz
Shortening &	
Flour to Coat Pan	

 Prep Time 10 Min

 Cook Time 50 - 60 Min

 Servings 5" x 9" Loaf

 Mesh Strainer for Sifting 1 ea

 Large Mixing Bowl 1 ea

 Wire Whisk 1 ea

 5" x 9" Loaf Pan/Baking Dish 1 ea

 Wooden Spoon/Rubber Spatula 1 ea

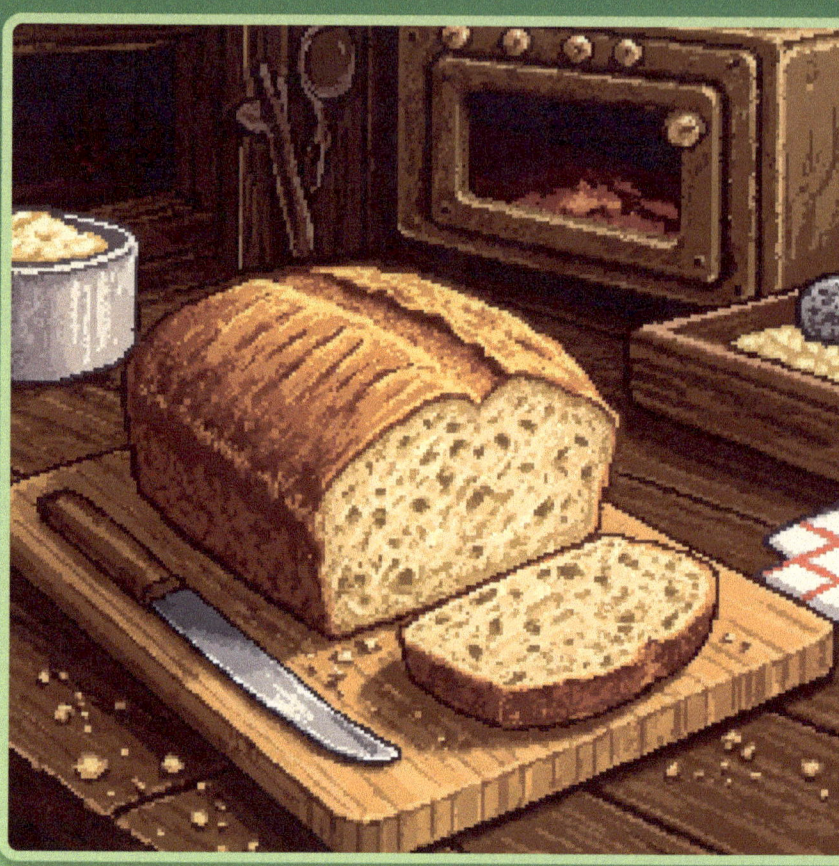

Cooking Directions

1   Preheat oven to 350.

2   Coat a 5" x 9" loaf pan with shortening and dust with
    flour. Shake out any excess flour.

3   Sift the flour into a large bowl. Add the sugar and beer
    and mix until well combined, so there are no lumps.

4   Transfer to the greased pan and bake for 50 - 60 min.
    until the bread is a light golden-brown.

5   Remove from oven and let rest in pan for 10 min. before
    removing and placing on a cooling rack. Let rest for 30
    min. before cutting into the loaf.

Fudgy Brownies

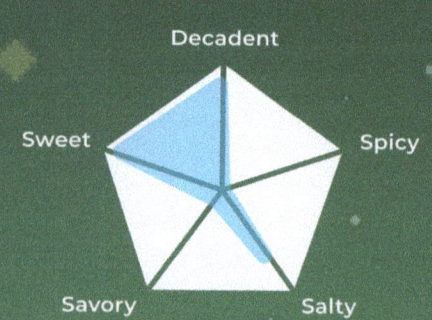

Decadent

Sweet
Spicy

Savory
Salty

This recipe is an old stand-by from my high school days. I first learned how to make brownies from scratch when I was a sophomore in high school, in one of the first cooking classes I ever took. They're simple, delicious, and easy to make.

If you want a larger batch, just use a 9"x13" baking pan and double the recipe. Simple as that.

Ingredients

Butter, Melted	½ C
White Sugar	1 C
Large Eggs	2 ea
Vanilla Extract	1½ tsp
Baking Cacao Powder	1/3 C
AP Flour	½ C
Salt	¼ tsp
Baking Powder	¼ tsp
Dark Chocolate Chips	½ C
Lard/Shortening & Flour for Pan	

Prep Time
15 Min

Cook Time
30 Min

Servings
16 Pieces

Large Mixing
Bowl
1 ea

Spoon for
tasting
1 ea

8" x 8" Baking
Dish
1 ea

Wooden
Spoon/Rubber
Spatula
1 ea

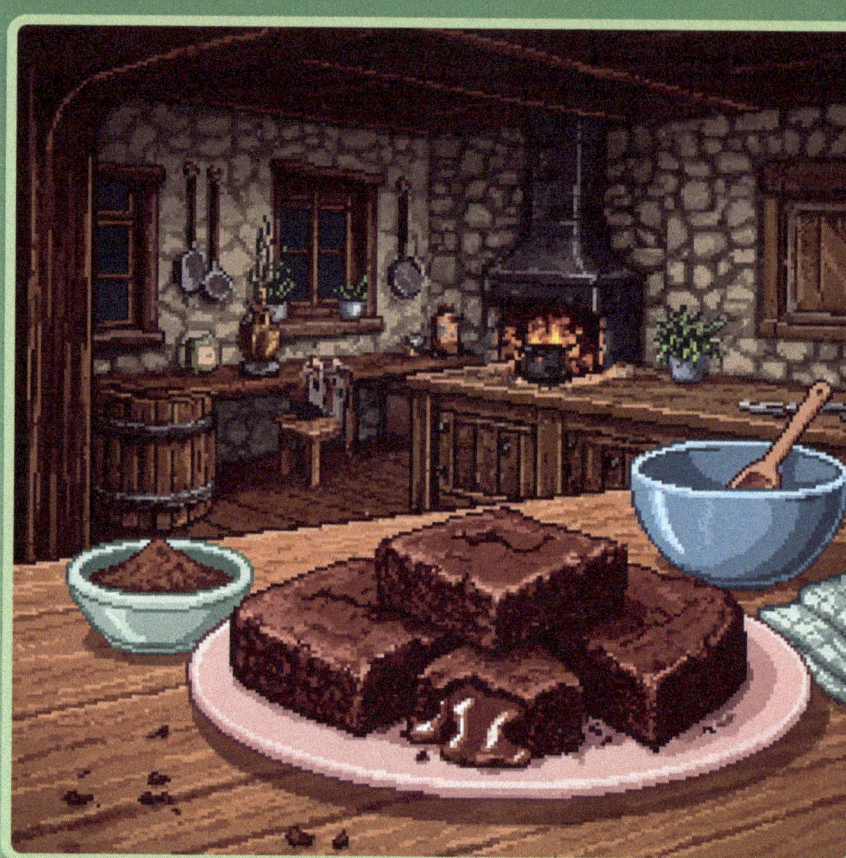

Cooking Directions

1   Preheat your oven to 350. Grease an 8" x 8"
    baking pan and dust with flour. Shake off
    excess flour from the pan.

2   In a large bowl, cream together the sugar, egg, and
    vanilla. In a separate bowl, sift the flour, cacao powder,
    salt and baking powder. Melt the butter in the microwave
    in 5 - 8 second long bursts. Once melted, add to the sugar
    mix and whisk to combine.

3   Add the dry ingredients to the wet and fold together
    until fully combined. Pour in chocolate chips and
    fold them in as well.

4   Transfer the batter to your baking pan. Place in
    oven and bake for 25 - 30 min. until the top is
    dry and the edges start to pull away from the
    sides of the pan. Remove from oven and let rest
    for 10 min. before cutting.

5   Cut the brownies into 16 even sized pieces and
    remove from pan. Enjoy hot, or store at room
    temperature, covered, for up to 4 days.

Recipe Tip

Try adding different kinds of chips to the filling, or chop up
some roasted nuts. You can't go wrong with brownies, so
make the variety you like the most.

Hot Water Crust

This pie dough is the key to making delicious English style pies, meat or otherwise. Try out a classic pork pie, meat and potato, or go hard with a mushroom & leek pie. The options of what can go inside a hot water crust pie are many, so get creative!

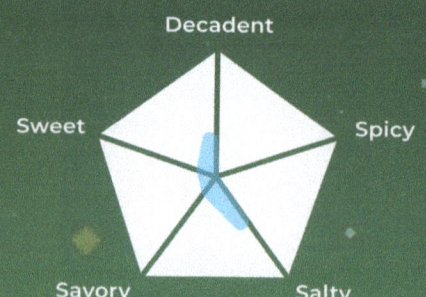

Ingredients

AP Flour	3½ C
Lard/Butter	½ C
Water	⅓ C
Salt	¾ tsp

 Prep Time
10 Min

 Cook Time
N/A

 Servings
6 XL Muffin Tins

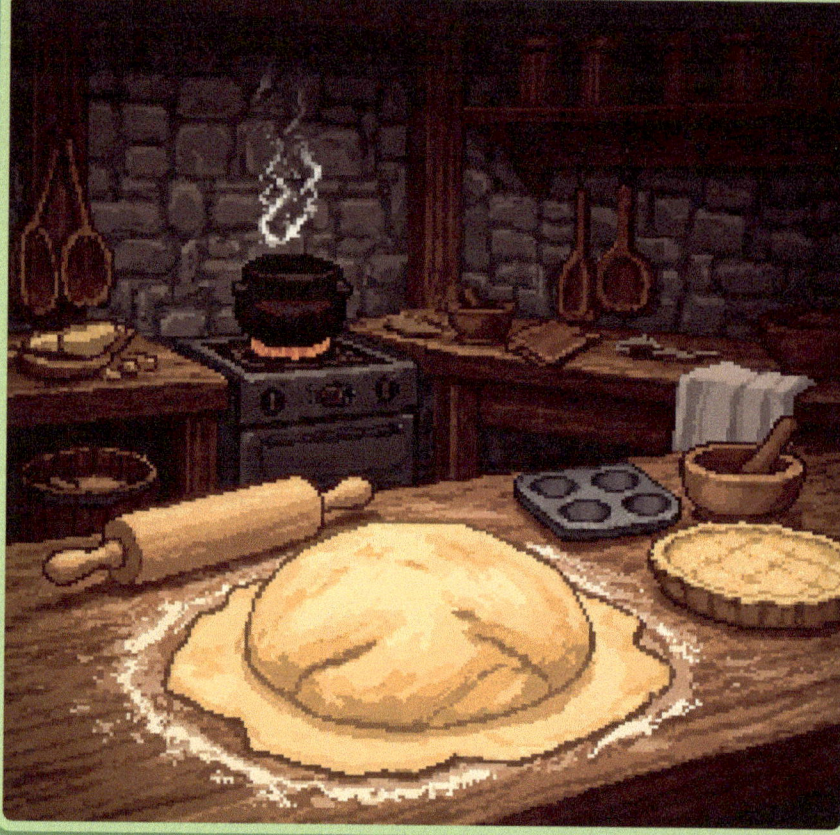

Cooking Directions

1 Place a small pot over High heat and add water and lard/butter.

2 Heat until boiling and lard/butter is fully melted. Cover and remove from heat.

3 Sift the flour and salt into a large bowl, then make a well in the center of the pile with your fingers.

4 Pour the water-fat mix into the flour and mix together with a wooden spoon or rubber spatula until the dough becomes shaggy.

5 Transfer the dough on to a floured surface and knead it until smooth.

6 Use at once, do not refrigerate.

LVLUPCookBook Channel

APPRENTICE

Growing and Improving

You've moved forward in your chosen Class, and tackled the challenges laid out for you to ascend to the rank of Apprentice. Congratulations!

Novice recipes are easier than they once were, and your skills have really begun to take form and develop.

There is still a ways to go, but you can look back with a sense of accomplishment and achievement. You may have already attempted a few Adept recipes, but if not that's ok.

There will be time for that soon enough...

LEVEL 10

Achievements Unlocked

Living Color • You understand how to sear a protein properly

Fork-Tender • You understand both Braising and Stewing

D'oh! • You've made mistakes, but you persevered and have reached a new rank!

Pop And Circumstance • You can now Sautee!

Bubbling Up • You know the difference between Boil and Simmer

Soups

Chicken Tortilla Soup

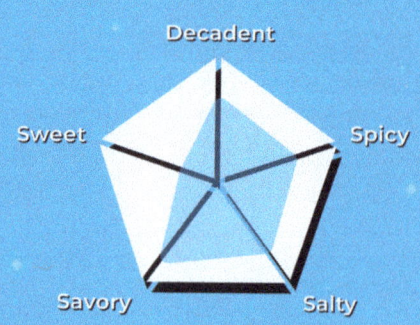

Decadent

Sweet

Spicy

Savory

Salty

I came up with this recipe out of the blue one evening while playing video games with my wife. It was one of those moments when inspiration strikes, and it's necessary to start writing immediately. When you are preparing the ingredients, think about what you'd like to add to the soup once it's done and served up at the table. Half the fun of it is the variety of toppings that work well with this dish!

Ingredients

Chicken Stock	64 Fl Oz
Black beans, Cooked or Canned	3 C
Chicken Thighs, Boneless, Skinless	4 ea
Vine Ripened Tomatoes, Diced OR	8 ea
14 oz Can of Diced Tomatoes	2 ea
Yellow Onion, Diced	1½ C
Green Bell Pepper, Diced	1 C
Carrot, Diced	½ C
Fresh Cilantro, Chopped	4 Tbsp
Garlic, Minced	2 tsp
Black Pepper	1 tsp
Cayenne Pepper	½ tsp
Nutmeg	½ tsp
Paprika	½ tsp
Chili Powder	1½ Tbsp
Coriander, Ground	2 tsp
Cumin	2 tsp
Oregano, Dry	2 tsp
Parsley, Dry	1 Tbsp
Salt	1 Tbsp
Bay Leaf	2 ea
Neutral Oil	2 Tbsp
Juice of 2 limes	

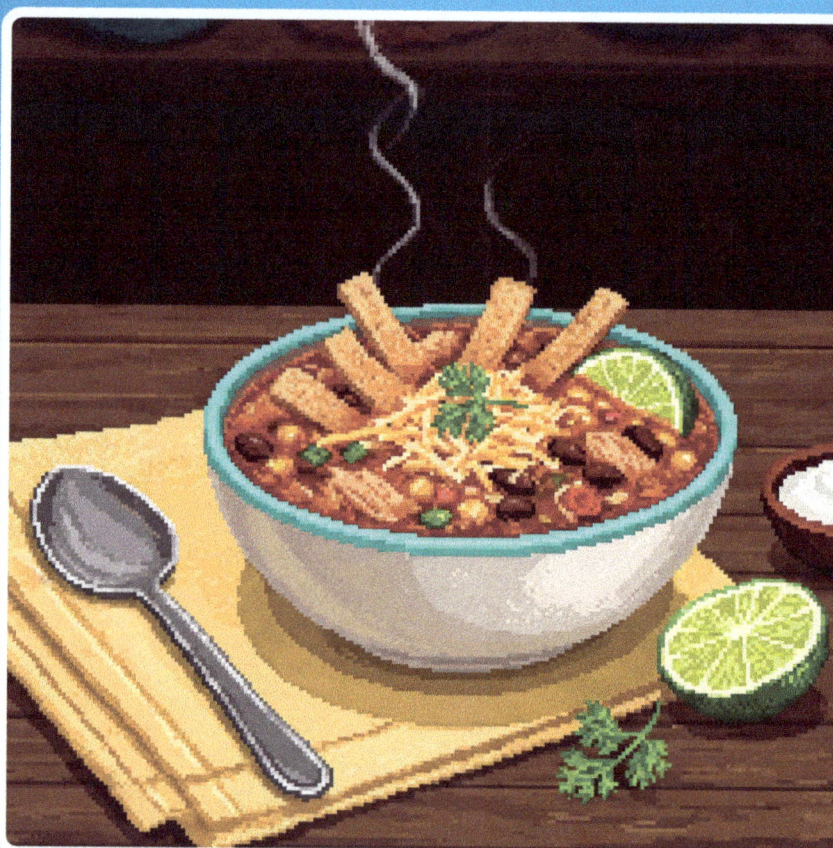

Prep Time
20 Min

Cook Time
35 Min

Servings
8 - 10 Bowls

Cooking Directions

1 Place a 6 - 8 Qt. pot over Medium High heat. When hot, add ½ of the oil. When oil is shimmering, place chicken thighs in pot. Cook for 2 - 3 min. per side, searing well.

2 Remove chicken from pot, set aside. Remove pot from heat, keeping leftover oil in pot, and turn off stove top. While chicken is cooling, cut and measure all other ingredients. Once cooled, cut the chicken into ½" cubes.

3 Return pot to Medium heat. Once hot, add the remaining oil. Then, add bell pepper, carrot, and onion one at a time, cooking each until soft before adding the next.

4 Add garlic and dry seasonings, cook for 1 min. stirring throughout. Pour in ¼ C of the stock and scrape up the brown bits (the fond) from the bottom of the pot. Add tomatoes, cilantro and beans. Stir well.

5 Add remaining stock to the pot and bring to a boil. Reduce heat to Medium Low to maintain a simmer. Cook, with lid on, for 25 minutes.

6 Uncover and add lime juice. Stir gently, then remove from heat. Serve Hot.

Recipe Tip

Great topping ideas include:
Fresh chopped cilantro, Crushed tortilla or corn chips, Shredded cheese, Diced avocado, Diced onion, and Sour cream. The options are limited only by your imagination!

Curry Chicken Soup

This recipe is versatile: any kind of curry paste can be used! Each has its own flavor profile and heat level. Try red curry paste for a good kick of heat, or yellow for an earthier and mellower flavor. The brightness and tang of green curry paste happens to be my favorite, and all of them can be found at Asian markets.

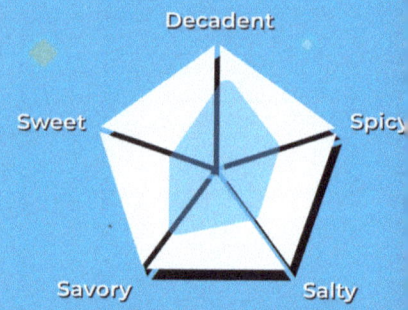

Ingredients

Chicken Thigh, ¾" Pcs	¾ C
Carrot, Small Dice	½ C
Bell Pepper, Small Dice	½ C
Yellow Onion, Small Dice	¾ C
Button Mushrooms, Sliced	6 ea
Ginger, Minced	2 tsp
Garlic, Minced	2 tsp
Turmeric	½ tsp
Black Pepper, Ground	¼ tsp
Green Curry Paste	2 Tbsp
Bay Leaf	1 ea
Chicken or Vegetable Stock	32 Fl Oz
Coconut Milk, Unsweetened	14 Fl Oz
Cilantro, Fine Chop	¼ C
Neutral oil	1 Tbsp
Juice of ½ a Lime	
Lime Wedges & Cilantro for Serving	

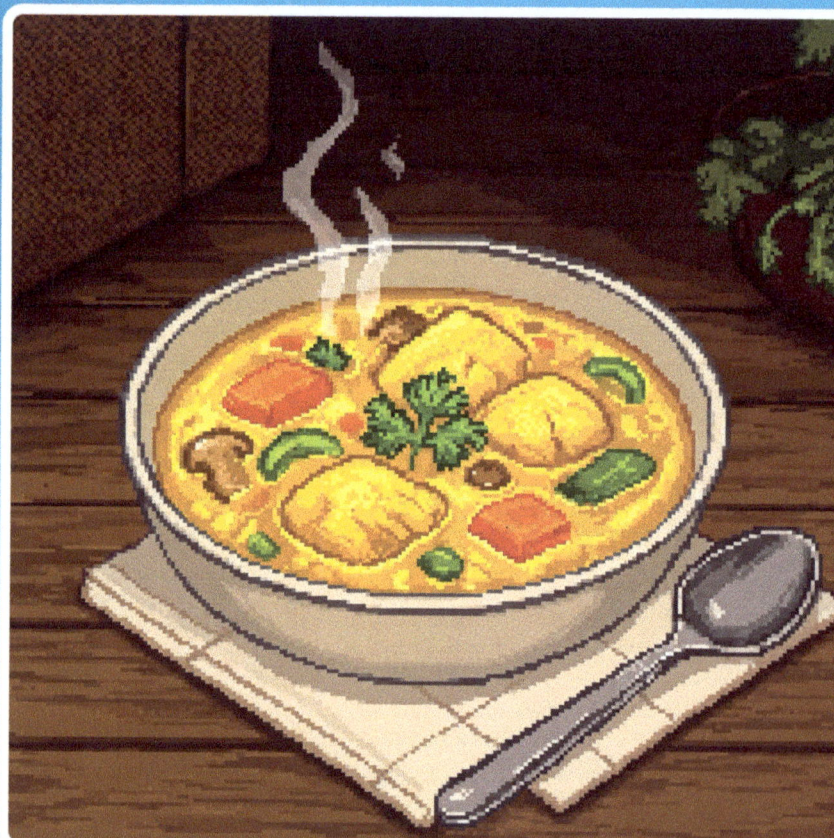

Prep Time
15 Min

Cook Time
45 Min

Servings
4 Portions

Cooking Directions

1   Place a 6 Qt. pot over Medium heat, add oil. When oil is shimmering add carrot, bell pepper, mushrooms, and onion one at a time, cooking each until soft before next.

2   Add ginger and garlic, cook until fragrant, about 1 minute.

3   Add spices and curry paste, stir well and cook for 2 - 3 minutes.

4   Add stock, stir well, and raise heat to High. Bring to a boil.

5   Add coconut milk, lime juice, and chicken. Stir well and bring back to a boil.

6   Reduce heat to Medium Low and simmer for 20 minutes, uncovered.

7   Remove pot from heat and stir in cilantro. Serve Hot.

Roasted Tomato Basil Soup

This Italian inspired soup is a delicious, grown up version of a classic. Top with more fresh basil, hot sauce, or finishing oil. Also, consider roasting some garlic cloves and using those to bring a depth of flavor to this soup that can be quite pleasing. Excellent accompaniments for this soup include a grilled cheese sandwich, a quesadilla, or garlic bread.

Decadent
Sweet
Spicy
Savory
Salty

Ingredients

Vine Ripened Tomatoes	8 ea
Garlic, Minced	1½ tsp
Chicken Or Vegetable Stock	24 Fl Oz
Heavy Cream	8 Fl Oz
Basil, Dry	½ tsp
Oregano, Dry	¼ tsp
Black Pepper, Ground	⅛ tsp
Salt	½ tsp
Bay Leaf	1 ea
Carrot, 3" Pc Peeled	1 ea
Corn Starch, For Slurry	1 Tbsp
Cold Water, For Slurry	1 Tbsp
Olive Oil	2 tsp
Large Bowl Of Cold Water	

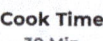

Prep Time
25 Min

Cook Time
30 Min

Servings
4 Bowls

Immersion Blender or Heat Safe Blender/ Food Processor

1 ea

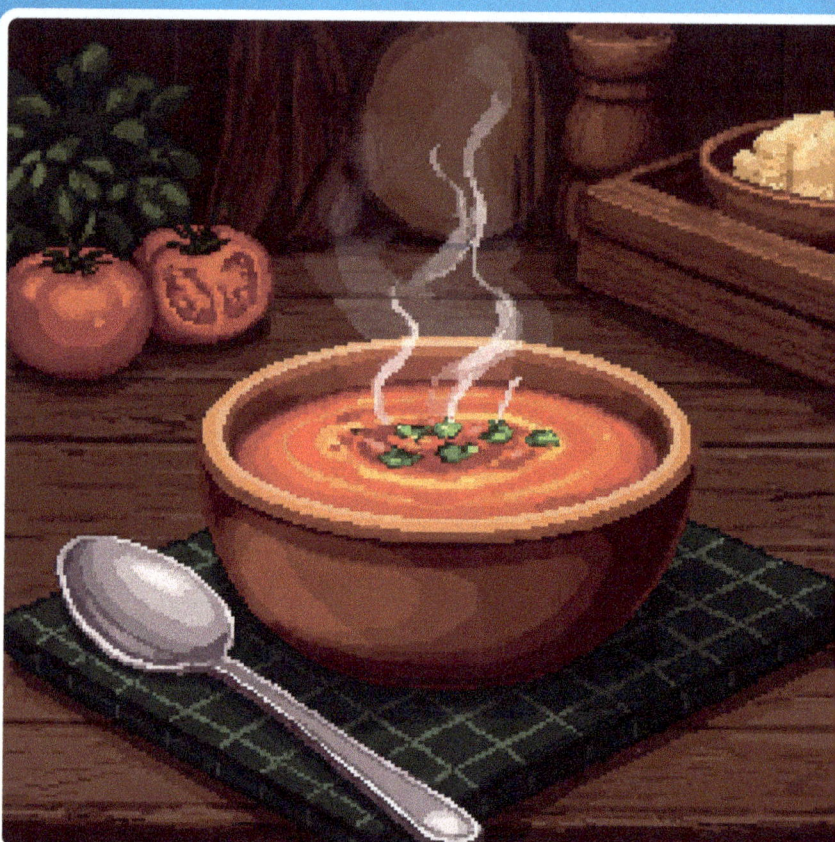

Cooking Directions

1   Preheat oven to 425. Fill a 6 - 8 Qt. pot ⅔ full with water
    and place over High heat. Cut an 'X' into each tomato,
    wrapping around the whole tomato. Be sure to cut only
    the skin, cutting as little into the flesh as possible.

2   When water is boiling, place the tomatoes in the pot and boil
    for 1 minute. Carefully transfer to a large bowl of cold water.

3   When cool, peel the tomatoes by gently pulling the skin off.

4   Cut tomatoes in half and remove the hard parts.
    Place 10 halves on a lined baking tray, cut sides up.
    Place in oven and roast for 15 minutes. Dice the
    remaining halves.

5   Turn broiler on High, and crack open oven door. Broil
    for 5-10 minutes until a good amount of char forms on
    the tomatoes.

6   Turn off oven, remove tray from oven, and let
    rest for 10 minutes.

7   Place a 4 Qt. pot over Medium heat. When hot, add oil.

8   When oil is shimmering, add garlic and cook for 30
    sec. Add all tomatoes, seasonings and stock. Raise
    heat to Medium High heat. Bring to a boil.

>>>> OVEN DIRECTIONS >>>>

9   When boiling, reduce heat to Medium Low to maintain a simmer. Cover, and cook for 15 minutes. Place the cornstarch and cold water in a small bowl, stir to combine and set aside.

10   Remove bay leaf from pot. Using an immersion blender or a heat safe blender/food processor, blend until smooth. Turn off stove eye while blending.

11   Raise heat to Medium, and return the soup to the pan if using a heat safe blender/food processor. When simmering, add the carrot piece and cover, cooking for 10 minutes.

12   Remove carrot from soup, then remix and add the Corn Starch slurry, stirring constantly. Let simmer and thicken for 2 - 3 more minutes. Remove pot from heat, serve Hot.

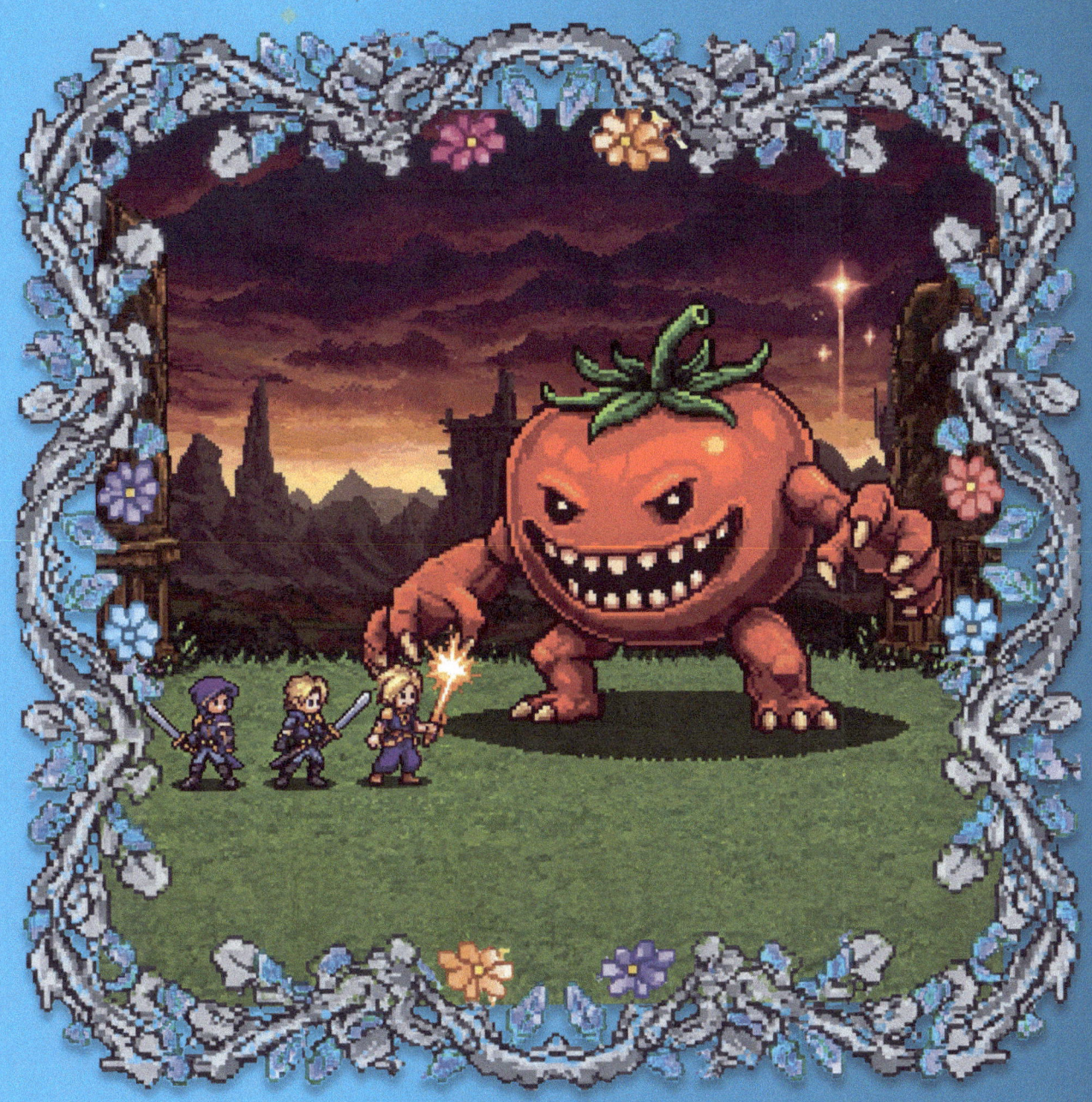

Sides & Appetizers

Buffalo Cauliflower

This recipe goes great with bleu cheese, ranch, or honey mustard dressings. Enlarge the recipe and it also works well as a healthy substitute for chicken wings. And served cold, they make a good addition to a Charcuterie board. Whether as passed hors d'oeuvres or a main entree, they are delicious!

Decadent
Sweet — **Spicy**
Savory — **Salty**

Ingredients

Lg Head Of Cauliflower, Cut Into Florets	1 ea
Large Eggs, Beaten	3 ea
Panko Bread Crumbs	1½ C
Paprika	1 tsp
Cayenne Pepper	¼ - ½ tsp
Black Pepper, Ground	⅛ tsp
Salt	¼ tsp
Hot Sauce	½ C
Butter, Melted	¼ C

Prep Time	Cook Time	Servings
15 Min	30 Min	4 Portions

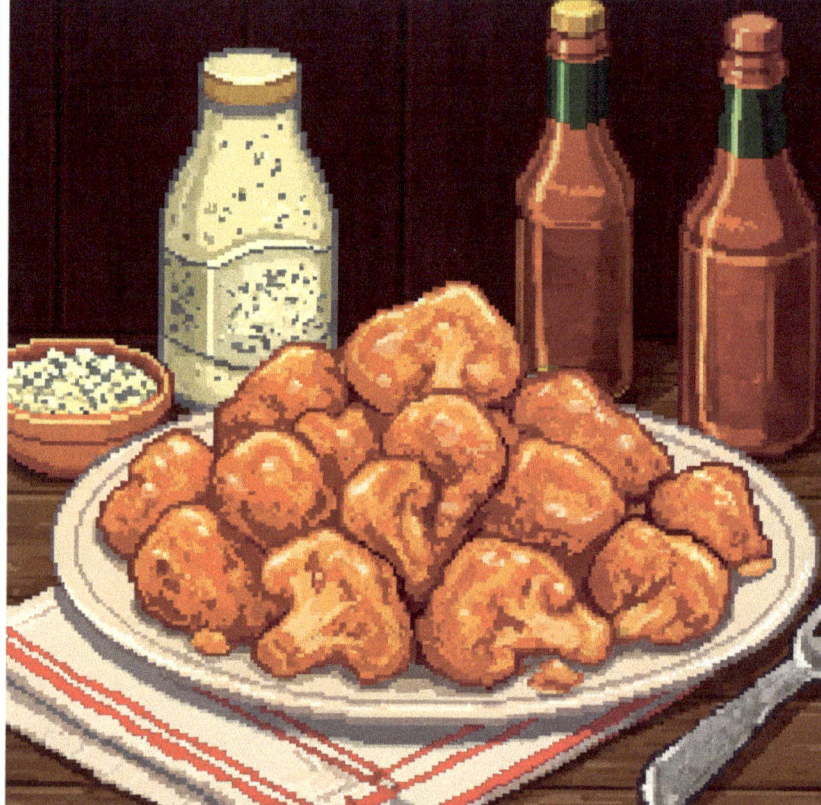

Cooking Directions

1   Preheat oven to 425. Line a baking sheet with parchment paper.

2   Place eggs in large bowl and whisk well. Add cauliflower florets and toss to coat well.

3   Combine the panko, paprika, cayenne, salt, and pepper in a separate large bowl. In batches, shake excess egg off each piece and toss cauliflower in the mix to coat well.

4   Place each floret on the baking sheet, making sure they aren't touching

5   Bake for 20 - 25 minutes, turning cauliflower halfway through cooking. While baking, melt the butter in the microwave or on stovetop. Place the butter and the hot sauce in a large bowl, whisk well to combine.

6   Once baking is done, remove cauliflower from oven. Transfer in batches to the bowl with hot sauce and toss well to coat.

7   Place tossed cauliflower back onto the baking sheet and bake for 5 minutes.

8   Remove from oven and let cool for 2 - 3 minutes. Serve warm.

Caribbean Jicama Slaw

Jicama is a variety of turnip of Central American origin, and has a neutral flavor with a very crunchy texture. It can be found in most grocery stores, and is often inexpensive. The crunch of the fresh vegetables contrasts nicely with the mouthfeel of the curried mayo, making an excellent topping for tacos or a side for broiled fish and pork.

You can simplify this recipe by using a large bore cheese grater, or a mandolin, to shred the vegetables, but this will yield a different texture than hand cutting. Doing this reduces the difficulty to Novice rather than Apprentice. Practice makes perfect though, so use this recipe to perfect your knife cuts; the Experience Points gained are well worth the effort.

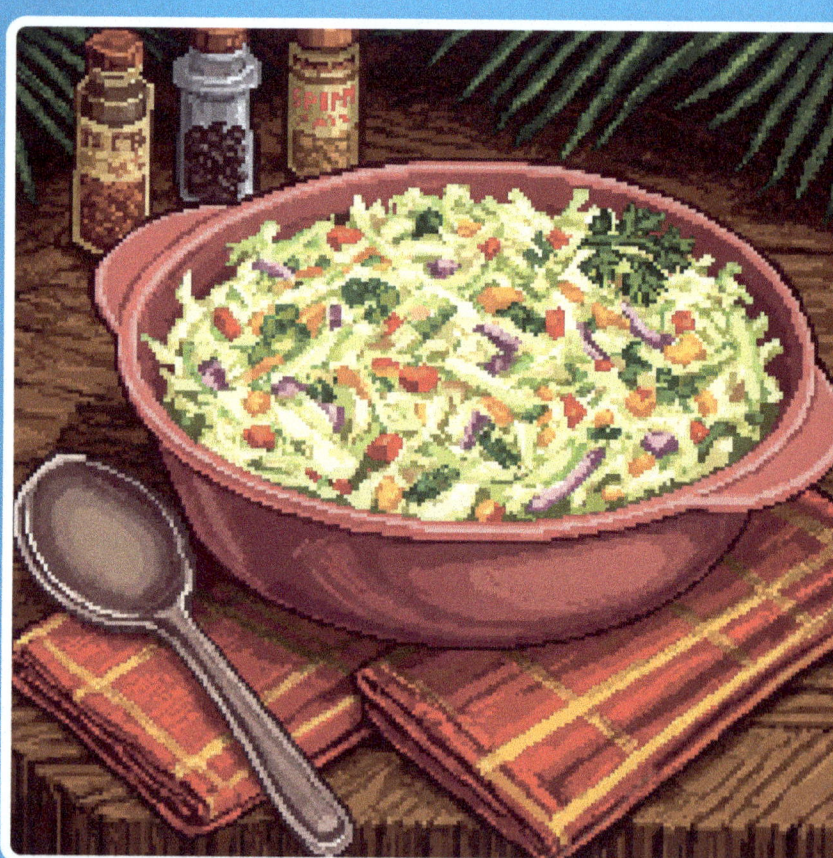

Ingredients

Jicama, Peeled, Thin Julienne	2 C
Carrot, Peeled, Thin Julienne	1 C
Bell Pepper, Thin Julienne	½ C
Turmeric	1 Tbsp
Cumin	¼ tsp
Nutmeg, Ground	⅛ tsp
Black Pepper, Ground	⅛ tsp
Salt	¼ tsp
White Sugar	½ tsp
Apple Cider Vinegar	1½ tsp
Garlic, Minced	1 tsp
Ginger, Minced	2 tsp
Mayo (Pg 145)	½ C

 Prep Time 20 Min

 Cook Time N/A

 Servings 6 - 8 Portions

 Mandolin 1 ea (Not Required)

 Large Bore Cheese Grater 1 ea

Cooking Directions

1   Cut and measure all ingredients.

2   In a large bowl, combine everything except the vegetables. Whisk well.

3   Add the vegetables and mix well. Cover tightly with plastic wrap or place in an airtight container.

4   Refrigerate for at least 2 hours, preferably overnight. Holds in fridge for 5 days.

Curried Chicken Wings

Decadent

Sweet — Spicy

Savory — Salty

These wings are delicious cold as well as hot. They make for an excellent addition to a charcuterie board, or as a healthy snack. They are not only good to make for party trays, but are also a great main course option.

Ingredients

Chicken Wings, Whole	8 ea
Ginger, Minced	2 tsp
Garlic, Minced	2 tsp
Soy Sauce	2 Tbsp
Cinnamon, ground	2 tsp
Honey	2 Tbsp
Turmeric	1 tsp
Garam Masala	1 tsp
Cumin	½ tsp
Neutral Oil	2 Tbsp
Juice & Zest of 2 Limes	

 Prep Time
5 Min + 2 Hr

 Cook Time
12 - 15 Min

 Servings
8 Wings

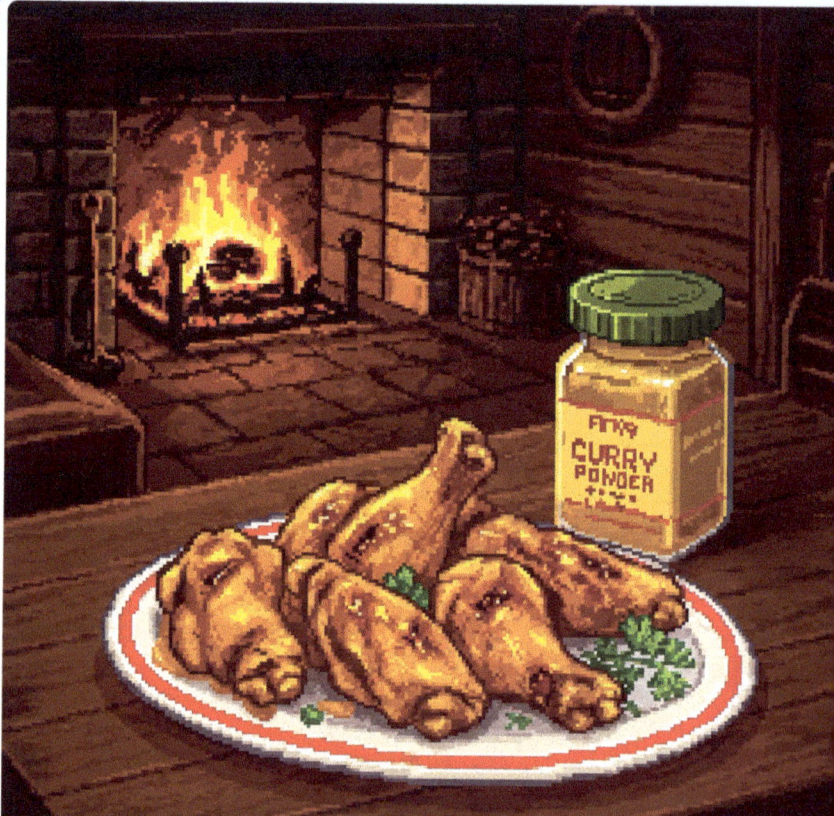

Cooking Directions

1   Place all ingredients except chicken wings in a bowl. Whisk until well combined.

2   Place the chicken in a gallon sized bag, or a shallow dish. Pour in the marinade and toss to coat. Place in fridge and let marinate for 2 hr. minimum, no more than 6 hr. Be sure to agitate the bag, or turn the chicken wings in the shallow dish, periodically to ensure proper marinating.

Broiling

1   Set broiler to High and adjust a rack so it is 6" - 8" from broiler. Remove chicken from marinade and let rest for 3 min.

2   Arrange chicken on a baking sheet lined with foil. Place on the upper rack.

3   Cook for 7 min., flip, and cook for 5 - 7 min. more until internal temperature is 165. Serve Hot.

Grilling

1   Remove chicken from marinade and let rest for 3 min. before cooking.

2   Grill chicken over Medium Hot coals for 5 - 6 min. per side, until internal temperature is 165. Serve Hot.

Nanny's Coleslaw

Decadent

Sweet — Spicy

Savory — Salty

This recipe has a special place in my heart. It's very simple but I find its delicate sweetness pairs well with anything that coleslaw would be served alongside. From BBQ, to Fried Chicken, to Beans and Cornbread, this side dish was a staple on my grandparents table. My grandmother, Nanny, would be requested to make it every time her church had a potluck or our family got together, and it was one of the first recipes I remember being taught and committing to memory.

You can use a large bore cheese grater to shred your vegetables, just like my Nanny did. But, you can also take this opportunity to practice those knife skills, working on your Chiffonade and mincing techniques. The hand chopping yields more Experience Points, but takes more time. Choose your path accordingly.

Ingredients

Green Cabbage, Finely Shredded	3 C
Carrot, Finely Shredded	½ C
Mayo (Pg 145)	¾ C
Apple Cider Vinegar	2 Tbsp
White Sugar	1½ Tbsp
Salt	¼ tsp

Prep Time
20 Min

Cook Time
N/A

Servings
6 - 8 Portions

Large Bore Cheese Grater
1 ea

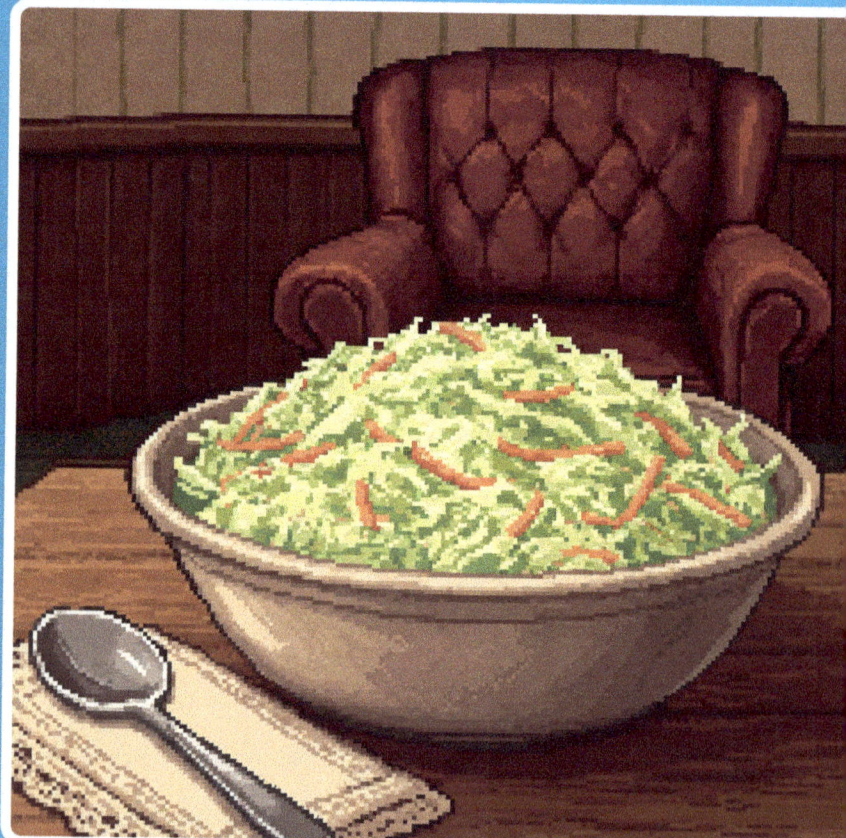

Cooking Directions

1   Combine all ingredients except vegetables in a
     large bowl and whisk well.

2   Add the vegetables and fold with a rubber
     spatula until well mixed. Cover tightly with
     plastic wrap or place in an airtight container.
     Let rest for 2 hr. minimum, overnight
     preferred. Holds for 5 - 7 days in fridge.

Roasted Garlic Polenta

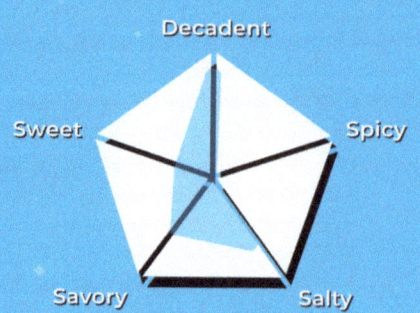

Sprinkling chopped green onions, grated parmesan cheese, or bacon bits onto creamy polenta is a simple way to elevate this side dish. Pretty much any topping you would enjoy on baked or mashed potatoes would go well with Creamy Polenta.

If you are planning on making fried polenta, pour your thickened polenta into a lined or lightly greased pan and smooth thick polenta so it is all even. Cool for 40-60 min. in the fridge until firm, then cut into desired shapes. Toss polenta pieces gently in seasoned flour and fry in oil temped to 350 for 3-4 minutes, until the edges are browned.

Ingredients

Water or Stock, Divided	32 Fl Oz
Yellow Corn Grits, Dry	1¼ C
Salt	1 tsp
Whole Garlic Bulb	1 ea
Olive Oil	½ Tbsp
Salt & Black Pepper For Garlic	

Prep Time
40 Min

Cook Time
15 - 20 Min
or 25 - 30 Min

Servings
4 Cups

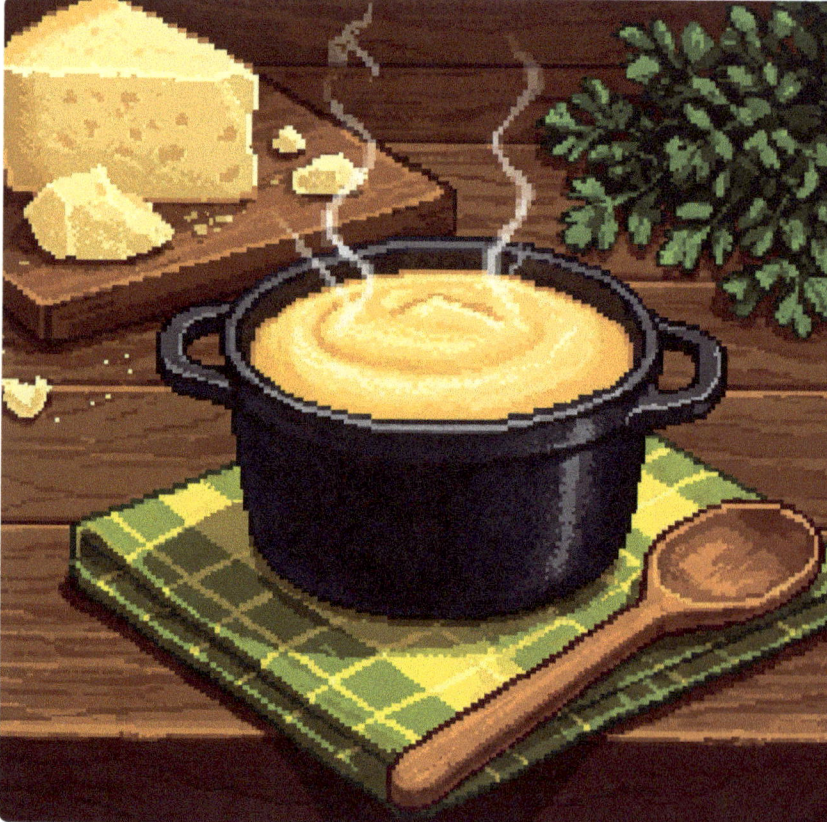

Cooking Directions

1   Preheat oven to 400. Cut the top off the bulb of garlic, and drizzle with olive oil, sprinkling with salt and pepper. Wrap tightly in tin foil, folding the foil up and twisting the top so the package looks like a tear drop.

2   Place in oven and cook for 40 minutes. Remove from oven and let cool for 15 - 20 minutes. When cool, remove the cloves from the bulb and mash into a paste.

3   In a 2 Qt. pot bring 16 Fl. Oz. of water/stock to a boil. When boiling, add 1 tsp. of salt. In a medium sized bowl, whisk the grits and remaining water/stock. Add the mixture to the pot. Stir continuously until completely combined. Add garlic paste and stir to combine fully. Cover and reduce heat to Low.

4   For creamy, looser polenta, cook for 15 - 20 min. stirring often. For thicker polenta (for frying) cook for 25 - 30 min. until the polenta starts to pull away from the pan as you stir it.

5   Serve Hot. Hold over lowest heat, covered, for up to 1 hr.

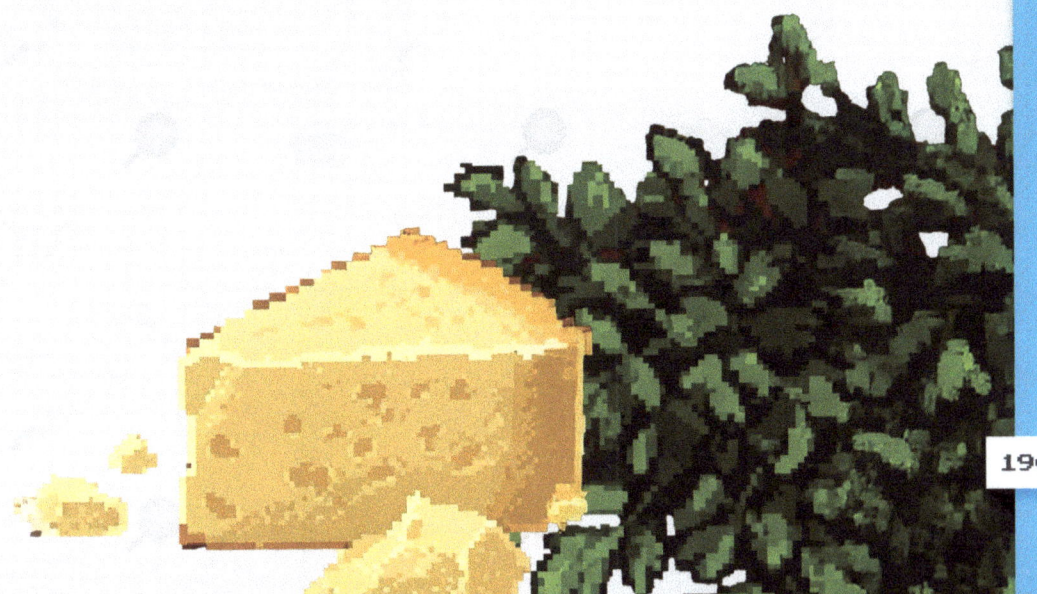

Vegetable Spring Rolls

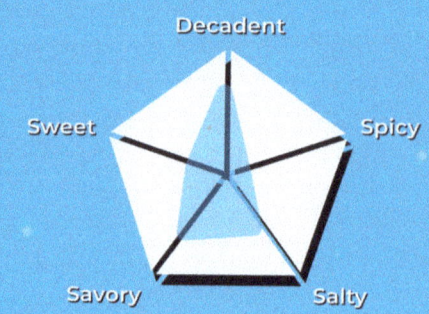

Decadent
Sweet
Spicy
Savory
Salty

Spring rolls are a delicious appetizer or side, and are deceptively easy to make. The rolling is the only challenging part, and once you get the hang of it, that too becomes easy. Serving these with some homemade Sweet Chili Sauce (Pg 155) or Teriyaki (Pg 253) will really make them pop!

Making spring rolls can take a bit of time, so making a large batch of them and freezing them is a good option.

Ingredients

Cabbage, Julienned (Nappa Or Green)	6 C
Carrot, Peeled, Shredded	1 C
Scallions, Chopped	4 ea
Bell Pepper, Thin Julienne	½ C
Neutral Oil	1 Tbsp
Soy Sauce	1 Tbsp
Rice Vinegar	2 tsp
Sesame Oil	1 tsp
Black Pepper, Ground	½ tsp
Garlic, Minced	2 tsp
Spring Roll Wrappers, Thawed	12 ea
Salt	⅛ tsp
Oil For Frying	2 C
Water For Rolling	

Prep Time	**Cook Time**	**Servings**
40 Min	15 - 20 Min	12 Rolls

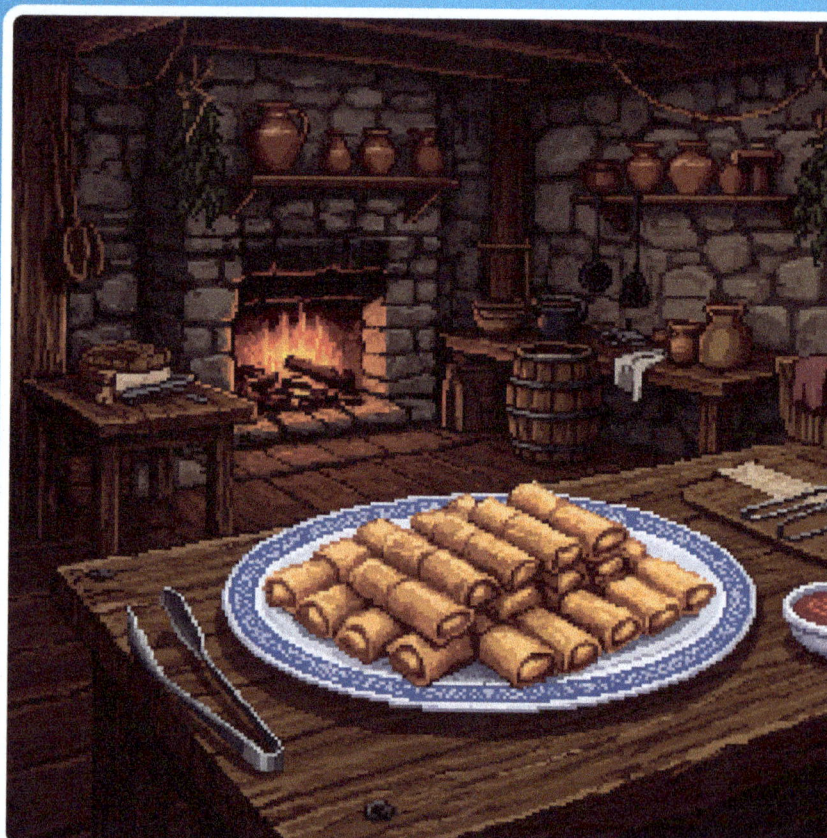

Cooking Directions
(Frying 15 – 20 Min)

1. Cut and measure all ingredients before starting. Remove the spring roll wrappers from the freezer and place in the fridge several hours before to thaw (I recommend the night before).

2. Place a large skillet over Medium High heat and add 1 Tbsp. of oil.

3. When oil is shimmering, add the garlic and cook for 1 min.

4. Add the remaining vegetables (except scallion pieces) and stir well. Cook for 8 - 10 min. until the cabbage is wilted and soft, but still a bit crunchy.

5. Add the soy sauce, rice vinegar, sesame oil and black pepper. Stir thoroughly.

6. Add the scallion pieces and the salt. Mix to combine and remove pan from heat. Transfer to a bowl to let the mix cool so it can be handled easily.

7. When the filling is cool, spread a sheet of the spring roll wrapper flat, laying it so it looks like a diamond, and scoop ¼ cup of the vegetable mix into the center of the wrapper.

8. Roll the 'bottom' corner up so it covers the filling, tucking the point under the filling.

>>>> FRYING CONTINUED >>>>

9   Bring the side corners to the center and roll up so there is about 2" of the remaining flap showing. Brush with a small amount of water and roll up to seal.

10 Repeat with remaining wrappers, making sure to cover the finished rolls to keep them from drying out.

11 Pour 2 cups of oil in a 3 - 4 Qt. pot and place over Medium-High heat. Using a thermometer to monitor the temperature, bring the oil up to 375. Keep track of how quickly it heats up, and adjust the heat setting accordingly to make sure it will hold the proper temperature without getting too hot.

12 Cook the spring rolls, 2 - 3 at a time, until the wrapper is golden brown, 4 - 5 min. Be sure to agitate the rolls often to ensure even cooking.

13 Remove cooked rolls from the pot and place on a paper towel to soak up excess grease. Let rest for 5 min. before serving.

Cooking Directions (Baking 13 – 15 Min)

1   Preheat the oven to 425. Follow the previous steps 1 - 10.

2   Brush your finished rolls lightly with oil, coating all sides evenly.

3   Place them on a baking sheet lined with foil, or on a wire rack in a lined baking tray.

4   Bake for 13 - 15 min. flipping halfway through.

5   Remove from the oven and let rest for 5 min. before serving.

Recipe Tip

Freeze the excess!
Once you roll them up, place them on a baking sheet lined with parchment paper and place in the freezer for 2 hr. until frozen through. Transfer your frozen rolls into a freezer bag and keep them for up to 3 months. To cook them, just place the frozen rolls in oil heated to 375 and cook until golden brown. If baking frozen rolls, simply brush with some oil and bake at 425 for 20 - 25 min.

Mains

All Purpose Braised Pork

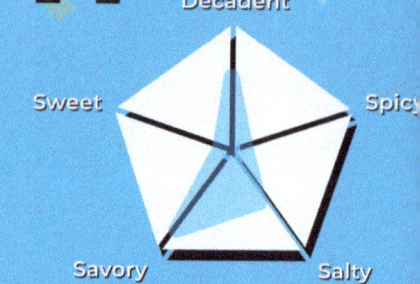

This recipe is the base for all kinds of dishes. Try reheating with taco seasoning for carnitas tacos, or filling for enchiladas and tamales. Mix the pork with some Sweet Heat BBQ sauce (see Pg 251) for delicious pulled pork sandwiches and platters. Try replacing the shredded chicken in Tortilla soup with pork for a more unctuous and earthy flavor. The applications are limited only by your imagination and your drive to experiment, and thankfully this recipe makes plenty of pork!

If you wish, you can retain the braising liquid but make sure to chill it overnight in the fridge so you can easily remove the fat from it the next day by straining away the solidified fat from the top. This liquid works well as a soup or stock base, and is packed with flavor.

Ingredients

Pork Butt Or Shoulder	5 - 6 Lb
Bay Leaves	2 ea
Oregano, Dry	1 Tbsp
Black Pepper, Ground	1½ tsp
Salt	¾ Tbsp
Parsley, Dry	2 tsp
Rosemary, Dry	1½ tsp
Ginger Powder	2 tsp
Nutmeg, Ground	1 tsp
Garlic Powder	2 tsp
White Sugar	2 Tbsp
Water or Stock	32 Fl Oz
Neutral Oil	2 Tbsp

  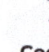

Prep Time
10 Min

Cook Time
3½ - 4 Hr (Oven)
6 - 7 Hr (Crock Pot)

Servings
4 - 4½ Lb

Small Food Processor
1 ea

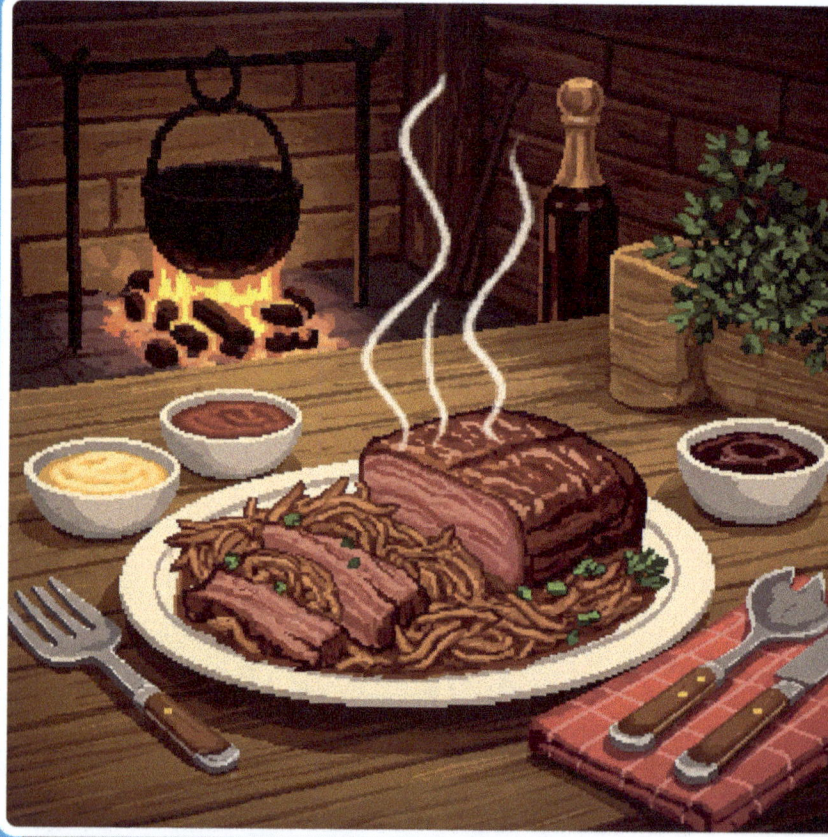

Cooking Directions
(Oven)

1   Place all herbs and spices (except the bay leaves) in a food processor and pulse 10 - 15 times to blend, if you have one. If not, no worries, just combine all seasoning ingredients and stir well.

2   Place pork on a large sheet of plastic wrap. Evenly rub the seasoning blend all over the pork. Place the bay leaves evenly apart on the pork as you wrap it tightly in the plastic. Place in the fridge on a plate and let rest for 4 hr. or overnight.

3   Preheat the oven to 300. Place a 4 - 6 Qt. pot, large enough to comfortably fit the pork, or a Dutch oven, over Medium High heat. Remove the pork from the fridge and unwrap, remove and retain the bay leaves. Once hot, add the oil to the pot.

4   When oil is shimmering, place the pork in the pot and sear on all sides, 2 - 3 mi. per side.

5   Once seared, pour the water or stock into the pot and add the remaining bay leaves to the pot. Bring the liquid to a hard simmer and if not using a Dutch oven cover the pot with aluminum foil, then the lid. If using a Dutch oven, simply place the lid on.

6   Transfer the pot into your oven and braise for 3½ - 4 hr. until a spoon can be inserted into the pork easily, and the meat pulls apart easily. Check on the liquid level halfway through, adding more if the level gets too low. Be careful of the steam when lifting the foil!

>>>> CONTINUED >>>>

7   Gently remove the pot from the oven. Remove the lid and aluminum foil, and transfer the pork to a large bowl or casserole dish. Be gentle, the pork will want to come apart easily. Remove bone and discard. Shred the pork, cool properly, and pack into airtight containers to store in the fridge. Holds for 5 days refrigerated, can be frozen for up to 30 days.

Cooking Directions (Crock Pot)

1   Follow the previous steps 1 - 4. Set your crockpot to Low.

2   Remove the pork from the pot and transfer to the crock. Pour your water/stock in the pot and scrape up any stuck on brown bits (the fond) from the bottom.

3   Place the bay leaves in the crock, then transfer the liquid from the pot to the crock. Cover and cook for 6 - 7 hr.

Recipe Tip

Try using leftover braising liquid in place of water when seasoning taco meat, or as an addition to the liquid when making pot roast or beef stew.

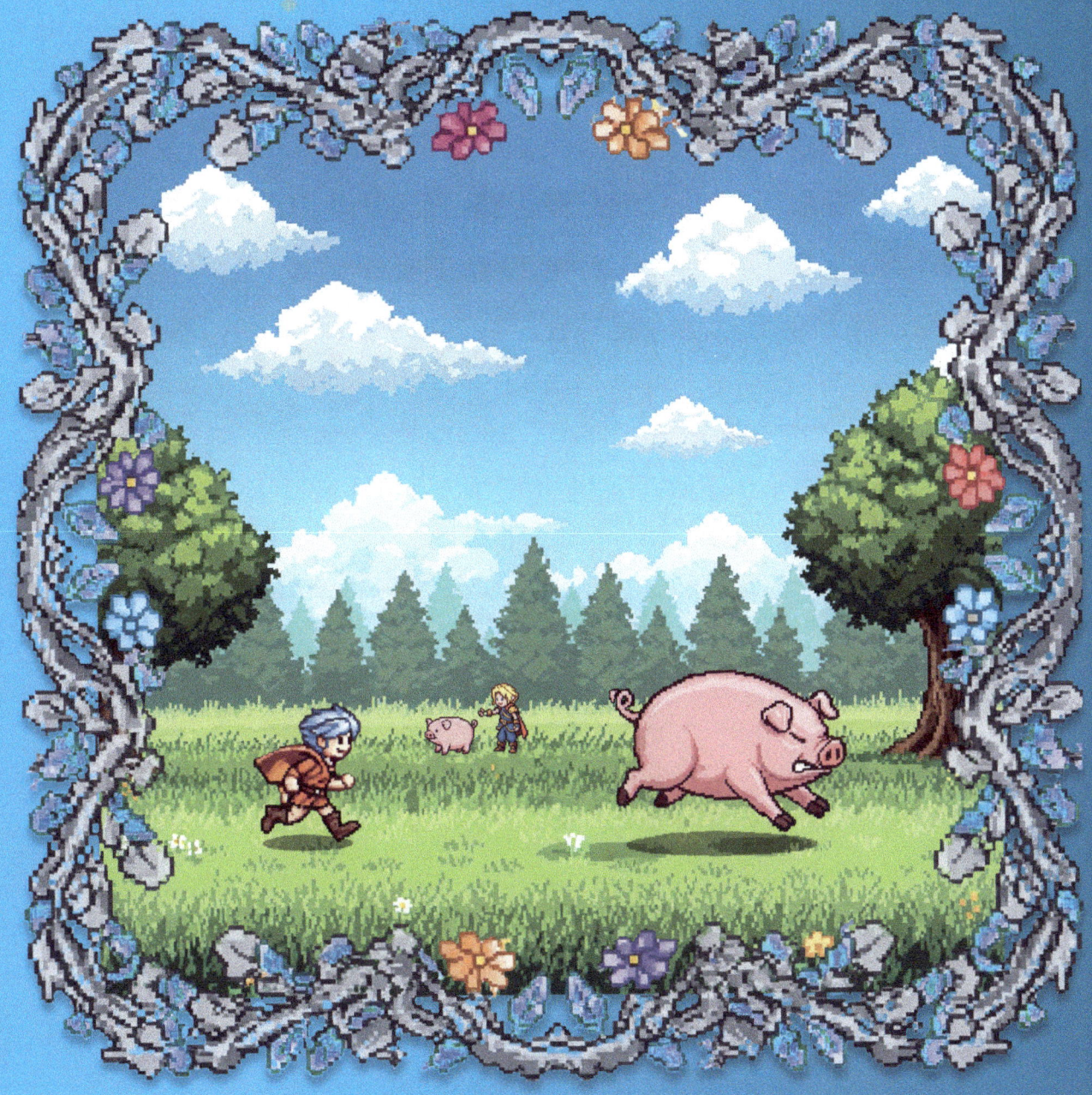

Char-Siu Pork

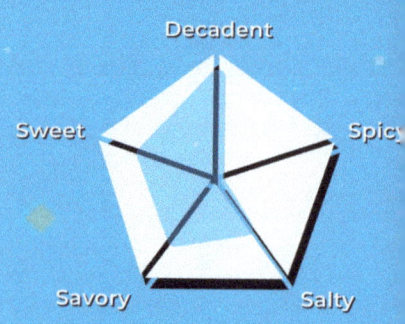

Decadent

Sweet

Spicy

Savory

Salty

This recipe is the secret behind those flavorful pieces of pork that are in the best egg rolls, fried rice, and lo mein. In fact, those are my top recommended dishes to make with this recipe, along with using this recipe for marinating racks of ribs before slow cooking them. It's a versatile dish, and you're encouraged to experiment with it. Don't be afraid to try out different combinations and discover your own preferred culinary fusions.

Ingredients

Pork Loin, Boneless	3 Lb
White Sugar	¼ C
Sesame Oil	½ tsp
Salt	2 tsp
White Pepper	¼ tsp
Mirin/Shaoxing Wine	1 Tbsp
Chinese Five Spice Powder	½ tsp
Soy Sauce	1 Tbsp
Hoisin	1 Tbsp
Brown Sugar	2 tsp
Honey	2 Tbsp
Hot Water (For Marinade)	1 Tbsp
Water (For Cooking)	12 Fl Oz

 Prep Time 15 Min

 Cook Time 40 Min

 Servings 3 Lb

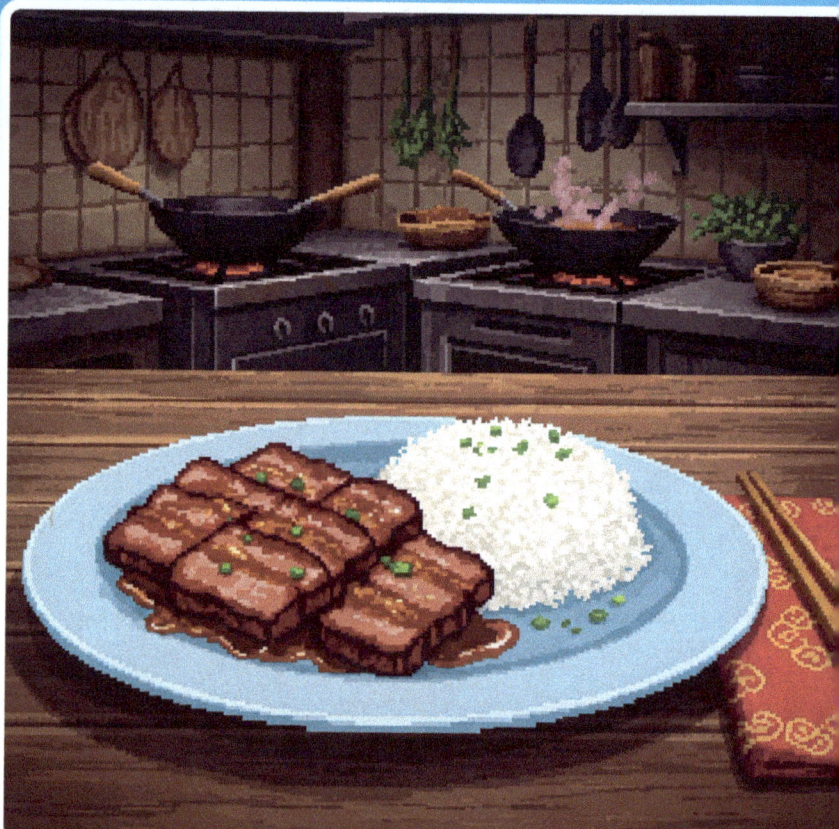

Cooking Directions

1 Cut pork lengthwise into strips about ½" thick, do not trim the excess fat.

2 Combine the remaining ingredients (except the 12 oz. of water) in a bowl large enough to hold the pork pieces. Set aside 2 Tbsp. of the marinade. Add the pork and toss well to coat. Cover with plastic wrap and refrigerate for 8 hr. minimum, overnight preferred.

3 Preheat oven to 475, move one rack into upper ⅓ of oven and one rack into the lower ⅓ of oven. Pour the remaining water into a roasting pan or oven safe dish and place on the lower rack in the oven during preheating.

4 Line a baking tray with foil, then place a wire rack in the tray. One at a time, remove the pork from the marinade, shake off excess marinade, and place on the wire rack.

5 Place the tray in the oven. Be careful of the steam when opening the oven door! Roast for 5 min. then lower heat to 375 and bake for 15 min. more.

6 Flip the pork and baste with the reserved marinade, then cook for 10 min. more. Remove from oven and let rest for 5 min. before serving. Will hold in fridge for 5 days.

Recipe Tip

This pork is tasty to eat as a main dish as well with a side of sautéed vegetables and white rice perhaps, or to use as a meat topping to level up a bowl of ramen or other hearty soup.

Chicken & Dumplin's

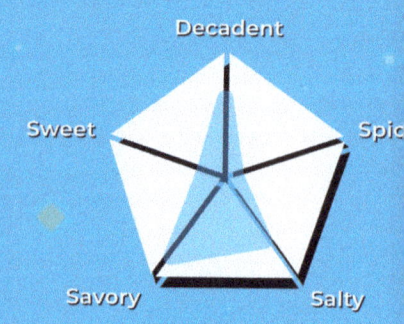

Decadent
Sweet
Spic
Savory
Salty

This recipe is inspired by one of the Sunday Dinner staples provided by my grandmother, Nanny. If you have a large crowd to feed consider doing things the way my Nanny did: buy a smaller, whole chicken and boil it in a large pot with seasonings to make your own broth and the shredded chicken at the same time. However, you can also make your life much easier and purchase a rotisserie chicken from the store and pull the meat you need from that. Either option works well, choose the one that works best for your time schedule.

Ingredients

Chicken, Shredded	3 C
Yellow Onion, Diced	¾ C
Celery, Diced	¾ C
Carrot, Diced	½ C
Garlic, Minced	2 tsp
Chicken Stock	64 Fl Oz
Bay Leaf	1 ea
Sage, Ground	1 tsp
Cumin	1 tsp
Salt	2 tsp
Black Pepper, Ground	¼ tsp
Coriander, Ground	1 tsp
Oregano, Dry	1 tsp
Paprika	1 tsp
Oil or Butter	4 Tbsp
AP Flour	4 Tbsp
Dumpling Balls/Strips (Pgs 263, 265)	8 oz

 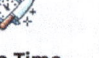

Prep Time	Cook Time	Servings
30 Min	20 - 25 Min	6 - 8 Bowls

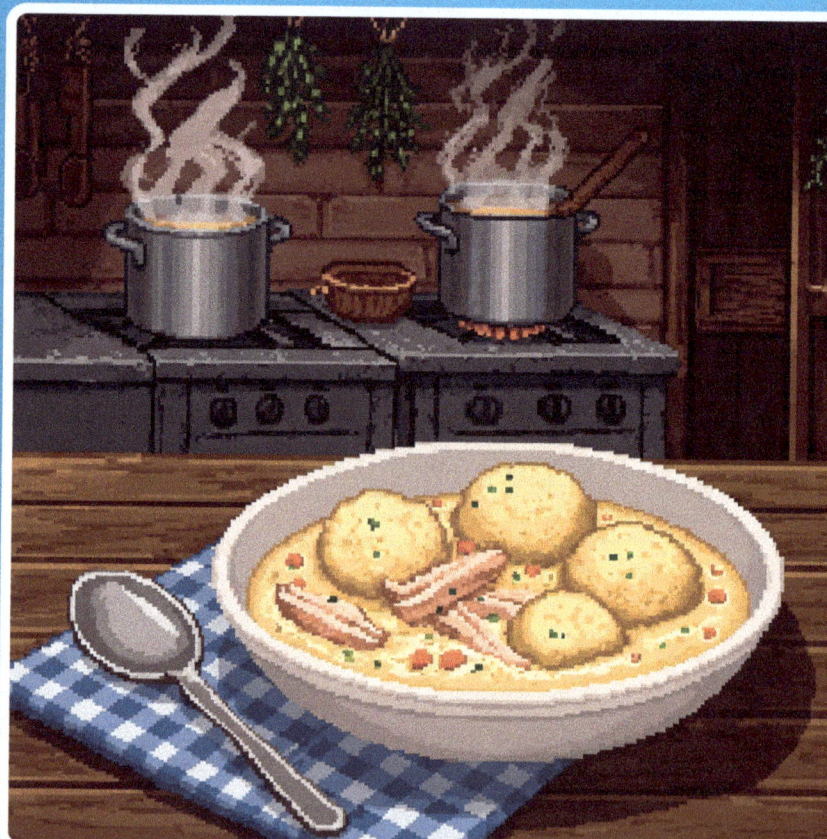

Cooking Directions

1   Place a 6 Qt. pot over Medium heat. When hot add oil.

2   When oil is shimmering, add the carrot, celery, and onion, cooking each until soft before adding the next.

3   Add flour and seasonings. Stirring constantly, cook for 2 - 3 minutes. This will bring your roux to the Blanc level.

4   Add 8 oz. of the stock and stir well, incorporating the roux and making sure there are no lumps. Add the remaining stock slowly, stirring throughout.

5   Raise heat to Medium High and add shredded chicken. Bring to a boil.

6   Lower the heat to Medium Low, cover the pot and simmer for 20 min.

7   Uncover and raise heat to Medium. Stirring gently, drop the dumplings (balls or strips) one at a time into the soup. Cook until the dumplings are floating at the top. Test a single dumpling to make sure they are fully cooked. You don't want to over or under cook them.

8   Remove pot from heat, serve immediately.

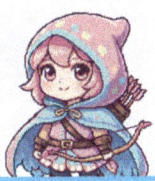

> **Recipe Tip**
>
> The two different dumpling recipes I have provided (Pgs 263, 265) both work well for this dish, and once you have learned them you should feel free to experiment with different flavorings for your dumplings. It's such a simple thing, but different flavors and types of dumplings completely change the profile of this dish.

Chicken Fajitas

Making fajitas at home seems intimidating; how do the restaurants get that unique flavor, and the loud sizzle when they bring out the pan? Now you too can make this magic happen at home! With this recipe, fajita night will quickly become a favorite to make and enjoy. And the leftovers are excellent for all kinds of dishes!

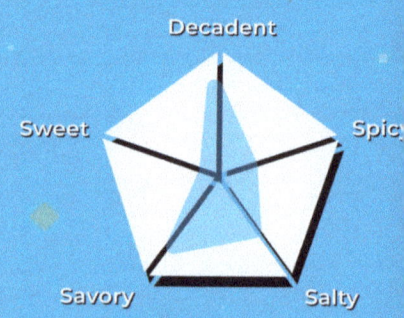

Decadent

Sweet — Spicy

Savory — Salty

Ingredients (Seasoning Blend)

Chili Powder	1½ tsp
Salt	½ tsp
Paprika	⅛ tsp
White Sugar	¼ tsp
Onion Powder	¼ tsp
Cayenne	⅛ tsp
Cumin	¼ tsp
Cornstarch	2 tsp
Ginger Powder	¼ tsp
Garlic Powder	¼ tsp
Black Pepper, Ground	¼ tsp

Ingredients (Fajitas)

Chicken Breast, Sliced Thin	1 ea
Green Bell Pepper, ½" Thick Julienne	1 ea
White Onion, ½" Thick Julienne	1 ea
Tomato Slices, ¼" Thick	5 ea
Mushrooms, Sliced	4 oz
Flour Tortillas, 5½"-6" Wide	8 ea
Avocado, Diced	1 ea
Monterey Jack Cheese, Shredded	1 C
Lettuce, Chiffonade	2 C
Neutral Oil	1½ Tbsp
Water	¼ C
Sizzle Sauce (Pg 153)	3 Tbsp
Salt & Pepper for Chicken	

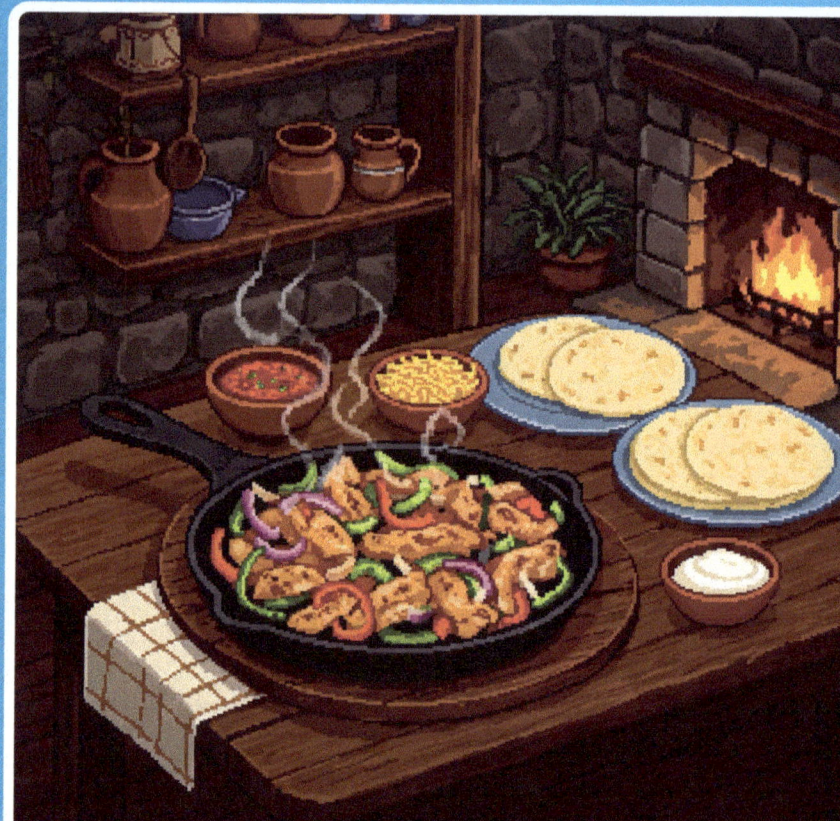

 Prep Time 15 Min

 Cook Time 25 Min

 Servings 8 Portions

Cooking Directions

1 Preheat your oven to 450 making sure there is a rack in the center of the oven. Place your sliced chicken in a bowl and sprinkle with salt and pepper, mix well to coat. Combine all seasoning ingredients, stir well, and set aside in a small bowl or ramekin.

2 Place a 12" - 14" oven safe (preferably cast iron) skillet over Medium High heat. When hot, add the oil.

3 When the oil is shimmering, place the chicken in the pan. Stirring once or twice, sear the chicken for 3 - 4 min.

4 Remove the chicken from the pan and set aside. Place the mushrooms and peppers in the pan and cook for 2 - 3 min. Then, add the onion and cook for 2 min. more.

5 Return the chicken to the pan and add the seasoning blend. Stir well to combine, then add the water, and stir until the water is evaporated.

6 Push the mix to the sides of the pan, creating an open space in the middle. Let the pan rest for 30 seconds, then sprinkle a little more oil on the pan and lay the tomato slices in the pan. Gently move the mix back over the tomatoes to cover them.

7 Place the pan in the oven and cook for 10 min. until the vegetables are soft.

8 Carefully remove the pan from the oven, place on the stove top over High Heat until the pan starts to pop. Add the Sizzle Sauce and stir well. Serve Hot with tortillas and desired toppings.

Chicken Parmesan

This is one of my favorite recipes to make from scratch at home. The savory tang of the sauce, the crunch of the parmesan laden breadcrumbs, and the saltiness of the cheese make for an irresistible combination. While this recipe is a little labor intensive, don't be intimidated by it; once you get into it, you'll see how simple it is.

Decadent

Sweet

Spicy

Savory

Salty

Ingredients

Large Chicken Breasts	2 ea
Pomodoro Sauce (Pg 151)	2 C
Provolone Slices	4 ea
Mozzarella, Shredded	½ C
Parmesan Cheese	¼ C
Breadcrumbs, Plain	1 C
AP Flour	½ C
Large Eggs	2 ea
Oregano, Dry	¼ tsp
Basil, Dry	¼ tsp
Salt	⅛ tsp
Black Pepper, ground	⅛ tsp
Neutral Oil	1 ½ C

 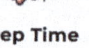

Prep Time
20 Min

Cook Time
30 Min

Servings
4 Portions

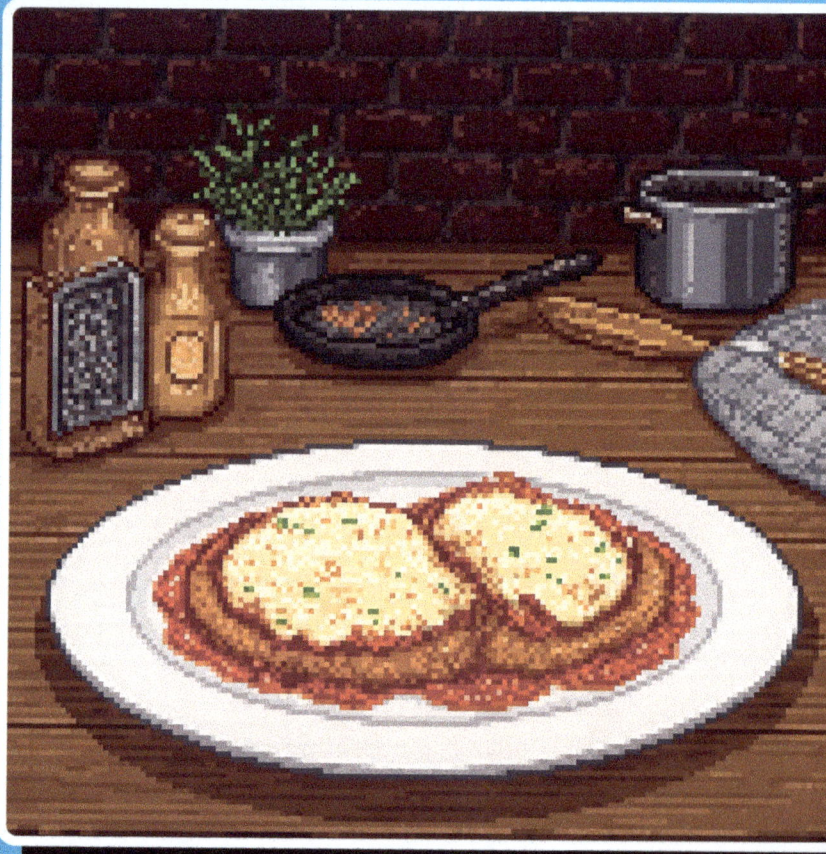

Cooking Directions

1   Place the Pomodoro in a small pot and set over Medium Low heat and cover. Remember to stir your sauce periodically throughout cooking, turning the heat to Low once it starts to bubble.

2   In a large bowl, combine the flour, ⅛ tsp. of salt, and the pepper. In a separate bowl, whisk the eggs together so they are well mixed. Finally, in a third bowl, combine the breadcrumbs, parmesan, basil, and oregano.

3   Take your chicken breasts and cut sideways all the way through as evenly level as possible. Cover the cutting board with plastic wrap, tucking the plastic under the bottom of the board on both sides. Using a mallet or a small pan, pound your chicken out so each piece is evenly ¼ - ⅜" thick.

4   Dredge a piece of chicken in the flour, coating both sides and shaking off excess. Next, dip the chicken in the egg, coating both sides and holding to drip excess egg off for a second. Finally, place the chicken in the breadcrumb mix and toss to coat, pressing the breadcrumbs gently into the breast, and setting aside on a plate or sheet pan. Repeat for remaining chicken pieces.

5   Place a 12" - 14" skillet with deep sides over Medium High heat and pour the oil in the pan. It should be between ¾ - 1" deep, and may require less or more oil depending on the size of your skillet. Using a thermometer to monitor the temperature, bring the oil to 350.

>>>> CONTINUED >>>>

6 When the oil is at 350 carefully place the chicken in the pan, placing as many as will fit in the pan without overlapping. Cook the chicken for 4 - 5 min. per side, flipping when the breading turns golden brown. While cooking, line a baking sheet with tin foil. Transfer the cooked chicken from the pan to the lined baking sheet, letting excess oil drip off of it for a few seconds. Repeat until all chicken is cooked.

7 Set your broiler to High and move a rack so it is 6" - 8" from the broiler. Leave the oven door cracked.

8 Spoon 3-4 oz. of Pomodoro onto each chicken piece. Then place ¼ of the mozzarella on each piece. Top with a slice of provolone and place the tray under the broiler. Broil for 2-3 min. until the cheese is melted and begins to develop small dark spots. Remove from oven. Let rest for 2 min. before serving. Serve Hot.

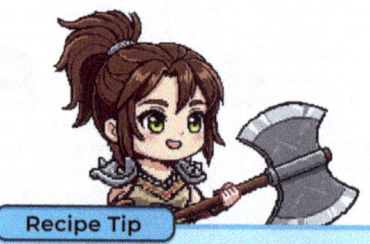

Recipe Tip

The chicken can be breaded and held in the fridge for up to 2 days in a covered container, and the pasta sauce can be made ahead of time and will hold for up to 5 days in an airtight container.

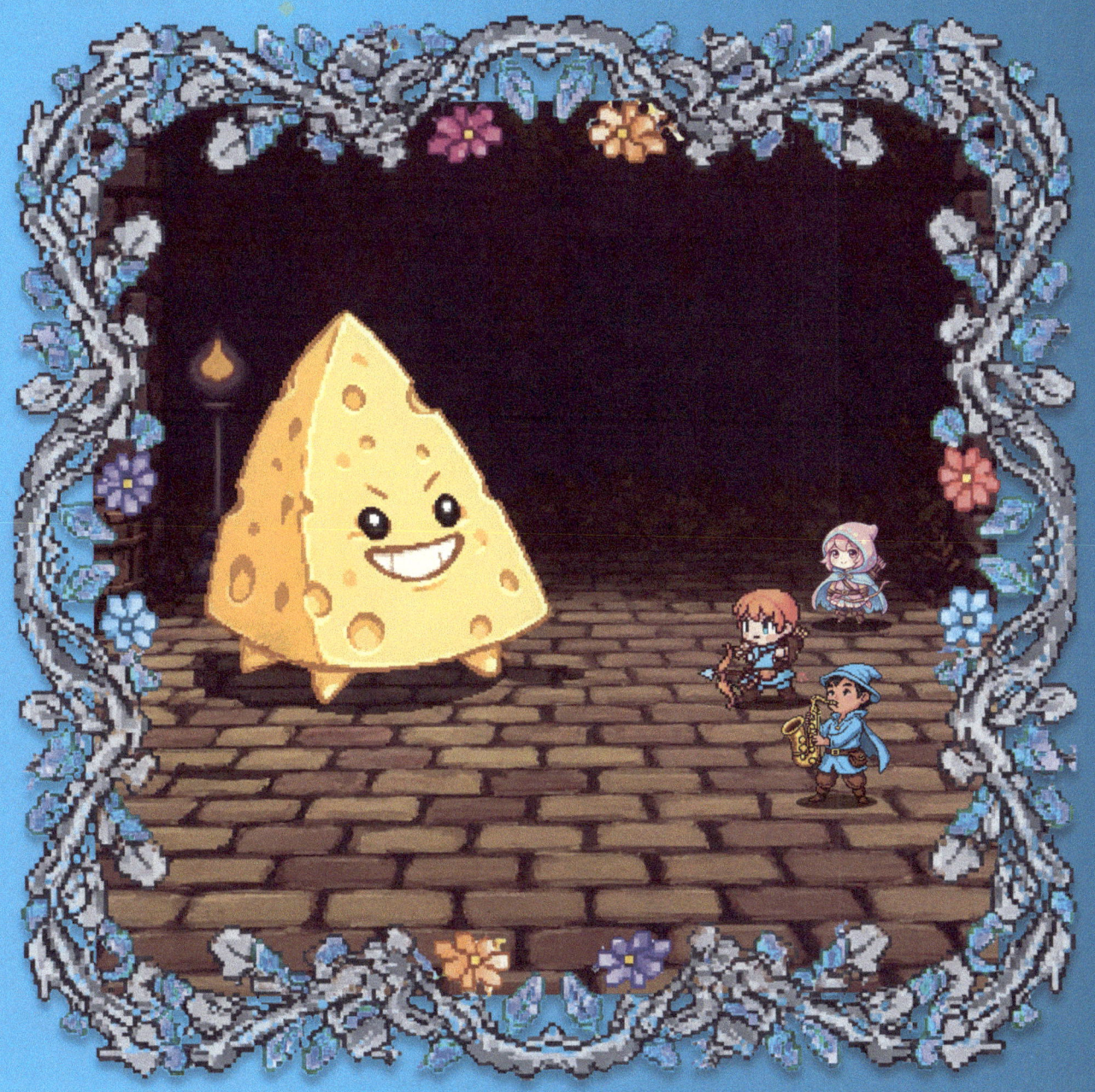

Classic Burger

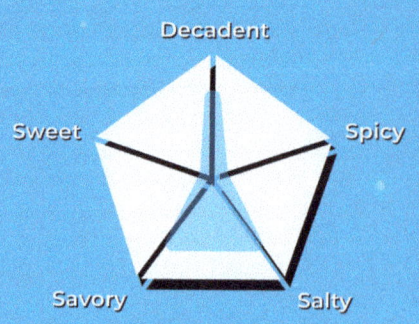

Decadent

Sweet

Spicy

Savory

Salty

If you are looking for a low-carb option, lettuce cups work very well in the place of buns. Carefully remove lettuce leaves from the head, being careful not to tear the lettuce as you peel them off. You'll need 2 cups, layered together, to place your burger in for structural support. To prevent things getting too messy, wrapping half of the burger in wax or parchment paper helps. This will ensure the back half of your burger doesn't fall out.

Keep in mind the consistency and texture of your toppings when layering the sandwich. It's advised to have toppings that are slippery (mayo, ketchup, tomatoes) on the bun and toppings with varying textures (onion, pickles, lettuce) should be in contact with the patty. This way, your burger won't fall apart as you eat it.

Ingredients

Ground Beef, 80/20	1 Lb
Yellow Onion, Diced	½ C
Lettuce, Hand Torn 1" Pcs.	1 C
Tomato Slices	4 - 8 ea
Pickle Chips	8 ea
Cheese Slices	4 ea
Buns	4 ea
OR	
Lettuce Cups	8 ea
Ketchup	
Mustard	
Mayo (Pg 145)	
Salt & Pepper for Patties	

Prep Time
15 Min

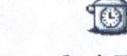
Cook Time
See Recipe

Servings
4 Burgers

Cooking Directions

1   Divide the beef evenly into 4 oz. portions and roll into balls. Press the patties so they are roughly ½" - ¾" thick. Do your best to make them as evenly shaped and level as possible. With your thumb, gently press into the middle of each patty.

2   Place a 12" - 14" skillet over Medium High heat. Generously apply salt and pepper to both sides of your patties. When hot, place the patties in the skillet, be sure not to overcrowd the pan.

3   Cook to desired doneness:

Rare - Cook for 2 min. and flip then cook for 1 - 2 min. more
Medium Rare – 3 min. and flip then cook for 1 - 2 min. more
Medium – 3 min. and flip then cook for 2 - 3 min. more
Medium Well – 4 min. and flip then cook for 2 - 3 min. more
Well Done – 4 min. and flip then cook for 4 min. more

4   After flipping, place the cheese on your patties to give it time to melt.

5   Toast your buns so they are only just brown. Alternatively, warm them up gently, but not toasted.

Build your burger as follows, from bottom to top:

Bottom Bun > Ketchup & Mustard > Pickle Chips > Diced Onion > Burger Patty, Cheese Side Down > Tomato Slice(s) > Lettuce > Mayo (on Top Bun) > Top Bun

Crispy Pork Belly

Crispy Pork Belly...What more is there to say? Tender, flavorful, crispy, all are proper descriptors for this dish. I advise searing them and tossing them in Teriyaki or Sweet Chili Sauce, or even Sweet Heat BBQ Sauce. Serve with sautéed vegetables and white rice, and you've got a decadent meal that is easy to fit into your schedule. Whether serving as a party snack, an entrée, or a topping for a rice bowl, this dish will make everyone ask for more.

Decadent

Sweet — Spic

Savory — Salty

Ingredients

Pork Belly, Skin Removed	8 oz
Paprika	½ tsp
Chinese Five Spice	½ tsp
Salt	⅛ tsp
Black Pepper, Ground	¼ tsp
White Sugar	1 tsp
Mirin/Shaoxing Wine	1 tsp
Neutral Oil, Or Reserved Lard	2 Tbsp

Prep Time
10 Min

Cook Time
6 Hr

Servings
8 oz

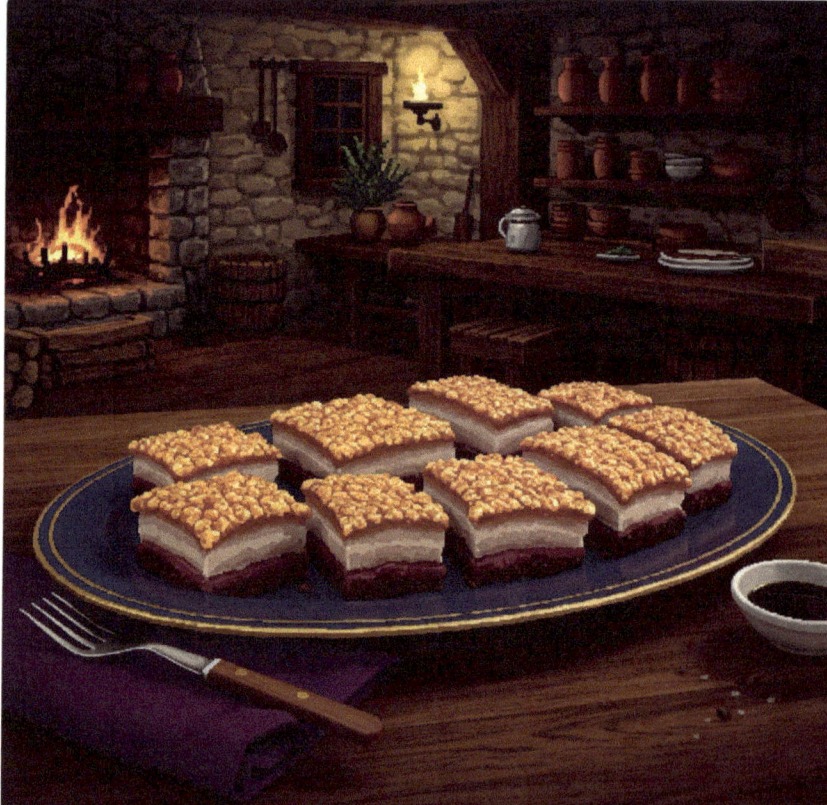

Recipe Tip

The chilled pork can be held for up to 3 days after slow roasting, so making it ahead of time and storing it is a great way to prep for the coming week.

Cooking Directions

1 Preheat oven to 200, make sure there is a rack in the center of the oven.

2 Using a sharp knife, carefully remove the skin from the pork belly by slicing in from the side. Be sure to cut as little fat as possible from the whole piece when removing the skin.

3 Once the skin is removed, cut shallow lines at an angle from one corner of the piece to another. Then, at an opposite angle, repeat from the opposite corner, cutting diamonds into the fat.

4 Place a pan over Medium heat. When hot, place the pork fat side down in the pan and sear for 8 - 10 min. A reasonable amount of fat should be rendered from the pork, and the surface of the fat side should be golden brown. If the pan starts to smoke, lower heat slightly to prevent burning.

5 Remove the pan from the heat and place the pork belly, fat side down, on the cutting board. Pour the Mirin/wine over it and rub it in. Sprinkle all your seasonings over the meat of the belly and rub them in as well. Pour the rendered fat into a heat safe container for use in other recipes.

6 Place the pork belly, fat side up, on a piece of foil large enough to wrap around the pork. Wrap the pork tightly, and wrap in a second layer of foil making sure that any seams are covered to prevent leakage.

> > > > CONTINUED > > > >

7   Place on a baking sheet and bake for 6 hr. Remove
    from oven and let rest on counter for 1 hr. before
    placing in fridge. Let chill for 8 hours to overnight.

8   Unwrap the chilled pork, scraping off any rendered fat
    stuck to the pork. Cut the pork into 6 equally thick
    slices, then cut those into 4 - 5 equally wide pieces.

9   Place a 10" - 12" skillet over Medium heat. When hot,
    add your oil or some reserved pork lard. When the
    oil is shimmering, lay your pork belly pieces in the
    pan and cook for 4 - 5 min per side. Make sure the
    meat is browned on both sides and thoroughly
    heated through.

10 Remove from pan and place on a paper towel to
    soak up excess grease. Serve Hot.

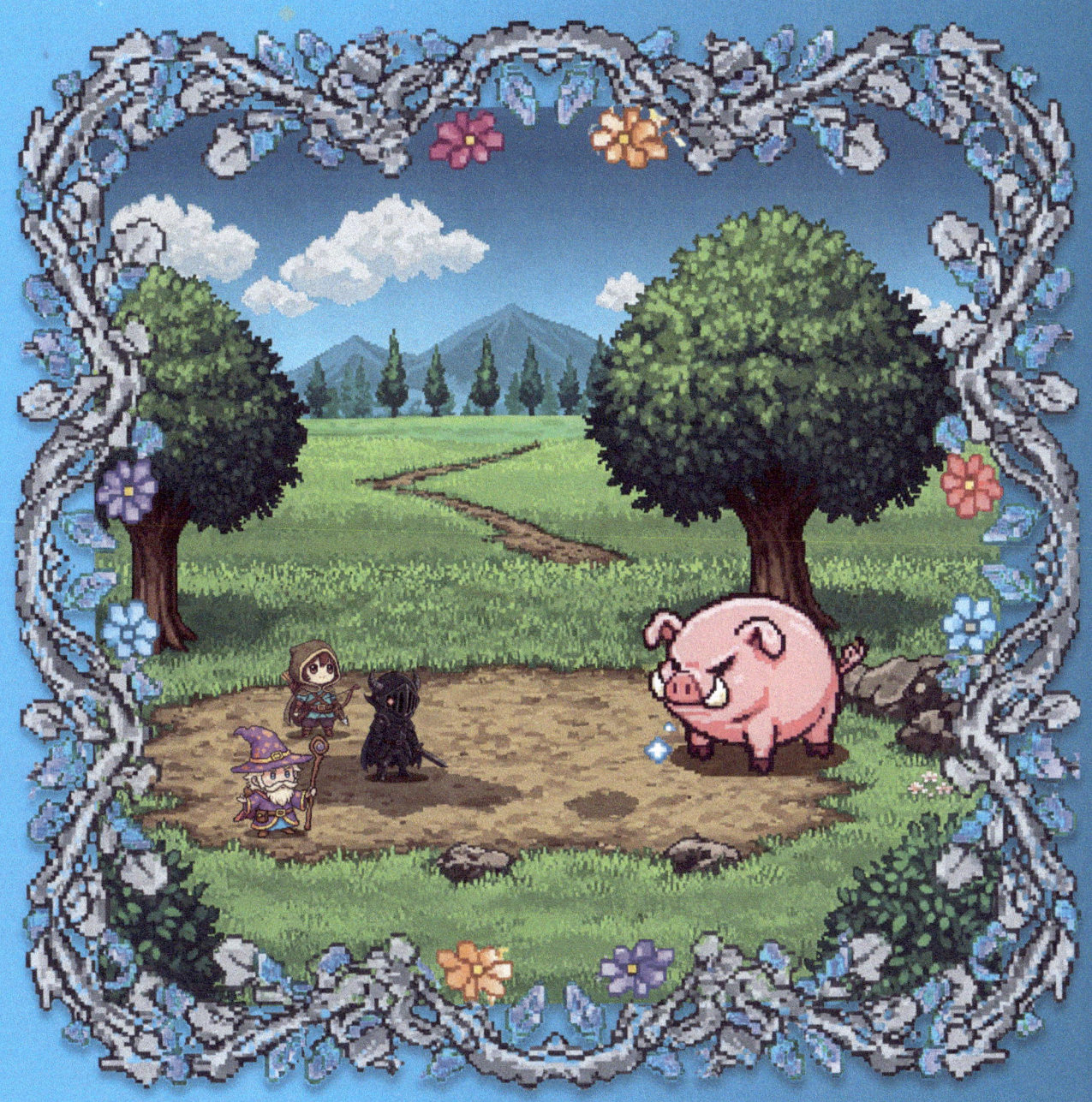

Fall Off The Bone Ribs

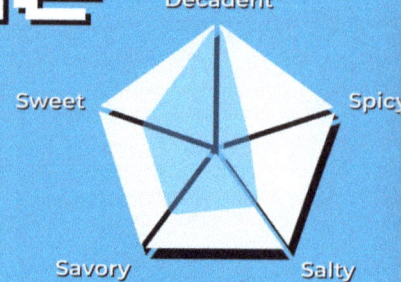

Decadent

Sweet

Spicy

Savory

Salty

I give full credit to my Uncle Jim for teaching me this simple method of making ribs long ago. They are always tender and have trouble staying on the bones. They make for a delightful meal any time of the year, but you can choose to alter the recipe slightly during the grilling season. No matter how you decide to cook them, these ribs won't disappoint.

Ingredients

Full Rack of Pork Ribs (Baby Backs)	1 ea
Cumin	½ tsp
Cinnamon	⅛ tsp
Coriander, Ground	¼ tsp
Black Pepper, Ground	¼ tsp
Salt	⅛ tsp
White Sugar	¼ tsp
Paprika	½ tsp
Oregano, Dry	¼ tsp
Chili Powder	½ tsp
Sweet Heat BBQ Sauce (Pg 251)	¾ C

Prep Time
5 Min

Cook Time
3 Hr

Servings
3 - 4 Portions

Recipe Tip

Try them grilled! Reduce the second cooking time by 30-45 min. Remove from the oven and let rest for 5 min. Then grill them over hot coals for 5 min. per side, brushing generously with BBQ sauce throughout.

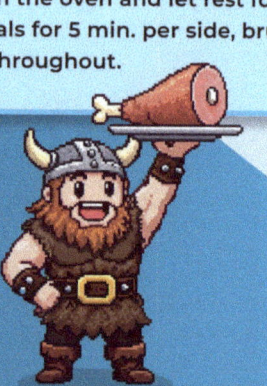

Cooking Directions

1   Preheat oven to 500. Mix all herbs and spices together in a small bowl. Cut the rack of ribs in half. Rub the spice mix into the rib halves, covering as much as you can. Wrap the rib halves in tin foil securely so no leakage occurs. Double wrap if needed.

2   Place the ribs on a lined baking tray and place in oven once preheated. Roast for 15 min.

3   Lower the oven heat to 285 (300 if not using a digital oven)

4   Bake for 2 hr. 45 min. Do not open oven door.

5   Remove tray from oven. Let ribs rest for 5 min. Set broiler to High and move the rack so it is 6" - 8" from the broiler.

6   Carefully remove the foil, exposing the top of the ribs. Broil the ribs for 5 min. to help form a char. Remove from oven, brush the ribs generously with BBQ sauce, then broil for 1 - 2 min. more to form a glaze.

7   Remove from oven and brush with any excess BBQ sauce. Serve Hot.

Italian Meatballs

Everybody enjoys a good plate of spaghetti and meatballs, and this recipe will hit that mark dead on. If you prefer larger balls than what this recipe makes, I advise forming them by hand. I use a 1 ½ Tbsp. scoop because that's the most commonly available size in stores. If you do make them larger, keep in mind they may take a bit more time to cook, so keep your thermometer at hand. Pairing these with your homemade Rustic Pomodoro (see Pg 151) makes a classic pasta dish that no one can resist.

Ingredients

Ground Beef, 85/15	½ Lb
Ground Pork	½ Lb
Scallion, Diced	1 ea
Yellow Onion, Diced	¼ C
Parsley Leaves, Fresh	¼ C
Garlic, Minced	1 tsp
Basil, Dry	½ tsp
Oregano, Dry	¼ tsp
Parmesan Cheese, Grated	2 Tbsp
Salt	½ tsp
Black Pepper, Ground	¼ tsp
Water	¼ C
Plain Bread Crumbs	⅓ C
Large Egg	1 ea

 Prep Time 30 Min

 Cook Time 15 - 20 Min

 Servings 20 Balls

 1½ Tablespoon Scoop 1 ea

 Stand Mixer 1 ea (Not Required)

 Food Processor 1 ea

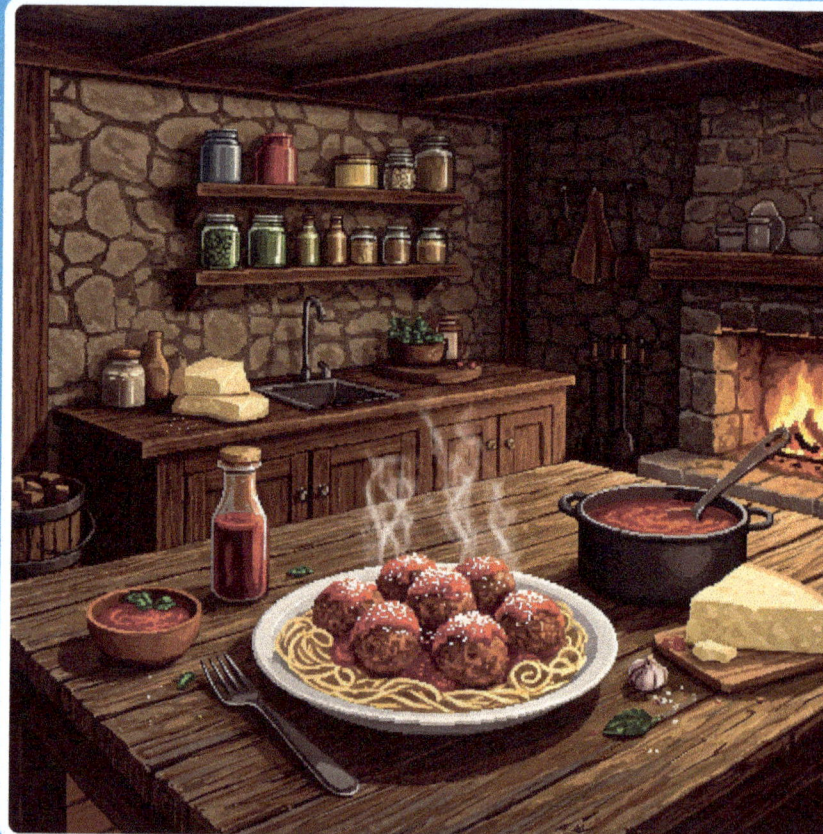

Cooking Directions

1   Preheat the oven to 350 and make sure a rack is in the center of the oven.

2   Place the scallion, onion, garlic, herbs, salt, and pepper in a food processor. Blend until thoroughly minced, almost a paste with no large chunks. If you don't have a food processor, make sure to mince all ingredients as finely as possible. Place both meats in a large bowl, and pour the onion slurry/transfer the finely cut ingredients into the bowl. Use the water to rinse out the processor and get the small bits left behind, and pour that in too.

3   Add the parmesan, egg, and bread crumbs, and mix with your hand or a wooden spoon to combine thoroughly. If using a stand mixer, mix on the first or second setting to thoroughly combine all ingredients. Mix until the meat feels smooth and slightly fluffy.

4   Line a baking tray with parchment paper. Using a 1½ Tbsp. scoop, or your hands, form the meat into golf ball sized balls and place on the tray. Don't keep the balls separate, having them touching will help them all cook evenly and stay moist. I advise placing them into rows of 4, starting in the center of the pan and then alternating which side you place the balls on, making 5 columns total.

5   Once all the meat has been transferred to the lined tray, place in oven and bake for 10 min. Then rotate the tray and bake for 8 - 10 min. more, checking the temperature with a thermometer after 8 min. Once the meatballs have reached an internal temperature of 155 remove them from the oven and let rest for 5 minutes before use/eating.

Kefta Kebabs

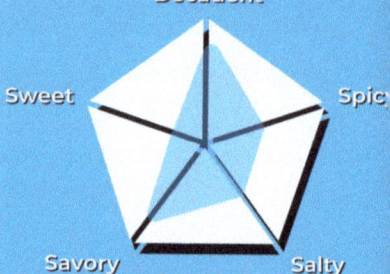

This traditional Middle Eastern dish is delicious served up as a sandwich wrapped in pita with vegetables and hummus or tzatziki, or as its own entree on a plate with baba ganoush, tabbouleh, grilled vegetables, or rice. It's fairly versatile, and it can be cooked in large batches and held in the fridge for up to 3 days as a quick lunch option, or a healthy snack.

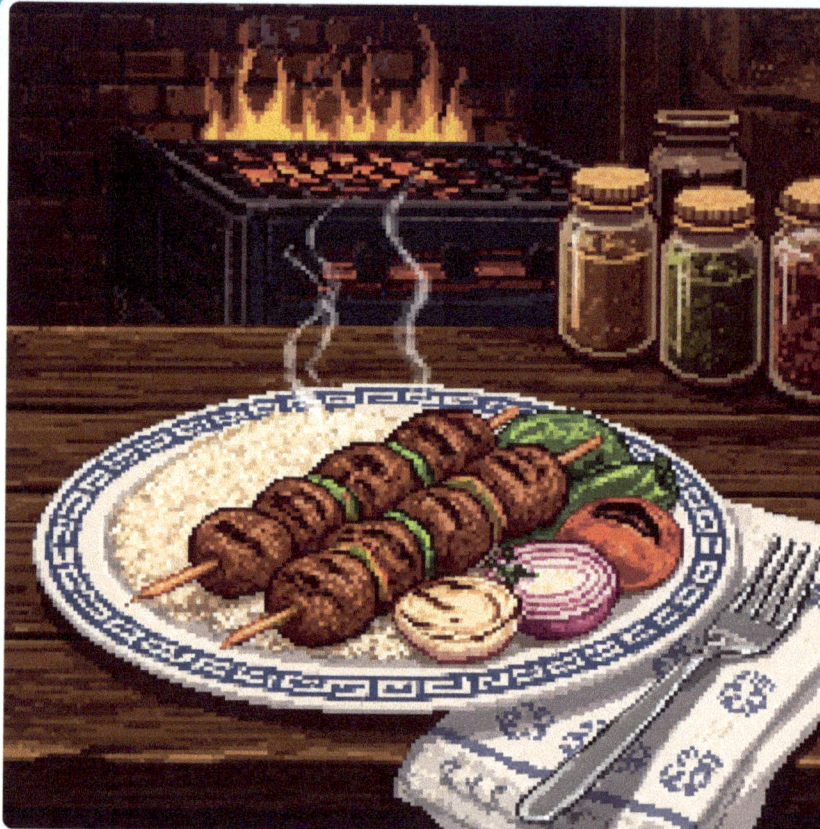

Ingredients

Ground Beef Or Lamb	2 Lb
Cumin	1 Tbsp
Coriander, Ground	2 Tbsp
Black Pepper, Ground	½ tsp
Cinnamon	2 tsp
Ginger, Ground	1 tsp
Cayenne	½ tsp
Parsley, Fresh, Finely Minced	6 Tbsp
Garlic, Minced	2 tsp
White Onion, Finely Minced	⅓ C
Salt	2 tsp

Prep Time
10 Min

Cook Time
7 - 10 Min

Servings
8 Pieces
4 oz ea

APPRENTICE

Cooking Directions (Broiling)

1 In a large bowl, combine the meat, onion, parsley, and seasonings. Mix by hand until smooth and well incorporated.

2 Set broiler on High and move an oven rack 6" - 8" from broiler. Form the mixture into balls weighing 4 oz. each, roughly 2" in diameter.

3 Flatten balls to 1½" thickness and place on a lined/greased baking pan.

4 Broil for 3 - 4 min. per side until internal temperature reaches 155.

Cooking Directions (Grilling)

1 Follow the above directions through step 2.

2 Spear 2 balls onto one skewer. Form the balls to keep the meat close to the skewer, long not wide.

3 Grill over Medium High coals (400 for a gas grill) for 3 - 4 min. per side, until internal temperature reaches 155.

Roast Beef Debris Po' Boys

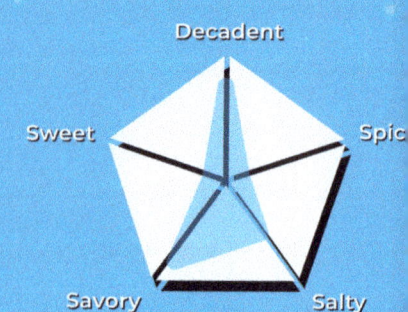

Decadent

Sweet

Spic

Savory

Salty

This recipe can be made up to 2 days in advance and held in the fridge. Just make sure you retain some of the braising liquid with the shredded beef to make sure it doesn't dry out. Also, I give instructions for making the beef on the stove or in the oven, but a crock pot works excellent for this recipe. Just place all braising ingredients in the crock, set to Low, cover, and cook for 6 hours. Simplicity.

Ingredients

Boneless Chuck Roast	1¾ - 2 lb
Beef Stock	24 Fl Oz
White Onion, Large Dice	½ C
Garlic, Minced	2 tsp
Worcestershire Sauce	2 tsp
Rosemary, Dry	1 tsp
Sage, Ground	½ tsp
Thyme, Dry	1 tsp
Oil	2 Tbsp
Loaf Of French Bread (Pg 371)	1 ea
Tomato Slices	8 - 12 ea
Lettuce, Chiffonade	2 C
Mayo (Pg 145)	¼ C
¼ of a White Onion, Thin Julienne	
Salt & Pepper for Seasoning Beef	

Prep Time
15 Min

Cook Time
3 Hr 15 Min

Servings
4 Sandwiches

Cooking Directions

1   Preheat oven to 350. Place an oven safe pot (with lid)
    just large enough to fit the roast in over Medium High
    heat. When hot, add oil.

2   Sprinkle the beef generously with salt and pepper on
    both sides. When the oil is shimmering, place the roast
    in the pot and sear for 2 - 3 min. per side.

3   Remove the roast from the pot and reduce the heat to
    Medium. Put the diced onion in the pot and cook for 2 min.
    stirring often. Add the garlic and cook for 30 seconds more.

4   Add 4 oz. of the stock to the pot and scrape up all the
    browned bits stuck to the bottom of the pot (the fond).
    Add the Worcestershire and the herbs, stirring well.

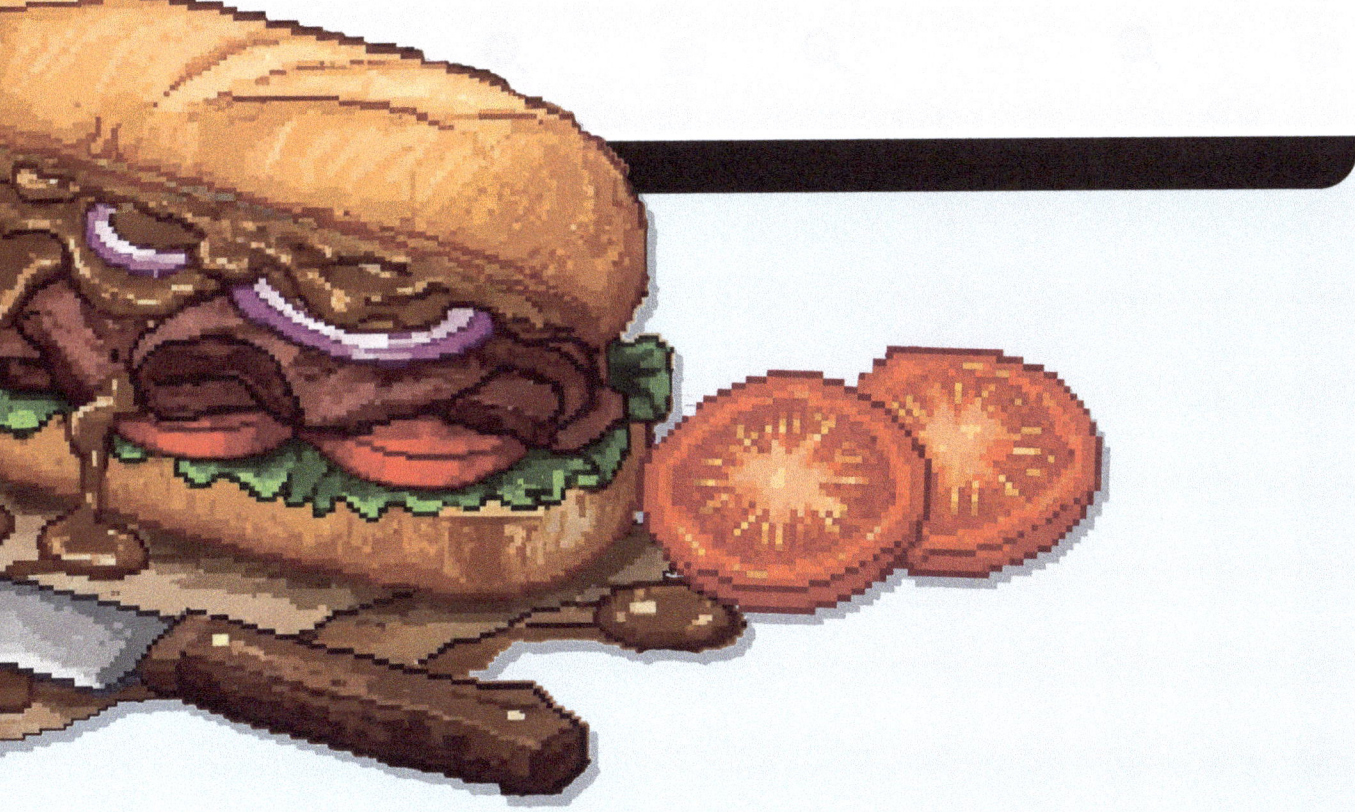

>>>> CONTINUED >>>>

5   Return the roast to the pot and add the remaining stock, enough so that the roast is between ½ and ¾ of the way submerged. Cover the pot tightly with foil before placing the lid on the pot. Bring the liquid inside to a simmer.

6   Turn off the heat and transfer to the oven. Cook for 2½ - 3 hr. until the meat can be pulled apart with a spoon. If you don't have an oven safe pot, just cover the pot with foil before placing the lid on, and once the liquid is simmering reduce the heat to Low and cook for the same amount of time.

7   Once the meat is tender enough, remove from the pot and place in a large bowl or dish. Using two forks, pull the meat apart, coarsely shredding it. Make sure there are no very large chunks of un-shredded beef. Return the beef to the pot with the braising liquid and cover, holding over Low until needed.

8   Cut your large loaf of French bread into 4 even pieces. Next, slice each piece in half long ways. Spread mayo on the 'top' piece of your bread. Using some tongs or a slotted spoon, remove roughly 6 - 8 oz. of meat from the pot and place evenly on the 'bottom' piece of bread, sprinkling with salt and pepper. On top of the beef lay down some onion slices, then your preferred number of tomato slices, then some shredded lettuce, then your top piece. If desired, spoon a small amount of the braising liquid over the beef when you put it on the sandwich.

9   Try not to eat the sandwich too fast!

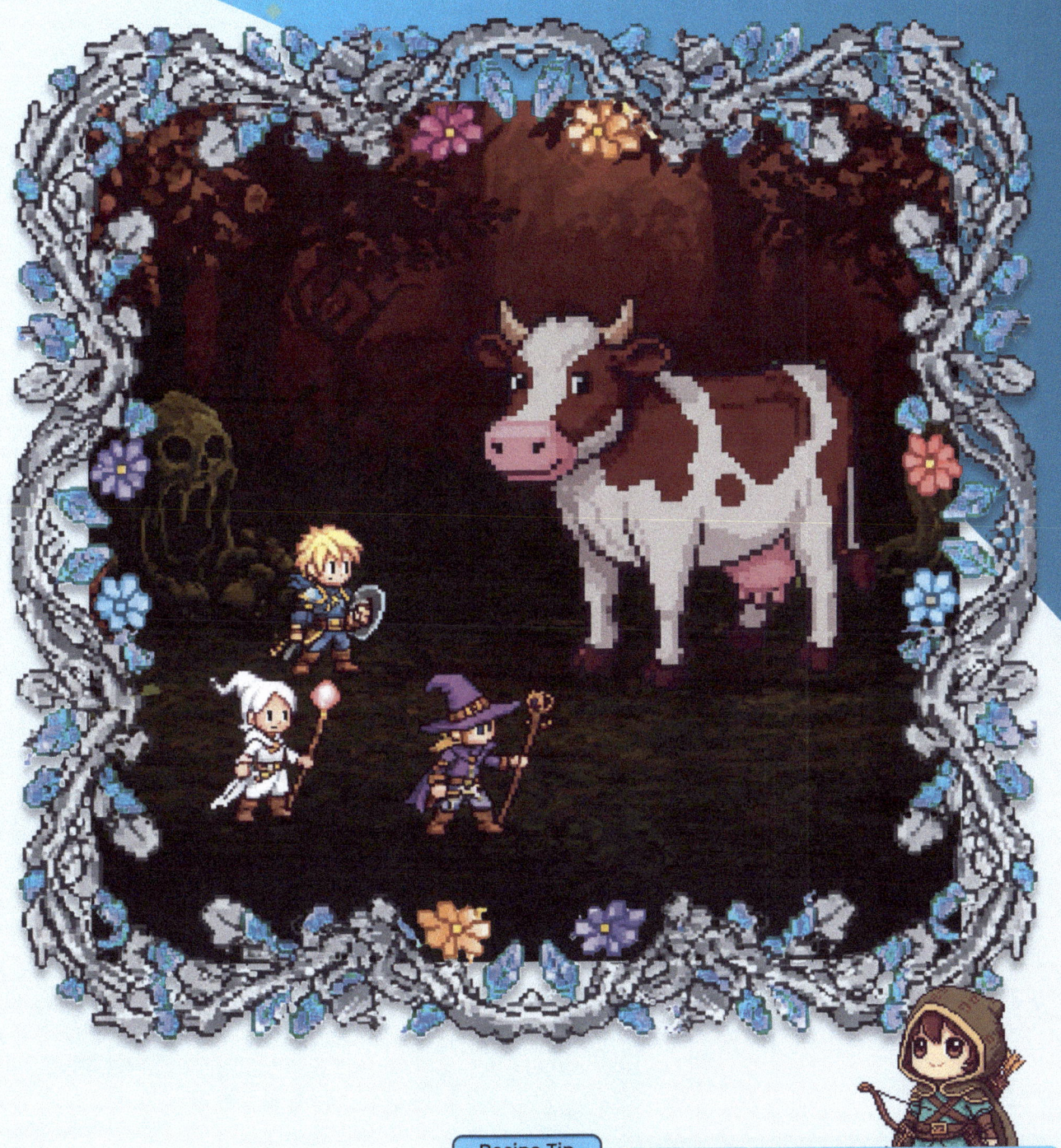

Recipe Tip

When choosing the bread for this recipe, if not making your own at home (see Pg 371), get one from the bakery that has a light and flaky crust, and a soft and airy inside. The right bread is essential for the enjoyment of this sandwich, so take it seriously. ▼

Roast Chicken with "Pan" Gravy

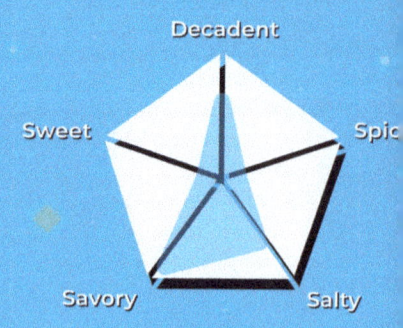

Decadent

Sweet

Spic

Savory

Salty

Roasting a whole chicken is Culinary Arts 101, and seems more difficult than it is. Don't be intimidated by the length of this recipe, or the prospect of trussing and carving up a chicken. The process is simple, and I'm confident you'll find it intuitive once you get started. As with all recipes, read it through at least twice to familiarize yourself with the steps, and visualize yourself performing them as you read.

The gravy recipe calls for using the drippings from the chicken and vegetables for the fat of the roux. Straining the vegetables in a colander over a bowl allows you to collect the drippings, measure out only what you need, and save the remainder for later use.

Ingredients (Chicken)

3 Lb Whole Chicken, Giblets Removed	1 ea
Carrots, 1" Rounds	2 ea
Celery Stalks, 1" Slices	2 ea
Yellow Onion, Lg. Dice	1 ea
Whole Garlic Cloves	4 ea
Rosemary Sprigs, Fresh	2 ea
Thyme Sprigs, Fresh	4 ea
Sage Leaves, Fresh	6 ea
Lemon Wedges	2 ea
Butter, Room Temp	2 Tbsp
Salt, Pepper, & Paprika (For Seasoning)	

Ingredients (Gravy)

Chicken Stock/Broth	16 Fl Oz
Garlic, Minced	1 tsp
Sage, Ground	⅛ tsp
Thyme, Dry	⅛ tsp
Salt	¼ tsp
Black Pepper, Ground	⅛ tsp
AP Flour	5 Tbsp
Drippings From Pan	6 Tbsp

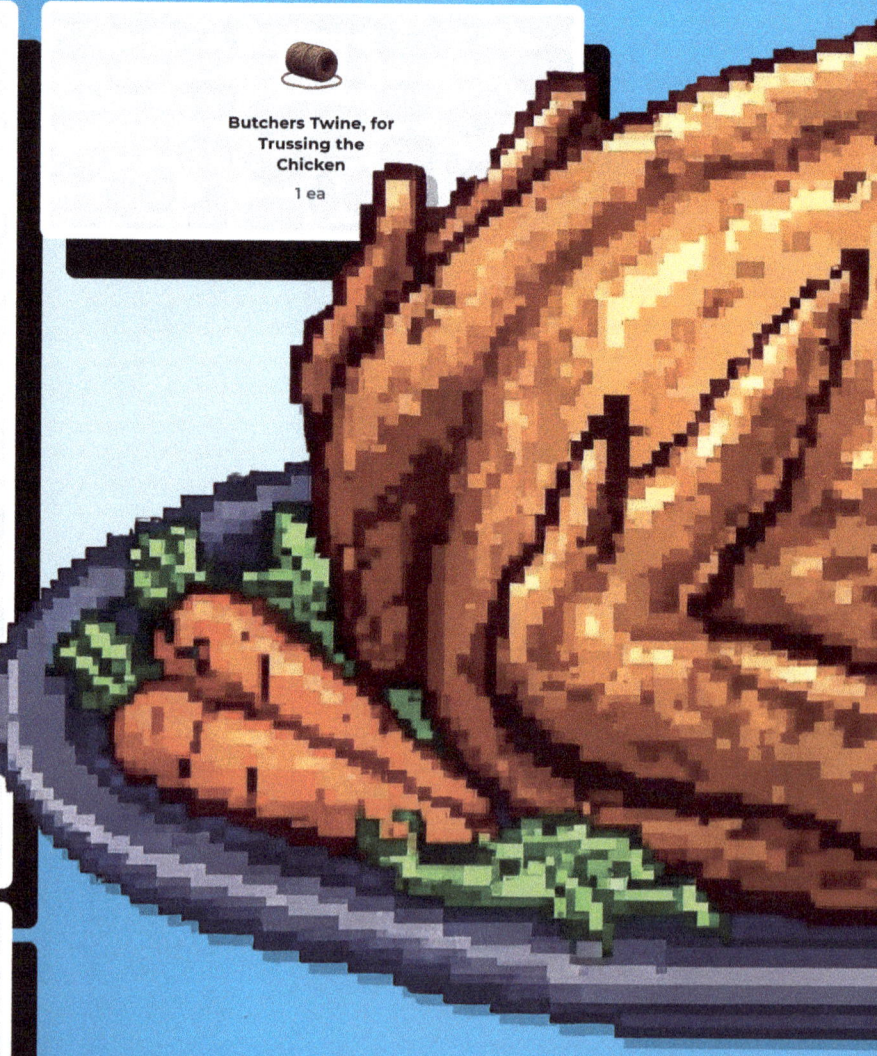

Butchers Twine, for Trussing the Chicken

1 ea

 Prep Time 20 Min

 Cook Time 1½ - 2 Hr

 Servings 1 Chicken 16 oz Gravy

Cooking Directions

1   Preheat your oven to 375.

2   Place the cut vegetables in a 9" x 13" roasting pan, mixing them up and spreading them out evenly. Take the fresh herbs, lemon wedges, and garlic cloves and pack them into the cavity of the chicken.

3   Pat the skin of the bird dry with paper towels. Truss the chicken by first tucking the wing tips back and under the wings. Then, holding the twine out with both hands wrap the twine around the ends of the legs twice and pull to bring them together. Form an 'X' with the twine and bring each end down over the thighs and under the chicken, crossing each end over to the other side to form another 'X' underneath. Then, bring the twine around the sides of the bird, over the wings, and meet them in the middle of the front of the chicken, where it's neck used to be. Gently pull the twine so the wings are held in place and knot together with a simple double knot. Trim off excess twine and make sure that the wings are tucked securely under the twine. This step, while not necessary, does help ensure an even cook for the whole chicken in the oven.

4   Use your fingers to gently pull the skin away from, but not tearing off, the chicken breast meat. Smear a small amount of butter under the skin of each breast, covering as much of the area as possible. Using your hands, smear the remaining butter all over the skin of the chicken. Sprinkle generously with salt, pepper, and paprika.

>>>> CONTINUED >>>>

5   Place the chicken on top of the cut vegetables and roast for 20 - 25 min. per pound. In this case, roast for 1 hr. to 1 hr. and 15 min. Make sure to check the temperature in both the inner thigh and the fattest part of the breast, ensuring the chicken has reached 165 internal temperature completely before removing from the oven.

6   When done cooking, carefully transfer the chicken to a cutting board to rest for 10 - 15 min. While the chicken is resting, strain the vegetables from the bottom of the pan over a large bowl.

7   Place a 1 Qt. pot over Medium Low heat. Measure out 6 Tbsp. of the pan drippings and place it in the pot. When hot, add the garlic and cook for 30 seconds. Add your flour and dry herbs. Stirring constantly, cook for 4 - 5 min. This will bring the roux to the Blond level. Add 4 oz. of the stock to the pot and stir well, working out any lumps in the roux.

8   Add the remaining stock and scrape up any stuck on bits (the fond) from the bottom of the pot. Whisk well until the roux is fully incorporated and bring to a simmer. Cook for 2 - 3 min. until it is thickened to coat that back of a spoon (nappe). Cover and reduce heat to Low.

9   By now your chicken should have rested for around 10 min. Hold your gravy over Low heat to let it rest for 5 min. more, then proceed to breaking the bird down.

> > > > CONTINUED > > > >

10   Using a sharp knife, cut the twine off and discard. First, cut through the skin connecting the thighs to the body. Pulling the thigh down, you'll see where the thigh bone joints into the hip. Pull the thigh away from the body so you can see the joint clearly. Pressing hard, cut through the cartilage of the joint. Repeat with the other thigh. If you like, you can also separate the leg from the thigh by laying it skin side down and looking for a tell-tale dark line between the leg and thigh. This line marks where the leg and thigh bones connect, and cutting down through it will reveal the joint, allowing you to cut through easily.

11   Next, gently pull a wing away from the breast until you can see the joint connecting the whole wing to the chest. Cut through the cartilage of the joint. Repeat for the other wing.

12   Finally, draw your knife down the center of the breast to reveal the thick cartilage plate in the middle of the two breasts. Making careful incisions, cut down the side of breast plate so that the breast comes away. Moving down, gently pull the breast away from the ribs, cutting through the meat as you do. When you reach the point where the back of the chicken begins, cut straight down to remove the breast from the carcass. Repeat with the other side.

13   Place your desired piece of chicken on a plate, and stir the gravy gently before spooning a generous helping onto the chicken and your plate. Serve Hot.

Roasted Buffalo Wings

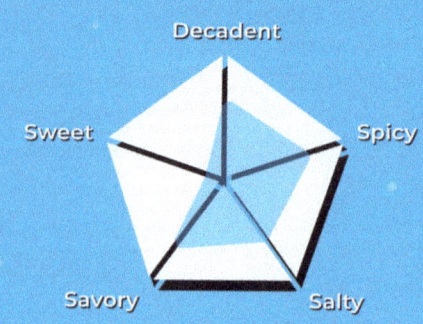

This recipe is not only much healthier than frying your chicken wings, it also has much less clean up. Steaming the wings first allows for the fat in the skin to melt out, and ensures your chicken stays tender and moist when roasting. Cooling them in the fridge for at least 1 hr. is also essential; this allows the chicken skin to dry out and guarantees a crispy wing.

Buffalo sauce is the traditional topping, but the options are nearly limitless. Try them tossed in Teriyaki (see Pg 253), hot olive oil and garlic with liberal amounts of parmesan cheese, or some Sweet Heat BBQ sauce (see Pg 251). Serve with crudité and dip it all in your own ranch or bleu cheese dressings (see Pgs 142, 131) for a delicious, completely homemade appetizer or entree.

A colander made to go into a pot for steaming vegetables is not hard to find, nor does it cost much. When selecting one, metal is the preferred substance. There are also large pots sold with colander inserts made to fit inside of them, and these work the best for this sort of recipe.

Ingredients

Whole Chicken Wings	8 ea
Butter	2 Tbsp
Hot Sauce	¼ C
Garlic, Minced	¼ tsp
Water for Steaming the Chicken	
A Pinch Each of Salt & Black Pepper	

  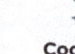

Prep Time
20 Min

Cook Time
35 - 40 Min

Servings
16 Wings

Large Pot w/Lid & Colander Insert

1 ea

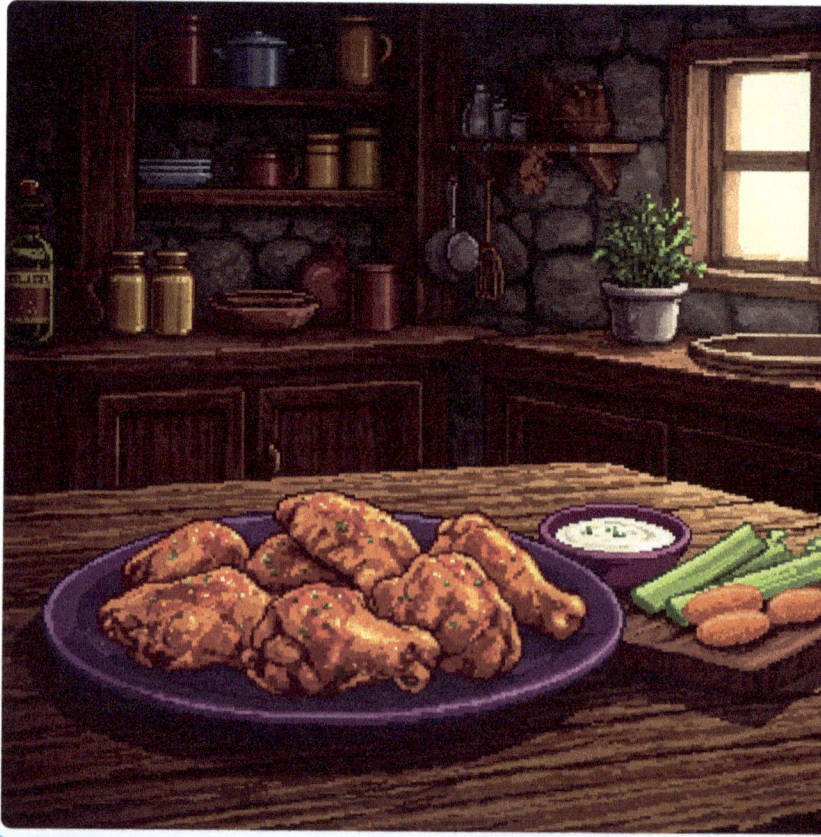

Cooking Directions

1   Using a sharp knife, separate the wingettes from the drumettes by cutting through the joint connecting them. Remove the wing tips as well (freeze these for stock!). Let rest on the counter during the next steps.

2   Place your heat safe colander/colander insert into the pot and fill it with water so that the level is about 1" - 1½" from the base of the colander.

3   Place over High heat and bring the water to a boil. When the water is boiling, place the chicken pieces on the colander in such a way that they are close, but not overcrowded. Work in batches if needed. Cover, reduce the heat so it maintains the simmer (Medium High), and steam the chicken for 10 min. They are done when you see bubbles appearing on and under the skin. Make sure that your water doesn't all evaporate.

4   Line a baking sheet with tin foil and then paper towels. Carefully remove the chicken from the pot with a pair of tongs and place on the paper towels. Discard the water. Transfer chicken to the fridge and let rest, uncovered, for 1 hr.

5   Preheat your oven to 425 and make sure there is a rack in the center of the oven.

>>>> CONTINUED >>>>

6 Take the chicken out of the fridge. Remove the paper towels, spray the foil with non-stick cooking spray, and place the chicken on the foil, skin side down. If available, spray a wire rack that fits in the pan with cooking spray (over the sink) and place the chicken on that, skin side down.

7 When oven is hot, place chicken in oven and roast for 20 min. Flip the chicken pieces over and roast for 15 - 20 more min. They're done when the skin is crispy and well browned. Remove from the oven and let rest for 2 - 3 min.

8 While the chicken is roasting, place a small pot over Medium heat. When hot, add the butter. When the butter is melted and stops bubbling, add your garlic and cook for 1 min. until fragrant. Add the hot sauce, salt, and pepper. Stir well to combine all ingredients. Remove from heat and leave uncovered.

9 When the chicken is done cooking and has rested, transfer it to a bowl large enough to toss them easily. Pour your hot sauce over the chicken and toss/stir to coat them evenly. Serve Hot.

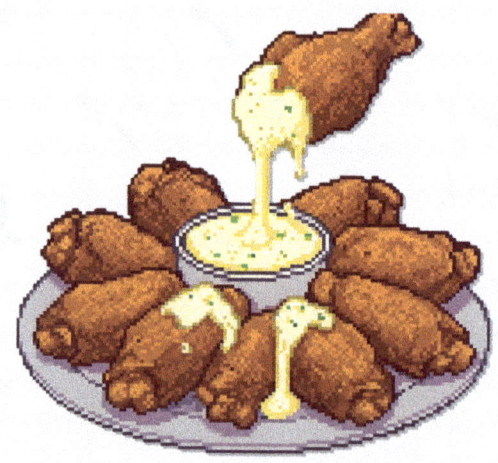

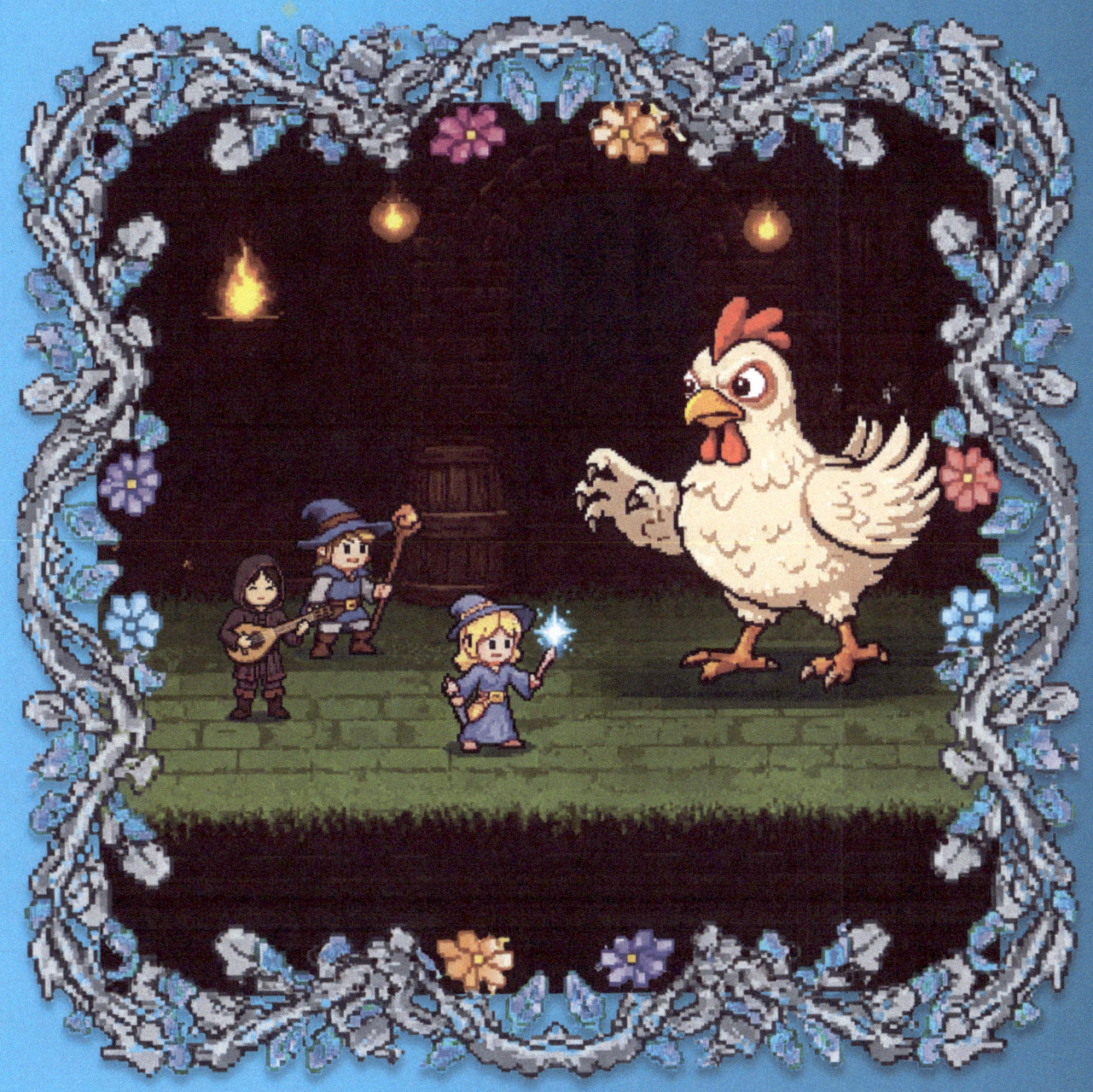

Skillet Pan Pizza

Almost everyone loves pan pizza, and this recipe allows you to make your very own at home for much less money than take out. I've given a recipe for a simple cheese pizza, but of course the fun with pizza is the toppings! Just be sure to slice any vegetables you want on the pizza thinly to make sure it doesn't get soggy, and fully cook ingredients like sausage or chicken before putting them on the pizza. Get creative, and have fun with it!

Decadent

Sweet · Spic[y]

Savory · Salty

Ingredients

Pizza Dough (Homemade/ Store Bought)	1 Lb
Passata (Or Plain Tomato Sauce)	¾ C
Shredded Mozzarella	12 oz
Garlic, Minced	1 tsp
Oregano, Dry	½ tsp
Basil, Dry	¼ tsp
Olive Oil	3 Tbsp
Cooking Spray For Pan	

Prep Time
5 - 15 Min

Cook Time
10 - 15 Min

Servings
2 - 4 People

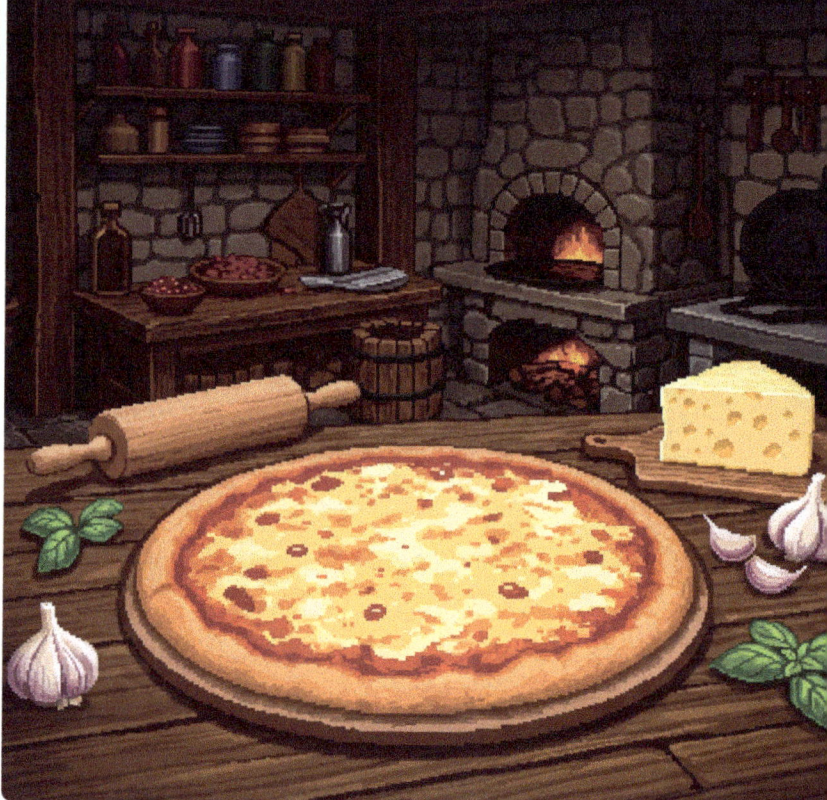

Recipe Tip

While mozzarella & provolone is the traditional blend for pizza, any cheese that gets stringy when melted will work well. Cheddar and Mozzarella works great for a BBQ pizza, Monterey and Pepper Jack is a great combo for a taco pizza. Get creative and have fun!

Cooking Directions

1   Preheat the oven to 425. Make sure an oven rack is in the center of the oven.

2   In a bowl, combine passata, garlic, and herbs to make the sauce. Stir well and set aside.

3   Coat a 12" - 14" oven safe skillet (large enough to fit the pizza round) in lard or cooking spray. If necessary, roll out the dough and form into 12" - 14" round.

4   Put ½ of the olive oil in the middle of the skillet. Press the dough gently to fully cover the surface of the pan. Brush the dough with the remaining olive oil, then top evenly with the sauce.

5   Cover generously with cheese.

6   Place the skillet over Medium High heat. Cook for about 3 minutes to preheat the pan and the dough. When you start to hear sizzling, remove the pan from heat.

7   Transfer the pan to the middle rack of the oven. Cook for 10 - 12 min. Until the cheese is bubbling and the crust is golden-brown.

8   Remove from oven and use a heat safe rubber spatula to make sure no part of the pizza is stuck to the pan.

9   Once you've made sure no part of the pizza is sticking to the pan, it should slide freely if you shake the pan a little. This will allow you to carefully slide the pizza out of the pan and onto a cutting board. Let rest for 3 - 5 min. before cutting.

Southwest Black Bean Burgers

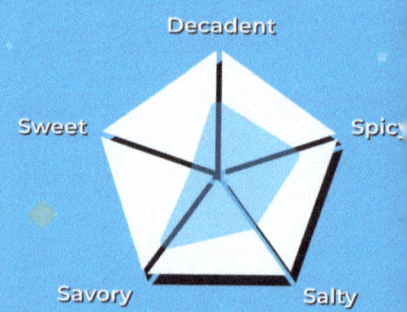

Decadent

Sweet

Spicy

Savory

Salty

These burgers are an excellent replacement for beef patties, and are much cheaper than buying premade black bean burgers from the store. They are simple to make, and freeze well once cooked. Simply double the recipe and cook the patties as instructed. Place the patties you want to freeze on a lined baking sheet in the freezer and let rest for 2-3 hrs until frozen solid. Then transfer them to a freezer bag and hold them for up to 3 months. When reheating, bake at 350 for about 25 min. flipping halfway through.

Using homemade Garlic Aioli is my preferred topping for these burgers, but like with all burgers, the toppings are limitless. So long as you keep the consistency and texture of your toppings and condiments in mind when layering them in the sandwich, you can put almost anything you want on them.

Ingredients

Black beans, Fully Cooked (Or Canned)	2 C
Red Bell Pepper, Diced	¾ C
White Onion, Diced	¾ C
Garlic, Minced	1 ½ tsp
Large Egg	1 ea
Chili Powder	1 Tbsp
Cumin	1 Tbsp
Paprika	1 tsp
Cinnamon	¼ tsp
Hot Sauce	1 tsp
Salt	¼ tsp
Black Pepper, Ground	⅛ tsp
Bread Crumbs, Panko, Plain	½ C
Buns	4 ea
Garlic Aioli (Pg 133)	¼ C
Tomato Slices	4 - 8 ea
Lettuce, Torn Into 1" Pcs	1 C
Neutral Oil, Divided	1 Tbsp

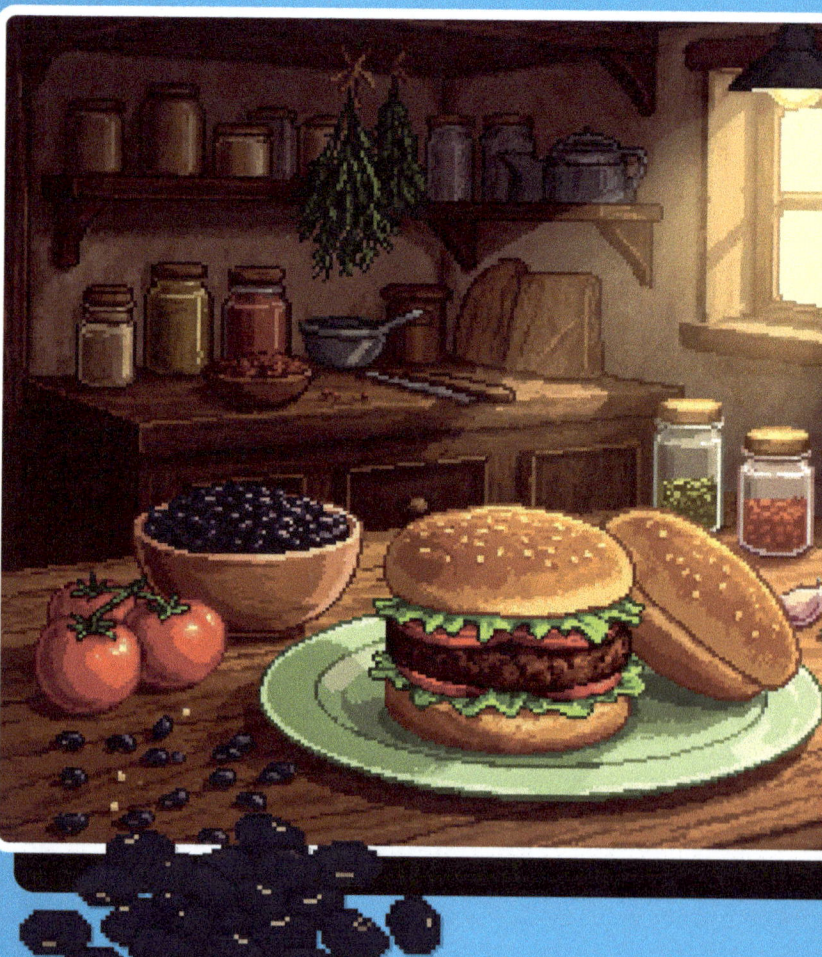

  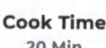

Prep Time	**Cook Time**	**Servings**
15 Min	20 Min	4 Burgers

Food Processor

1 ea

Cooking Directions

1. Place the black beans in a large bowl and mash with a fork or potato masher until pasted, with small chunks of black bean still visible. Place a 10" - 12" skillet over Medium High heat. When hot, add ½ Tbsp. of oil.

2. When the oil is shimmering, add ½ cup of the bell peppers, the onion, garlic, and seasonings in the pan. Cook for 3 - 4 min. until the vegetables are soft. Transfer the vegetable mix to a food processor. Blend until finely chopped, but not a slurry or paste. If you don't have a food processor, mince the vegetables as finely as possible. Transfer to the bowl with the beans and fold to combine.

3. Place your hot sauce and the egg in a separate bowl and mix together until the egg is completely mixed together.

4. Transfer the egg mixture to the bowl with the bean mix and fold to combine. Add the bread crumbs and mix until well combined and the mixture becomes tacky and holds together.

5. Form the mix into 4 even sized patties, roughly ½" thickness. Set aside on a plate or baking tray lined with parchment paper.

   If Grilling: Grill over High heat (450 - 500 for a gas grill) for 6 - 8 min. per side or until the patties are 145 internal temperature.

   If Pan Searing: Place a large skillet over Medium High heat. When hot, add the other ½ Tbsp. oil. When the oil is shimmering, place the patties in the pan and cook for 6 - 8 min. per side until they reach an internal temperature of 145.

   If Baking: Preheat your oven to 375 and make sure a rack is in the center of the oven at the start of the recipe. When hot, place the patties on a baking sheet lined with parchment paper and place in oven. Bake for 20 min. flipping halfway through, and make sure they reach an internal temperature of 145.

6. Build your burgers as follows, bottom to top:
   Bottom Bun > Garlic Aioli > Bell Pepper > Black Bean Patty > Lettuce > Garlic Aioli (on top bun) > Top Bun

Dressings & Sauces

All-Purpose Stock Gravy

Decadent

Sweet

Spicy

Savory

Salty

This is a multi-use recipe that's minimalist and basic on purpose. Follow these steps to make any kind of gravy you may want to accompany your dish. Making a Pork roast? Chicken or Pork Stock works great. Cooking up some Fried Chicken? Try using Beef stock for a delightful depth of flavor. Making some Black Bean burgers? Try out Vegetable stock to turn them into open faced sandwiches.

Mother Sauce: Espagnole or Veloute

Ingredients

Stock (Any Variety)	16 Fl Oz
Garlic, minced	1 tsp
Salt	¼ tsp
Black pepper, ground	⅛ tsp
Sage, ground	⅛ tsp
Thyme, dry	⅛ tsp
Butter/Oil	2 Tbsp
AP Flour	2 Tbsp

Prep Time
5 Min

Cook Time
8 - 10 Min

Servings
16 oz

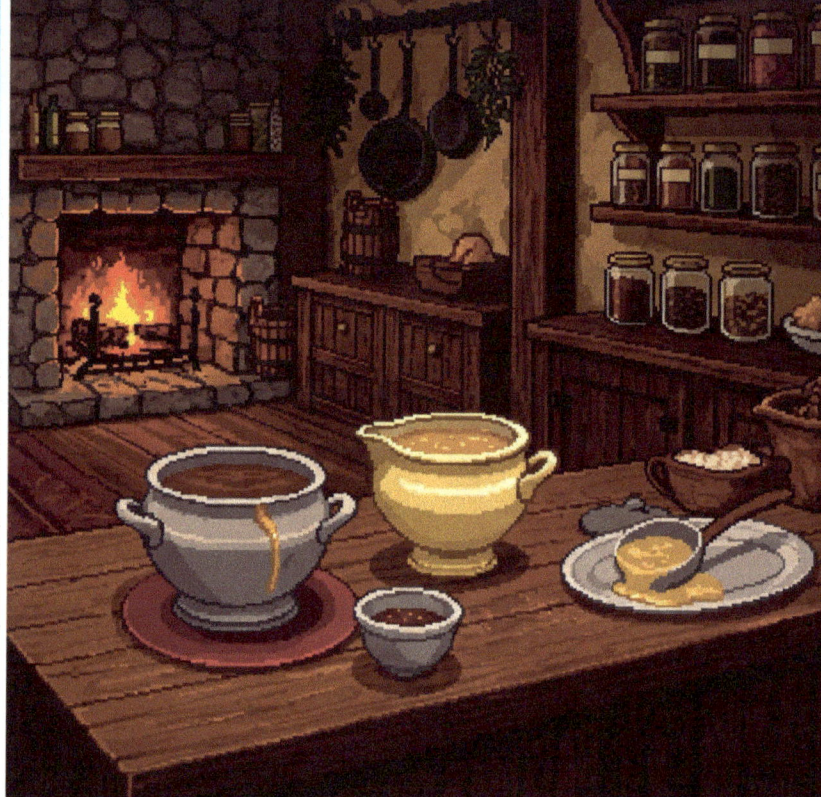

Cooking Directions

1   Place a small pot over Medium heat. When hot, add the butter/oil.

2   When the butter stops bubbling, or the oil starts shimmering, add the garlic. Cook for 1 min.

3   Add the flour and seasonings; mix well. Stirring frequently, cook your roux for 4 - 5 min. This will bring it to the Blond level.

4   Add 4 oz. of the stock and stir well, working out any lumps in the roux. When smooth, add the remaining stock and be sure to scrape up any bits stuck to the bottom of the pot.

5   Bring to a simmer and reduce the heat to Medium-Low. Cook for 2 - 3 min. or until desired consistency is reached.

6   Remove pot from heat and transfer gravy to a heat safe container. Cool completely before covering. Holds in fridge for 5 days. Reheat gently before use.

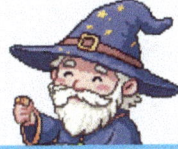

Recipe Tip

The versatility of this recipe is what makes it so special, and you should feel encouraged to play around with it, and develop your own personal gravy preferences.

Bolognese Sauce

This recipe is a staple of Italian cuisine. It's not only a great sauce for spaghetti or linguine, but is also needed to make Lasagna Bolognese or Stuffed Shells Bolognese. The sweetness of the Pomodoro blends well with the unctuous nature of the beef. Get creative and enjoy this recipe to the fullest!

Mother Sauce: Tomato

Ingredients

Ground Beef, 80/20	1 Lb
Salt	½ tsp
Black Pepper, ground	¼ tsp
Garlic Powder	½ tsp
Carrot, minced	2 Tbsp
Yellow Onion, minced	2 Tbsp
Water/Stock	8 Fl Oz
Pomodoro Sauce (Pg 151)	3 C
Butter/Oil	1 Tbsp

   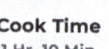

Prep Time
10 Min

Cook Time
1 Hr 10 Min

Servings
32 oz

Decadent

Sweet   Spic

Savory   Salty

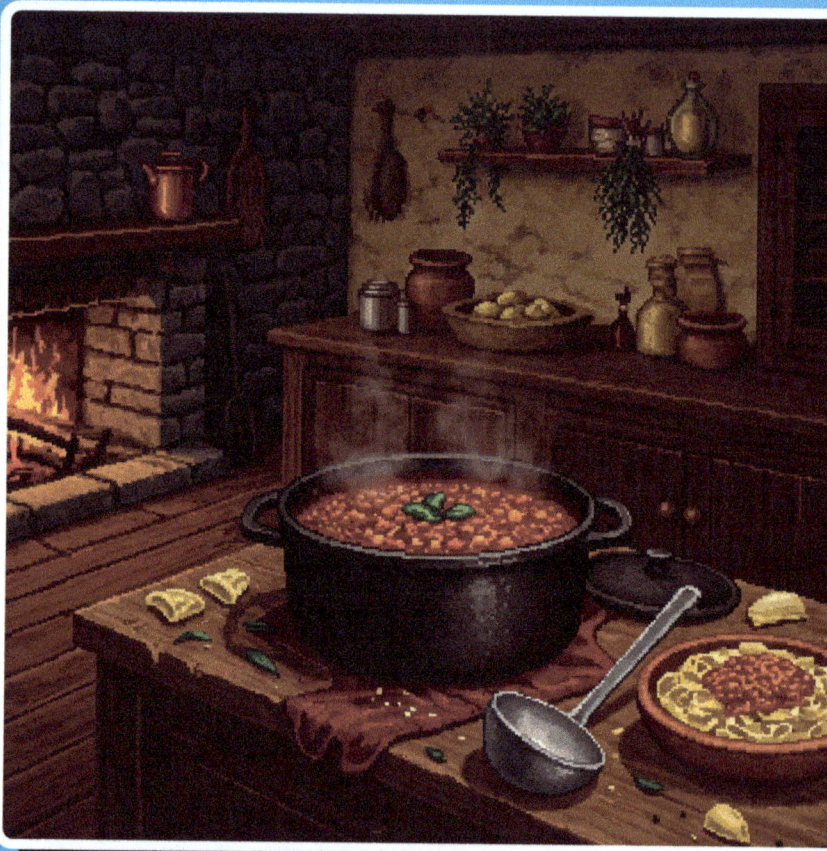

Recipe Tip

Sharp eyed chefs will notice this recipe is just a combination of the 'Fluffy Ground Beef' and 'Rustic Pomodoro Sauce' recipes. Making these two items ahead of time is a great way to prepare yourself for a quick and easy meal when you need it.

Cooking Directions

1   Place a 10" - 12" skillet/pot (with lid) over Medium High heat. When hot, add the butter/oil.

2   When the butter stops bubbling, or the oil starts to shimmer, add the ground beef and break it into large pieces.

3   Add the vegetables, and seasonings. Stir to combine.

4   Pour in the water/stock and cover. Bring to a simmer and reduce heat to Medium Low.

5   Cook, covered, for 1 hour. Add more liquid if needed to prevent it all from evaporating.

6   When done cooking, remove the pan from the heat and uncover. Using a potato masher, break apart the large pieces of meat until they are small and evenly sized.

7   Strain the meat in a colander over a large bowl in the sink. Let drain for 1 - 2 minutes.

8   While the meat is draining, place the Pomodoro in the skillet/pot you cooked the meat with. Place the pan/pot over Medium heat.

9   When simmering, add the beef to the Pomodoro and stir well to combine.

10   Serve Hot with your preferred pasta. Cool completely before placing in an airtight container and moving to th fridge. Will hold for 5 days.

Campagnolo Sauce

Decadent

Sweet

Spicy

Savory

Salty

Campagnolo is Italian for 'farmer' or 'countryman'. In this context it means 'of the countryside'. The use of mushrooms, onions, and peppers brings an earthiness that compliments the spicy sausage well. Either lump sausage or sliced links may be used, choose whichever suits your sense of aesthetics better. If using links, I advise partially cooking them before slicing. Giving the sauce more time to simmer allows the flavors to meld together in a very pleasant way, so it's something to consider.

Mother Sauce: Tomato

Ingredients

Pomodoro Sauce (Pg 151)	3 C
Italian Sausage (Hot)	8 oz
Yellow Bell Pepper, Diced	¼ C
Mushrooms, Quartered	½ C
Yellow Onion, Diced	¼ C
Garlic, Minced	1½ tsp
Oregano, Dry	¼ tsp
Parsley, Dry	½ tsp
Black Pepper, ground	⅛ tsp
Salt	½ tsp
Parmesan Cheese, Grated	2 Tbsp
Olive Oil (Optional)	1 Tbsp

Prep Time
5 Min

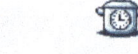
Cook Time
3 Min

Servings
¼ Cup

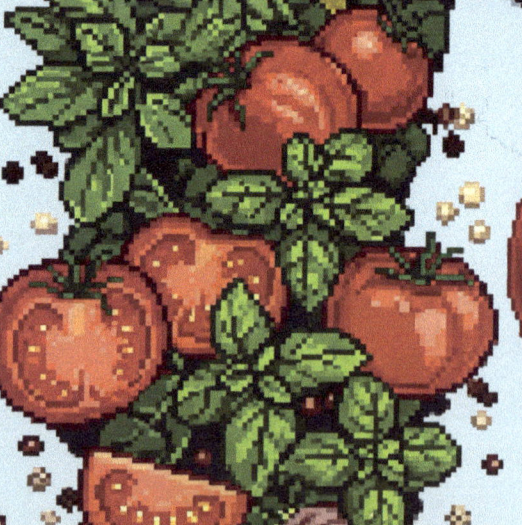

Cooking Directions

1   Using your hands, tear the sausage into 1" pieces and form into solid shapes, or roll them into balls. If using links, slice into ½ - ¾" thick pieces. Set aside.

2   Place a 2 - 3 Qt. pot over Medium-High heat. When hot, put the sausage pieces into the pot and cook for 2 min., stir, and cook for 2 min. more, searing well on two sides. Remove sausage from pot and set aside.

3   If the sausage did not have enough fat to make a layer on the bottom of the pot, add the olive oil and bring to a shimmer. Add the garlic and cook for 1 min.

4   Add the bell peppers and onion. Cook for 2 min. Then, add the mushrooms and cook for 2 min. more. Be sure to scrape up the brown bits (the fond) stuck on the bottom of the pot.

5   Return the sausage to the pot and then add the Pomodoro. Stir well and bring to a simmer.

6   Add the remaining ingredients and stir. Lower the heat to Low and cover. Let the sauce simmer for 10 min. at minimum, up to 1 hour.

7   If not using immediately, place in an airtight container and refrigerate. Holds in fridge for 5 days.

Fra Diavolo Sauce

The name of this dish translates to "Devil's Brother" and the liberal use of red pepper flakes should give you an idea why. I find that using Pomodoro as a base adds an element of sweetness that doesn't work to lessen the heat, but rather, give it balance and almost highlight the heat.

Pairing this sauce with seared shrimp or scallops is the traditional way to use it, but it also works well with chicken. Topping with chopped, fresh basil is a good way to not only make your dish attractive, but it also adds an herby sweetness that further highlights the heat this sauce brings.

Mother Sauce: Tomato

Ingredients

Dry White Wine (Pinot Grigio)	½ C
Pomodoro Sauce (Pg 151)	2 C
Parsley, Dry	½ tsp
Garlic, Minced	2 tsp
Oregano, Dry	½ tsp
Black Pepper, Ground	¼ tsp
Salt	½ tsp
Yellow Onion, Half Moon Slices	½ C
Red Pepper Flakes	1½ tsp
Olive Oil	2 Tbsp

 Prep Time 5 Min

 Cook Time 15 - 20 Min

 Servings 16 oz

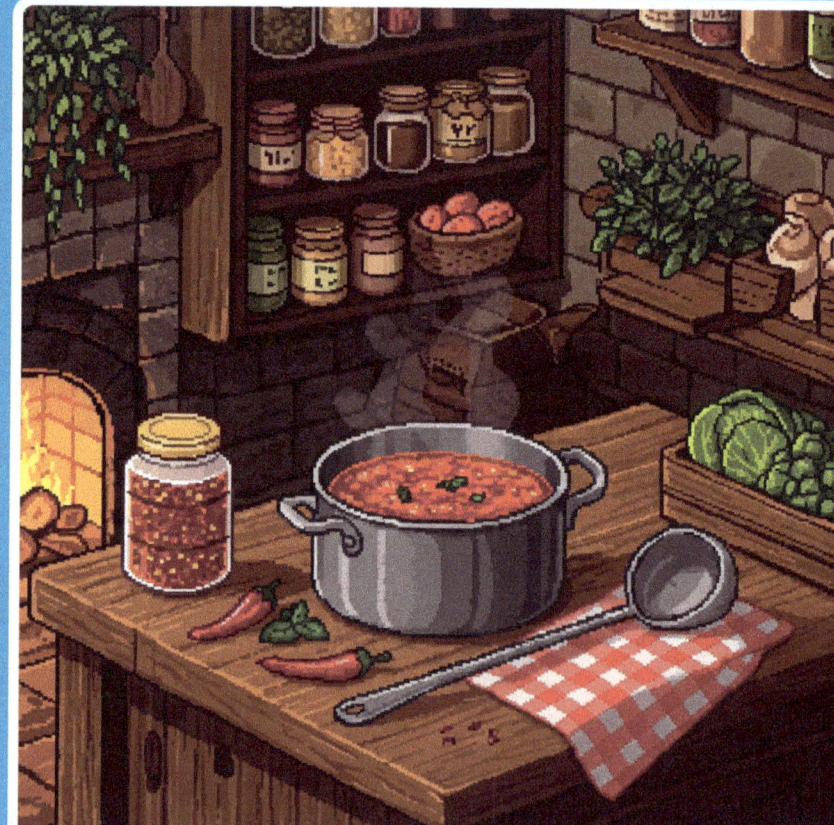

Cooking Directions

1 Place a 10" - 12" skillet over Medium High heat. When hot, add the olive oil.

2 When the oil is shimmering, add the onions and cook for 2 - 3 minutes, until slightly soft.

3 Add the garlic and cook for 1 min. until fragrant.

4 Add the wine and bring to a simmer. Cook for 3 - 4 min. reducing by half.

5 Add the Pomodoro sauce. Be careful as it may splatter. Bring it to a simmer.

6 When simmering, lower the heat to Medium Low and add the remaining ingredients, stir to combine.

7 Cook for 10 min. for flavors to combine. Use immediately or cool properly and store in airtight container and refrigerate. Will hold for 5 days in fridge.

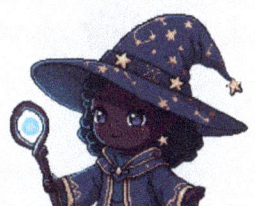

Recipe Tip

If you really like to feel the heat, try substituting the pepper flakes for chopped Calabrian peppers, and use the oil the peppers are packed in instead of olive oil.

Pumpkin Cream Sauce

Decadent

Sweet — Spicy

Savory — Salty

This sauce takes me back to my childhood. I grew up in a small town in New Hampshire, called West Chesterfield. Every October there's a festival in the neighboring town of Keene: Pumpkin Fest. The whole town, and the surrounding towns, become obsessed with autumn, and particularly pumpkins in the weeks leading up to it. Pumpkin lattes (even before they were all the rage), pumpkin tarts, pumpkin centric entrees at the local restaurants, all of them delicious. And this recipe is an homage to that atmosphere.

It's possible to do some prep work far in advance of cooking it. Follow steps 1-3, but instead of moving on to the next step, remove the seasoned puree from the pan and let cool on the counter. When cooled you can put it in an airtight container to hold it in the fridge for up to a week. Or, you can place a clump of it on a sheet of plastic wrap and roll it up into a tube, twisting off the ends. Wrap this package in foil so it holds its shape, and it can be frozen for up to 3 months. When you need to use it, just transfer it from the freezer to the fridge and let rest for 24 hours. Then you can add it to simmering milk and pick the recipe up from there.

Mother Sauce: Bechamel

Ingredients

Pumpkin Puree, Unsweetened	¾ C
Milk	16 Fl Oz
Garlic, Minced	1 tsp
Sage, Ground	¼ tsp
Nutmeg, Ground	⅛ tsp
Black Pepper	⅛ tsp
Salt	¼ tsp
Olive Oil, Divided	2½ Tbsp
AP Flour	1½ Tbsp
Parmesan Cheese, Grated	2 Tbsp

Prep Time
5 Min

Cook Time
10 - 15 Min

Servings
16 oz

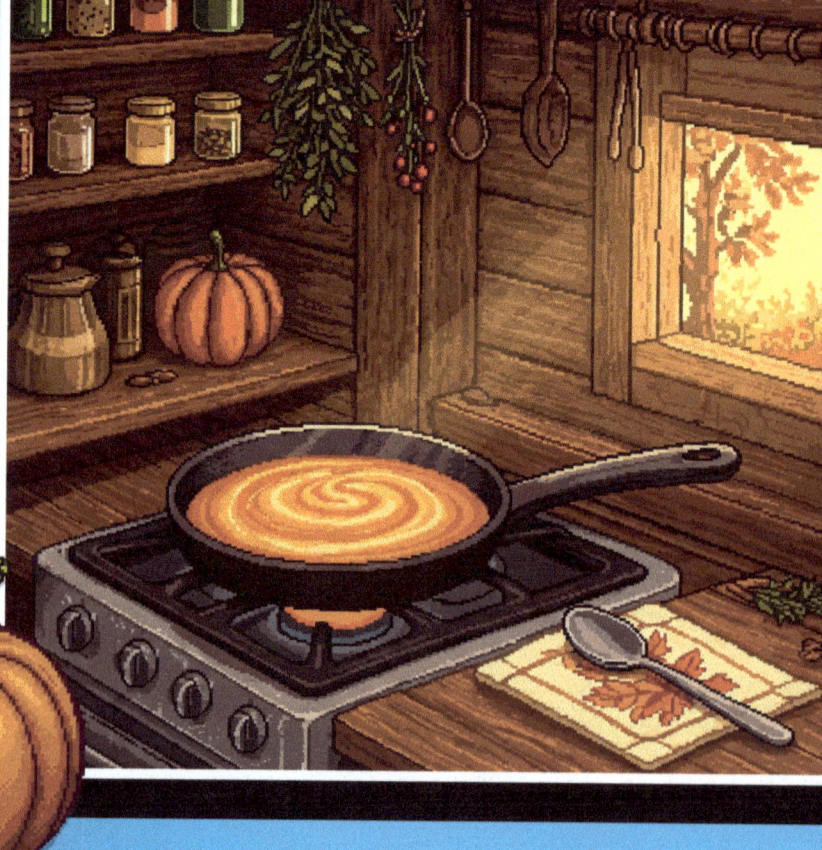

Cooking Directions

1   Place a 1 Qt. pot over Medium High heat. When hot, add 1 Tbsp. olive oil.

2   When the oil is shimmering/the butter has stopped bubbling, add the garlic to the pan and cook for 1 min.

3   Add the pumpkin puree, sage, and nutmeg. Stir well and cook for 2 - 3 min. until the pumpkin is dry and slightly clumpy.

4   Remove the pumpkin from the pan, set aside. Add the remaining olive oil. When shimmering, add the flour and mix well. Cook for, 2 - 3 min. bringing your roux to the Blanc level.

5   Pour in 8 oz. of the milk and whisk until no lumps remain in the roux. Add the rest of the milk and pumpkin puree, and whisk until fully combined.

6   Whisking all the while, bring to a simmer and lower the heat to Medium Low. Cook and reduce for 5 - 10, until it coats the back of a spoon (nappe).

7   Add the salt and pepper, stir, then add the parmesan cheese while whisking. Serve Hot.

APPRENTICE

Sweet Heat BBQ Sauce

This recipe is everything a BBQ sauce should be; it has an acidic tang, a bit of a kick, and a sweetness that lingers on the tongue. It glazes perfectly on grilled and broiled meats, and works well as a dipping sauce. Also, try mixing it in with ranch or bleu cheese dressing to make a unique salad or sandwich topping.

The red pepper flakes are kept to ¼ tsp. because I find that too much heat can take away from the enjoyment of the flavors of smoked or slow roasted meats. However, everyone has a different palate, so if you know that you enjoy really hot sauces, I'd say increase the amount to ½ or even ¾ tsp. Just keep in mind that red pepper flakes get hotter as they rest in the food when it cools.

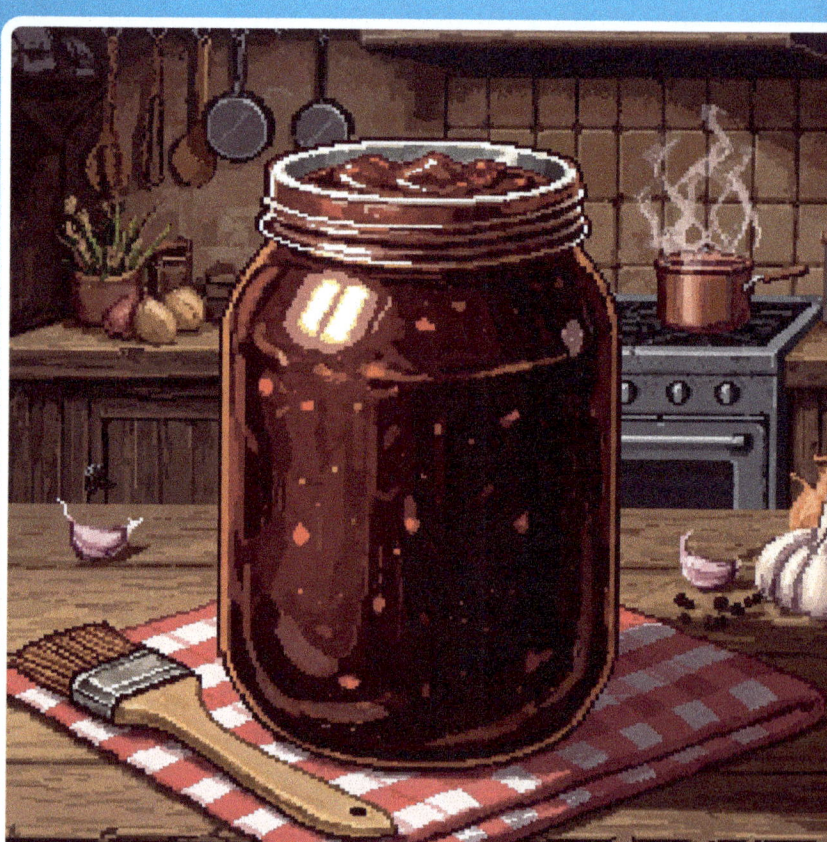

Ingredients

Plain Tomato Sauce (Canned)	28 oz
Yellow Mustard	¼ C
Water	16 Fl Oz
Apple Cider Vinegar	8 Fl Oz
Honey, Or Corn Syrup	1 C
Dark Brown Sugar, Packed	⅓ C
White Onion, Minced	1½ C
Black Pepper, Ground	1 Tbsp
Chili Powder	1 Tbsp
Salt	½ tsp
Cumin	¼ tsp
Cinnamon	¼ tsp
Red Pepper Flakes	¼ tsp
Garlic, Minced	1 tsp

 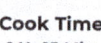

Prep Time	Cook Time	Servings
10 Min	1 Hr 15 Min	64 oz

Immersion Blender/Heat Safe
Blender or Food Processor
(Not required)
1 ea

Cooking Directions

1   Whisk together the tomato sauce, mustard and water in a 3 - 4 Qt. pot.

2   Add the remaining ingredients (except the honey and red pepper flakes) and whisk again to incorporate.

3   Place the pot over High heat and bring to a boil, whisking often. When boiling, add the honey and whisk well. Reduce the heat to Low or Medium Low to maintain a simmer for 1 hr.

4   Add the red pepper flakes and simmer for 5 min.

5   Remove from heat and let cool for 1 hr. stirring every 10 - 15 min.

6   Transfer sauce to a blender, or use an immersion blender, and blend until smooth. This step is not required, but it does help to smooth out the texture if you do it.

7   Store in airtight containers and refrigerate. Holds for 4 weeks in fridge.

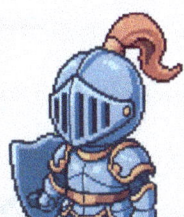

Recipe Tip

Having more time to stew allows for more capsaicin to be extracted and dispersed throughout the sauce, so if you really want to bring the heat, add them halfway through cooking instead of at the end.

Teriyaki Sauce

APPRENTICE

Decadent

Sweet

Spicy

Savory

Salty

This sauce is my answer to the overly sweet teriyaki sauces offered in so many establishments in America. While there is supposed to be a sweet element to teriyaki, it's meant to be balanced with salty and unctuous flavors in the sauce. This sauce works excellent for stir fries, glazing chicken, pork and seafood, and even as a dipping sauce. Try altering the values slightly in the recipe to craft your own ideal version of the sauce. Perhaps you want it much hotter? Or maybe you prefer it sweeter? It's up to you to decide, but with this recipe as a base, you can't go wrong.

Ingredients

Soy Sauce	½ C
Mirin/Shaoxing Wine	¼ C
Water	¼ C
Fish Sauce	1 tsp
Sesame Oil	1 tsp
White Sugar/Honey	2 Tbsp
Garlic, Minced	1 tsp
Scallions, Thinly Sliced	2 Tbsp
Ginger, Minced	1 tsp
Red Pepper Flakes (Optional)	⅛ tsp
Cornstarch, For Slurry	1 Tbsp
Cold Water, For Slurry	1 Tbsp

Prep Time
10 Min

Cook Time
5 - 10 Min

Servings
8 oz

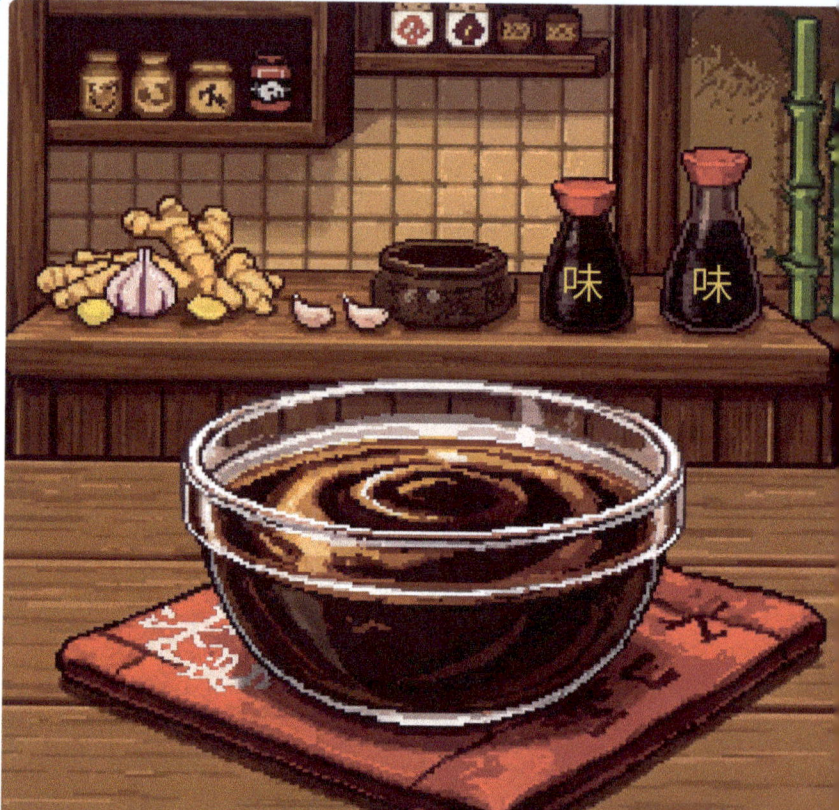

Cooking Directions

1   Combine all ingredients, except cornstarch, in a small pot. Whisk vigorously to combine. In a small bowl, combine the cornstarch and cold water fully.

2   Place over High heat and bring to a boil. Do not reduce at all.

3   Whisking constantly, add the slurry to thicken the sauce so it coats the back of a spoon (nappe). You may not need all the slurry, so add it slowly.

4   Remove from heat and cool for 20 - 30 minutes, whisking often, before transferring to an airtight container to refrigerate. Holds for 14 days.

5   Gently reheat before use in recipes.

Terry's Pesto

Decadent

Sweet — Spicy

Savory — Salty

My wife's mother loved to make her own pesto, and it was part of some of my wife's favorite dinners growing up. Using walnuts instead of pine nuts creates an earthier and more robust flavor in the pesto. Whether combining with cream to make a pasta sauce, heating it up in a pan and tossing some tortellini in it, or mixing it into your cold pasta salad, this sauce is a great way to brighten up your meal.

Ingredients

Fresh Basil Leaves, Packed	2 C
Parmesan Cheese, Grated	½ C
Olive Oil (More If Needed)	⅓ C
Walnut Pcs	½ C
Garlic Cloves	4 ea
Lemon Juice	1 Tbsp
Salt	⅛ tsp
A Pinch Of Black Pepper	

Prep Time
5 Min

Cook Time
N/A

Servings
12 oz

Medium to Large Food Processor
1 ea

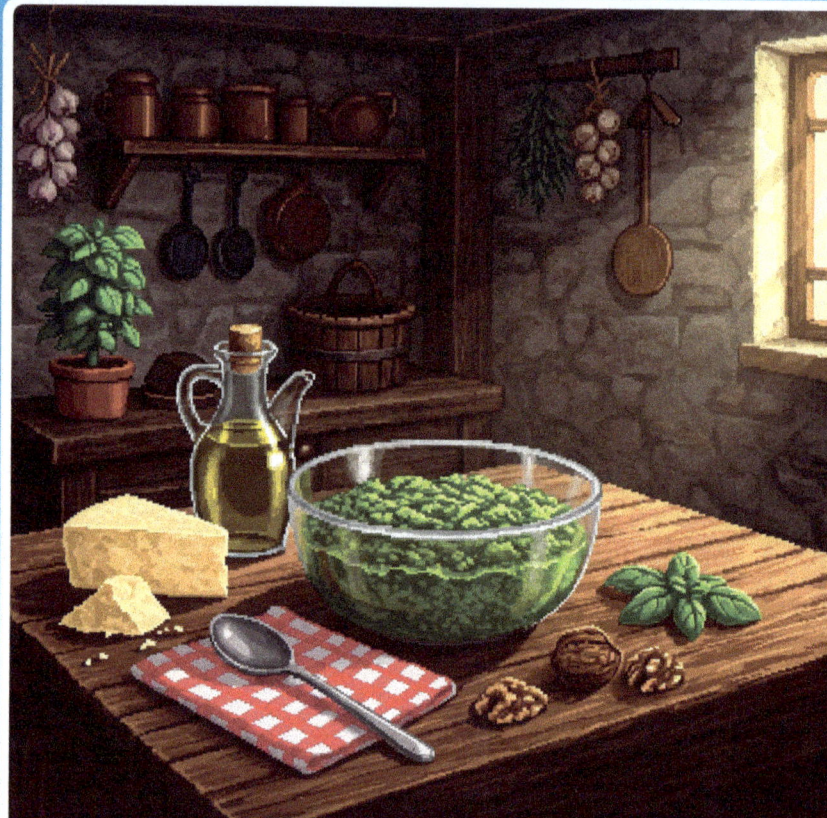

Cooking Directions

1   Place all ingredients, except the olive oil, in a food processor. Pulse 15 - 20 times.

2   Add ½ of the oil and blend for about 10 seconds. Add the remaining oil and blend until smooth. If the mixture is too chunky, add more olive oil 1 Tbsp. at a time until smooth.

3   Transfer to an airtight container and refrigerate. Holds in fridge for 3 days.

Desserts & Baking

Apple Crisp

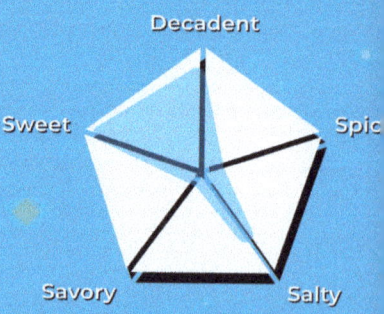

This is another classic dish straight from my childhood, a staple of the autumn months. When I was growing up in New England every family had their own Apple Crisp recipe. This particular recipe is courtesy of my wife's step-grandmother, and is delightful. If you've never had Apple Crisp before, you're in for a real treat. Serve it warm with a scoop of vanilla ice cream and brighten up any autumn day.

Ingredients (Filling)

Apples, Peeled & Sliced	8 C
AP Flour	1 Tbsp
White Sugar	1 C
Lemon Juice	2 Tbsp
Water	3 Tbsp
Cinnamon	1 Tbsp
All Spice, Ground	¼ tsp
Ginger, Ground	½ tsp
Butter/Shortening for Greasing The Pan	

Ingredients (Crumble)

AP Flour	1 C
Dark Brown Sugar, Packed	1 C
Baking Soda	¼ tsp
Quick Cook Oats	1 C
Salt	⅛ tsp
Butter, Melted	¼ C

Prep Time
15 Min

Cook Time
40 - 45 Min

Servings
9" x 13" Pan

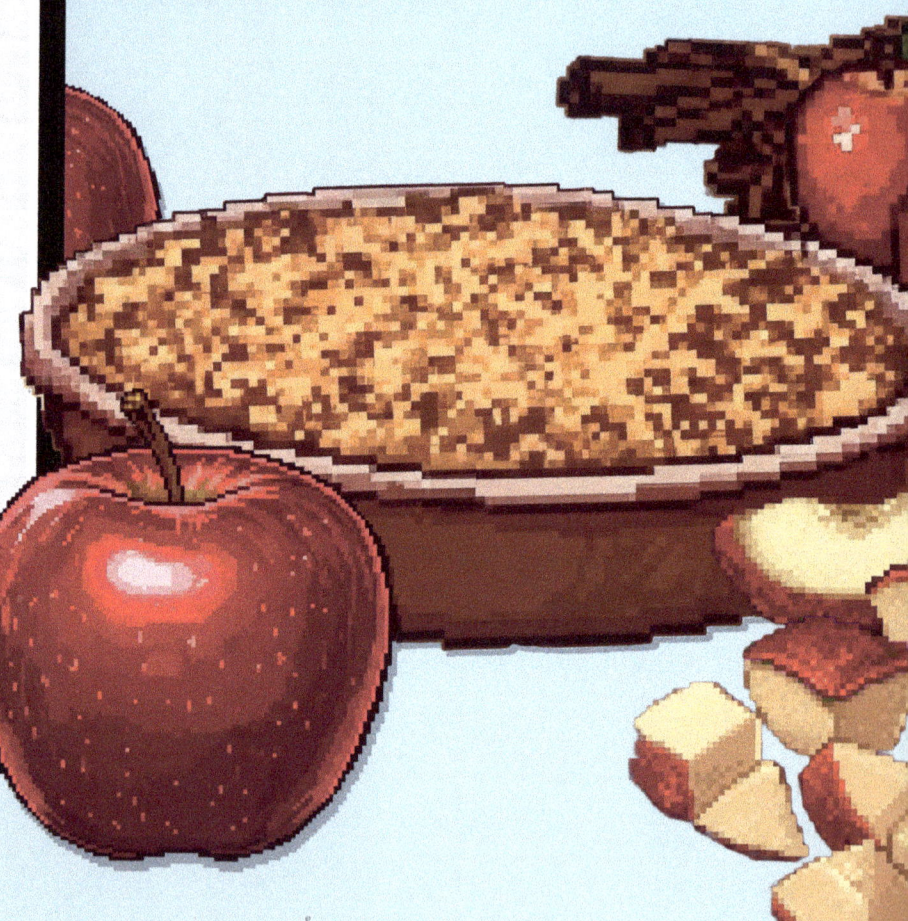

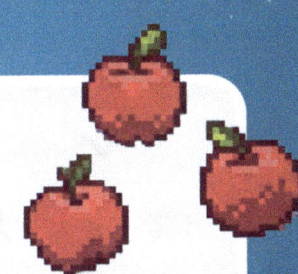

Cooking Directions

1   Preheat your oven to 350. Using butter or shortening, grease the sides and bottom of a 9" x 13" baking dish.

2   Place all of the filling ingredients in a large bowl and stir thoroughly to combine, making sure all apple slices are coated. Transfer to the greased baking dish.

3   The same bowl, place the Crumble ingredients with the butter going in last. Stir together with a fork until chunky and grainy. Distribute in an even layer over the filling.

4   Bake in the oven until the crumble is a rich golden brown and the filling is bubbling, 40 - 45 min.

5   Remove from oven and let rest for 10 min. before serving.

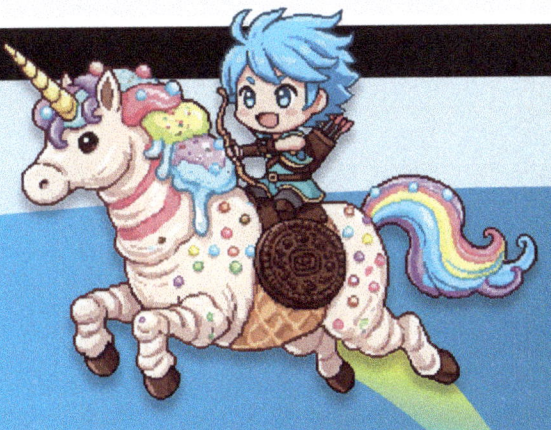

Recipe Tip

If you'd rather make a smaller portion of this recipe, simply cut it in half and bake it in an 8"x 8" square baking pan. The cooking time will remain the same, and it will be just as delicious!

Chunky Chocolate Chip Cookies

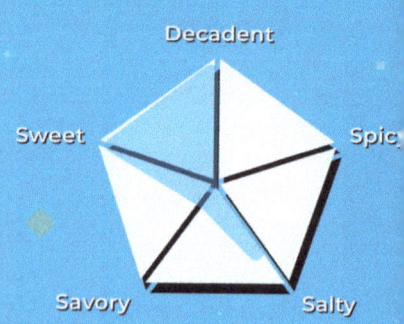

Chunky chocolate chip cookies are beloved by nearly everyone, and the use of dark chocolate chips and toasted pecans make these cookies stand out. The touch of cinnamon is essential to bring out the flavors of your chocolate and the nuts. Try them with different types of chips, adding various spices, or even adding 1 cup of pumpkin puree to your wet ingredients when creaming them together. The options are limitless with this recipe as a base.

Don't feel like making all 48 cookies? Simply line a baking sheet with parchment paper and scoop out dough balls onto it, making sure they are as close as they can be without touching. Place in freezer for 1-3 hr. until frozen solid. Transfer dough balls to a large freezer bag and return to freezer. Will hold for up to 2 months. To bake frozen dough balls, set the oven to 335 and bake for 11-13 min. until lightly golden brown with slightly darker edges.

Ingredients

Butter, Room Temperature	1 C
White Sugar	1 C
Dark Brown Sugar, Packed	1 C
Large Eggs, Room Temperature	2 ea
Vanilla Extract	2½ tsp
Baking Soda	1 tsp
Hot Water	2 tsp
Salt	½ tsp
AP Flour	3 C
Cinnamon	½ tsp
Toasted Pecans, Chopped	½ C
Dark Chocolate Chips	3 C

Prep Time
20 Min

Cook Time
10 Min

Servings
48 Cookies

1½ Tablespoon Scoop
1 ea

Stand Mixer
1 ea
(Not Required)

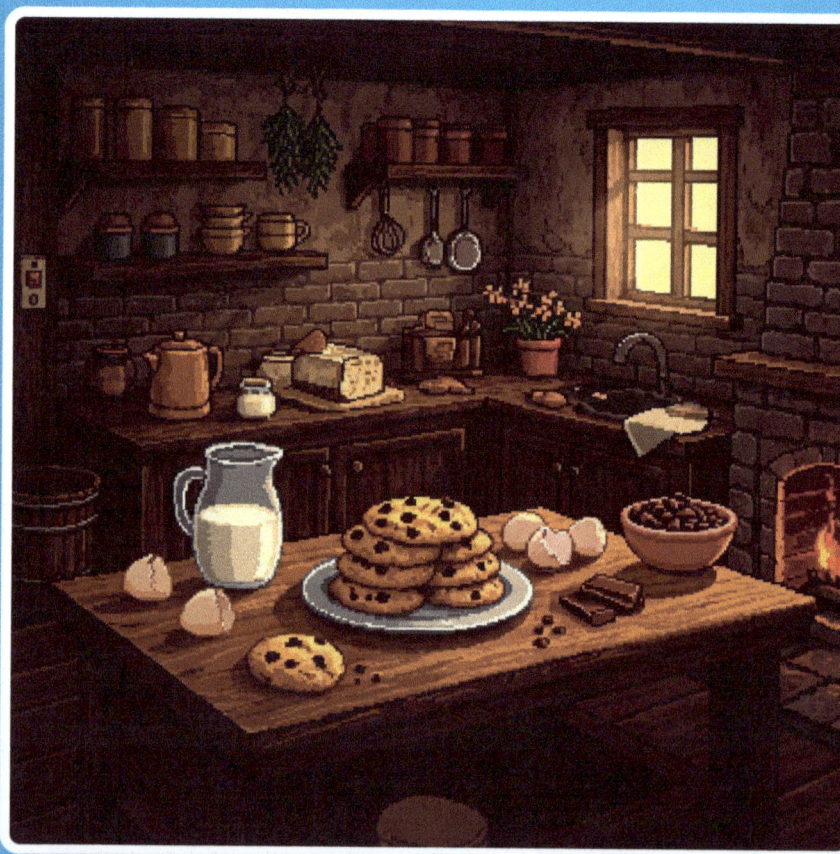

Cooking Directions

1   Preheat your oven to 350, making sure there is a rack in the center of the oven. In a large mixing bowl, beat the butter, both sugars, and vanilla extract together until smooth. In a separate bowl, sift together your flour, salt, and cinnamon. Set aside.

2   Add the eggs one a time to the bowl with your sugar in it, beating until fully incorporated between each. Dissolve your baking soda in the hot water. Add to the batter, and beat to combine.

3   In batches, add the flour to your wet ingredients and mix together with a wooden spoon. If using a stand mixer, beat them together on a low setting until just combined. Be careful not to over-mix or the cookies will not rise properly.

4   Add your chocolate chips and pecans, and stir them in so they are evenly distributed throughout the dough. Stop using stand mixer at this point to prevent over-mixing.

5   Using a 1½ Tbsp. scoop, or a spoon, form balls and place them 2" apart from one another on an ungreased baking sheet or pan. In between batches, store the dough in the fridge.

6   One pan/sheet at a time, bake in the oven on the center rack until the cookies are a light golden brown, with the edges being slightly darker, usually 9 - 10 min. I advise setting a timer for 8 min. and checking on the cookies then, since every oven bakes differently.

7   Remove baking sheet from oven and let cookies cool for 2 min. on the pan before transferring to a wire rack to cool completely. Eat warm, or store at room temperature, in an airtight container, for up to 5 days.

Classic Dumplin' Balls

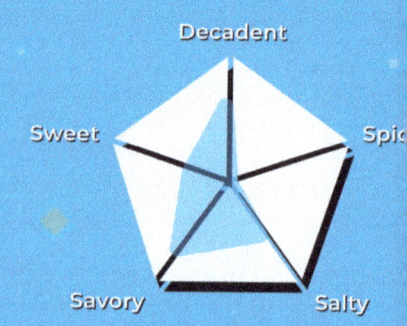

Decadent

Sweet Spic

Savory Salty

These classic dumplin's are the gold standard for chicken and dumplin's, and beef stew. They turn any dish into one that will stick to your ribs and comfort you. Try adding herbs in small amounts to help them stand out, or minced garlic to give them a deeper flavor. They take a bit longer to cook than flat sheet dumplin's, so you want to keep an eye on them. When they are overcooked they get a little dry. Once the majority of your dumplin's are floating in your soup, that's when they are done. These dumplin's also soak up much more liquid than the sheet kind, so keep that in mind too.

Ingredients

AP Flour	1 C
Cold Butter, Cubed	4 Tbsp
Milk	3 Tbsp
Large Egg, Beaten	1 ea
Salt	½ tsp
Black Pepper	¼ tsp
Sage, Ground	¼ tsp
Baking Powder	1 tsp

Prep Time
5 Min

Cook Time
5 - 7 Min

Servings
8 oz of Dough

1½ Tablespoon Scoop
1 ea

Dough Cutter
1 ea
(Not Required)

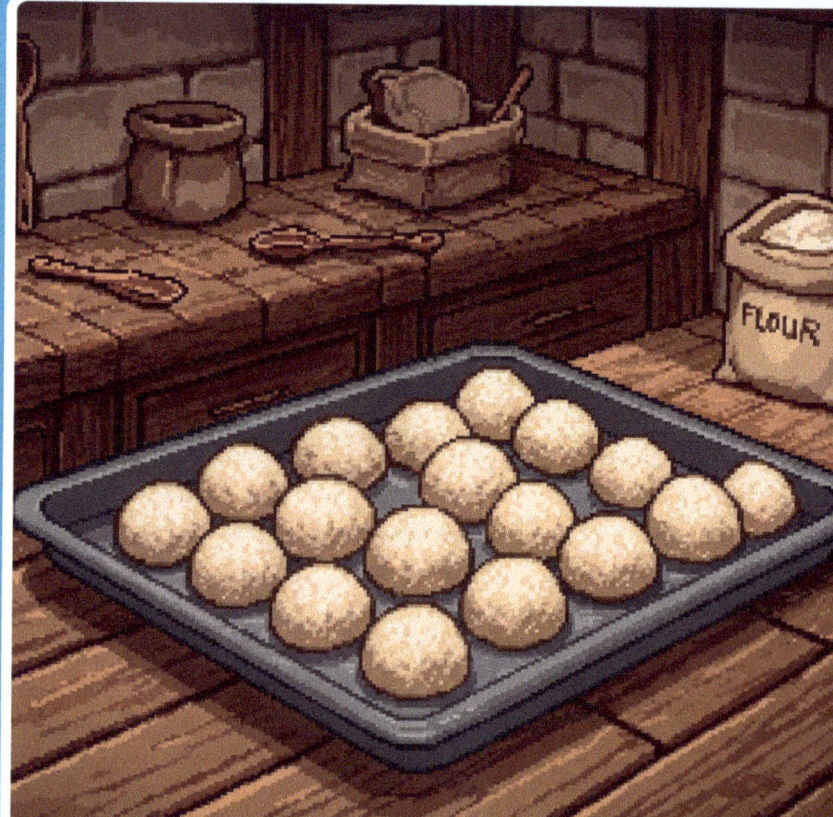

Cooking Directions

1   Sift the flour, salt, pepper, sage, and baking powder into a large bowl.

2   Add the butter cubes. Using a dough cutter, or your hands, blend with the flour until the mixture becomes grainy. Then, using your hands, rub the grains together until the dough is clumped and there are few grains left.

3   Whisk the milk and egg together in a small bowl. Pour into flour bowl, stirring with a rubber spatula or wooden spoon until fully incorporated. This takes a bit of work, but don't be discouraged!

4   Cover with plastic wrap pressed down onto the dough and refrigerate until needed, at least 10 min.

5   Using a ½ Tbsp. scoop, or a spoon, form the dough into evenly sized balls. Drop the balls into simmering liquid, and cook for 5 - 7 min. until all the balls are floating. If not using immediately, place in an airtight container and refrigerate. Will hold for 2 days in fridge, and 1 month frozen in a freezer bag.

Ginger-Sage Sheet Dumplin's

Decadent

Sweet

Spic

Savory

Salty

This dumplin' recipe is the perfect addition to homemade Chicken & Dumplin's. The ginger and sage add a subtle flavor to the soup that can't be beat. I encourage you to try various combinations of herbs and spices in your dumplin' dough to find your favorite kinds. These sheet dumplin's make for a nice textural change to stews and soups, and as they are thinner than ball dumplin's they only take about 2-3 minutes of cooking until they are floating and ready to eat.

Ingredients

AP Flour	1 C
Baking Powder	¼ tsp
Salt	⅛ tsp
Black Pepper, Ground	⅛ tsp
Ginger Powder	¼ tsp
Sage, Ground	½ tsp
Butter, Cold & Cubed	1 Tbsp
Milk	¼ C

Prep Time
10 Min

Cook Time
5 Min (in Soup)

Servings
8 oz

Rolling Pin
1 ea

Dough Cutter
1 ea

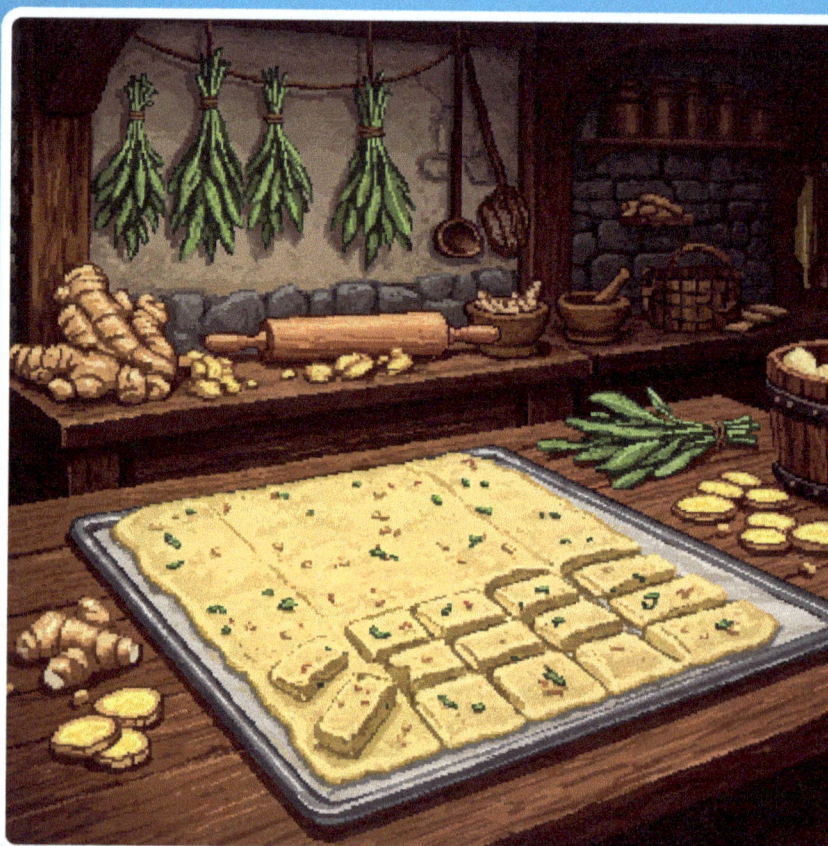

Cooking Directions

1   Sift the flour, baking powder and salt together in a large bowl.

2   Add the ginger, pepper, and sage. Mix together with a fork. Then, add the butter cubes.

3   Using a dough cutter, or your hands, incorporate the butter into the flour mix, working it until the dough becomes grainy and crumbly.

4   Add the milk 1 - 2 Tbsp. at a time, mixing with a wooden spoon or your hand as you do, until the dough is solid and no longer shaggy. It may not require the full ¼ cup of milk.

5   Transfer the dough onto a floured surface and press into a rectangular shape.

6   Roll the dough out into a rectangle that is ⅛" - ¼" thick.

7   Let rest at room temperature for 10 min.

8   Cut the dough into strips roughly 1" wide and 3" long. If not using immediately, gently toss in flour and shake excess flour off pieces before placing in an airtight container. Will hold in fridge for 2 days, and can be frozen for 1 month in a freezer bag.

Snickerdoodle Cookies

This classic recipe is a go-to when bringing cookies for a gathering, as they don't have any allergy reactions and are universally enjoyed by adults and children alike. What more is there to say? Snickerdoodles are great!

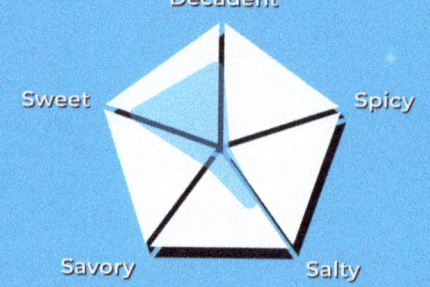

Decadent
Sweet
Spicy
Savory
Salty

Ingredients

Butter, Room Temperature	½ C
Shortening/Lard	½ C
White Sugar	1½ C
Large Eggs, Room Temperature	2 ea
AP Flour	2 ¾ C
Vanilla Extract	2 tsp
Cream Of Tartar	2 tsp
Baking Soda	1 tsp
Salt	¼ tsp
White Sugar, For Dusting	3 Tbsp
Cinnamon, For Dusting	2 tsp

Prep Time
20 Min

Cook Time
20 - 30 Min

Servings
24 Cookies

1½ Tablespoon Scoop
1 ea

Stand Mixer
1 ea
(Not Required)

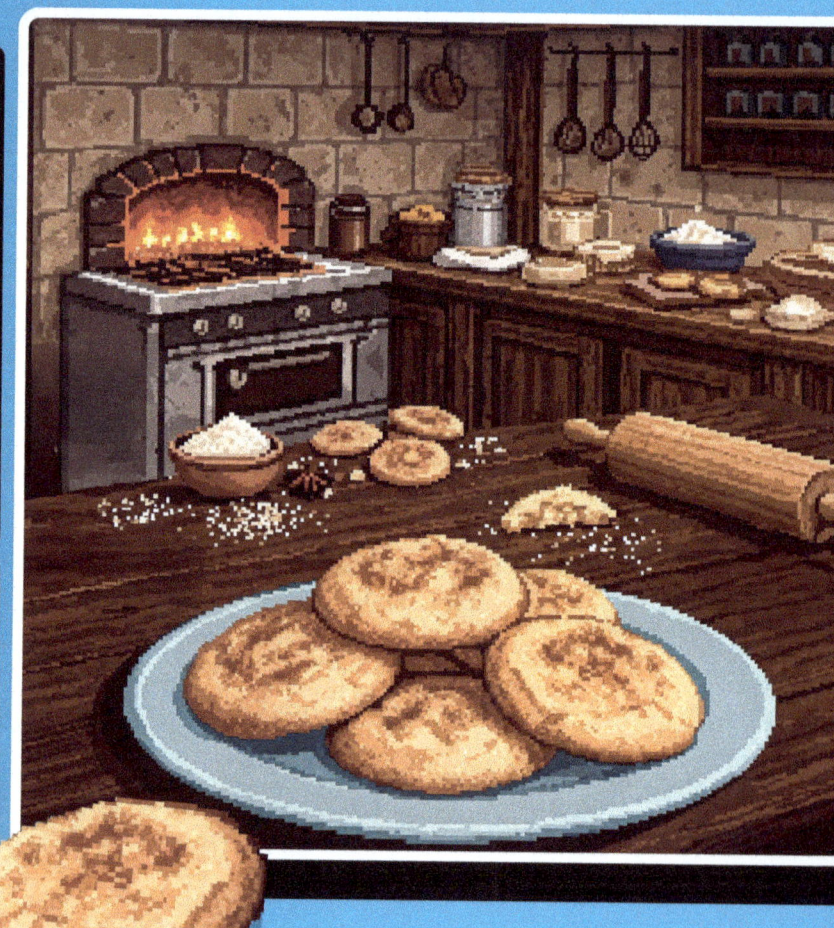

Cooking Directions

1   Preheat oven to 400.

2   Place the butter, 1½ C of sugar, and shortening/lard in a large mixing bowl. If using a stand mixer use a low setting, or by hand mix together until creamed.

3   Add the vanilla and eggs and mix for 30 - 45 seconds until well combined.

4   Sift the flour, tartar, salt and baking soda together into a medium sized bowl.

5   In small batches, add the flour mixture to your wet ingredients, mixing on low speed or by hand between each batch.

6   Mix until all dry ingredients are fully incorporated, but be careful not to over-mix. Otherwise your cookies won't rise well.

7   Using a 1½ Tbsp. scoop, or a spoon, form the dough into even balls. Set aside.

8   Once all dough has been formed, mix the sugar and cinnamon for dusting together. Rolls the balls into your dusting mix.

9   Line a baking sheet with parchment paper and set the dough balls 2" - 3" apart from each other.

10   Bake for 8 - 10 minutes, so they are set but not hard.

11   Remove from oven and let rest on the pan for 1-2 min. before transferring to a rack for cooling. Repeat until all dough balls are baked, storing the balls that aren't being baked in the fridge between batches.

LVLUPCookBook Channel

ADEPT

A Road Less Travelled

You are now a competent and actualized cook. You know what you are about, and are now ready to face the more complex challenges to hone the skills you learned as a Novice and shaped as an Apprentice.

The rank of Adept is not easily achieved, and you're on the path to unlocking your true potential.

Don't be dissuaded by mistakes you make while climbing through this rank. You've come so far, and you should look back at all the recipes you have crafted and learned with pride.

Now is the time where if you feel you want to branch out into a different class, do so. If not, then tackle the Adept challenges with the same zeal that brought you here.

LEVEL 20

Achievements Unlocked

Not Just For Breakfast
- You've made several gravies, and know the difference between a sauce and a gravy

Roux Apprentice
- You know several types of roux and how they are used

Dual Wielding!
- You can now make at least 2 recipes in tandem

Mix It Up!
- You can now craft your own seasoning blends

If At First You Don't Succeed...
- You've refined your methods to cook in a smoother flow

...Fry, Fry Again
- You've fried multiple foods, and know the difference between Shallow and Deep frying

Soups

French Onion Soup

This French classic never fails to please. Caramelizing the onions well is the key to developing that specific flavor that is so addictive. I find that using a blend of stocks is also a necessity for truly great French Onion Soup. Duck and beef is my preferred combination, but since duck stock can be hard to come by (and expensive) in stores, chicken works as a good substitute. Using fresh herbs and a proper Bouquet Garni is a must. Most stores will sell a mix of herbs they label as 'Poultry Blend' and this will have all the herbs I listed in the recipe. It not only works perfectly for this soup, but also for making your own stocks at home.

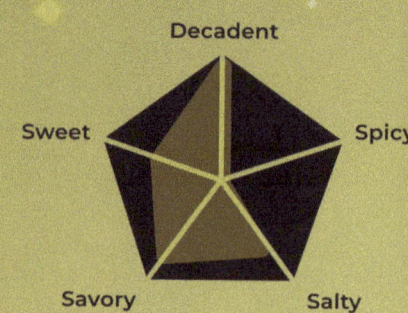

Ingredients

Large Red Onion, ¼" Rings	1 ea
Large Yellow Onion, ¼" Julienne	2 ea
Large White Onion, ¼" Julienne	2 ea
Red Wine	8 Fl Oz
Beef Stock	32 Fl Oz
Chicken or Duck Stock	32 Fl Oz
Rosemary Sprigs, Fresh	3 ea
Parsley Sprigs, Fresh	8 - 10 ea
Sage leaves, Fresh	4 ea
Thyme sprigs, Fresh	5 ea
Bay Leaf	1 ea
Black Peppercorns, Whole	½ Tbsp
Butter	2 Tbsp
Onion Base	1 Tbsp
Gruyere/Swiss Cheese, Shredded	1 C
Bread Rounds, Dried	12 ea
8 x 8" Square of Cheesecloth	
10" Butchers Twine	
Salt to Taste	

Prep Time	Cook Time	Servings
10 Min	70 - 90 Min	6 - 8 Bowls

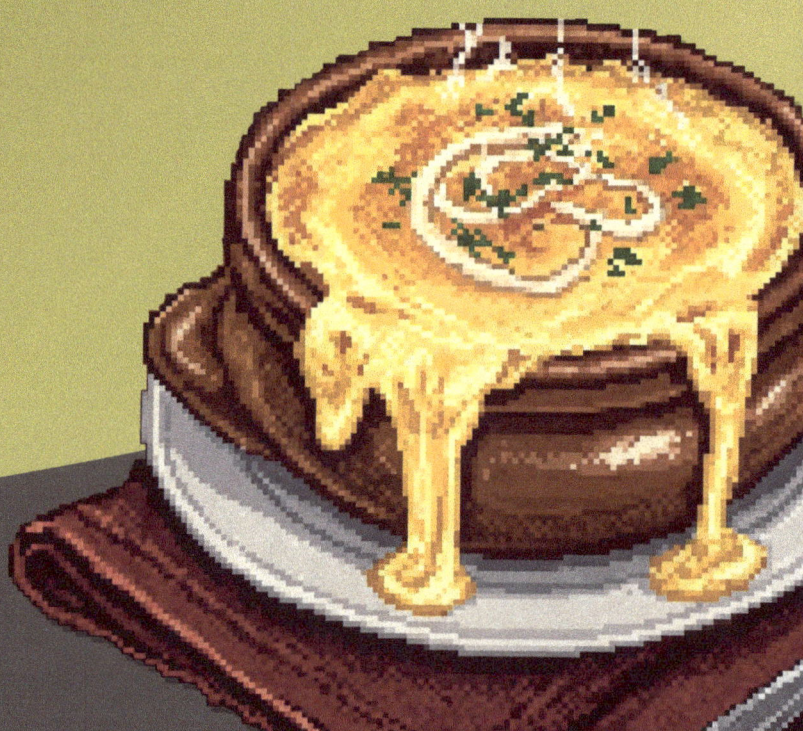

To Serve:

Set broiler in oven to High, and move a rack so it is 6" - 8" away from broiler, keep oven door open throughout. Place 6 - 8 oz. of soup in an oven safe bowl or crock. Set 1 or 2 bread rounds on top of soup, then cover the bread with shredded cheese. Place under broiler and cook until the cheese is melted and bubbling. Carefully remove bowl/crock from oven and place on a plate lined with a heat resistant trivet.

Alternatively, before putting soup in any bowls, set the broiler to high and move a rack so it is 6" - 8" away from broiler. Place the bread rounds on a baking sheet, and cover each piece with a thick layer of shredded cheese. Place tray under the broiler, and broil until the cheese is melted and bubbling. Remove tray from oven. Place 6 - 8 oz. of soup in a bowl, then place 1 - 2 pieces of the bread on top of the soup.

Cooking Directions

1. Place the herbs and peppercorns into the center of the cheesecloth square. Wrap up and tie the top together with the twine, using a simple double knot and leaving 7" - 8" of twine free. This is your Bouquet Garni.

2. Place a 6 - 8 Qt. pot over Medium heat. When hot, add butter and melt until butter no longer bubbles. Add onions and a pinch of salt. Stir well. Reduce heat to Medium Low, cover, and cook until well caramelized (dark brown), about 30 - 40 minutes, stirring roughly every 5 minutes. Lower heat slightly if onions begin to burn at all.

3. Once onions are caramelized, place the Bouquet on top of the onions and tie the free end of the twine to a handle of the pot. This will ensure you can easily remove the Bouquet later.

4. Mix the onion base into 8 oz. of the beef stock, set aside. Raise the heat under the pot to High.

5. Add the wine and beef stock-onion base mixture, stir well and cook for 5 minutes to reduce by ¼ - ½. Add remaining stock and bring to a boil. Reduce heat to Medium Low and cover.

6. Simmer for 30 minutes minimum. If simmering longer, be sure to periodically check on the soup, adding water if the soup reduces too much. Serve Hot.

Roasted Red Pepper Soup

This delightful soup is great for spring time lunches and dinners, and reheats well so making it ahead of time is a great way to free up your schedule. Topping with fresh cilantro, a sprinkle of cinnamon, or a twist of lemon juice is an easy way to liven up the already flavor packed aspects of this soup.

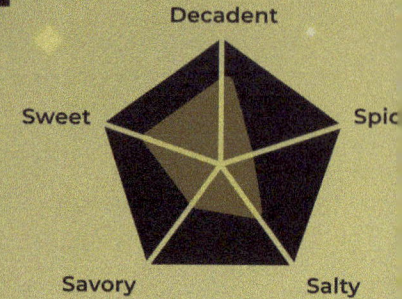

Decadent

Sweet

Spicy

Savory

Salty

Ingredients

Yellow Onion, Diced	1½ C
Zucchini, Diced	1 C
Red Bell Pepper	3 ea
Sun dried Tomatoes, Julienne	¼ C
Chicken Or Vegetable Stock	16 Fl Oz
Coconut Milk, Unsweetened	14 Fl Oz
Garlic, Minced	1 tsp
Coriander, Ground	1 tsp
Cumin	1 tsp
Salt	1 tsp
Black Pepper, Ground	¼ tsp
Paprika	½ tsp
Bay Leaf	1 ea
Neutral Oil	1 Tbsp

Prep Time
40 Min

Cook Time
35 Min

Servings
4 - 6 Bowls

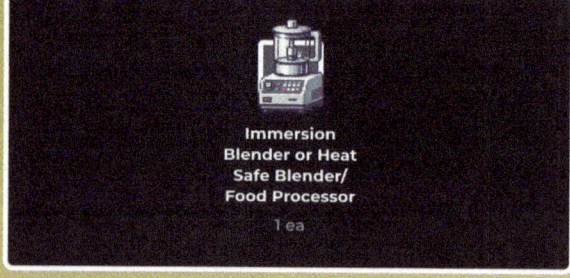

Immersion Blender or Heat Safe Blender/ Food Processor
1 ea

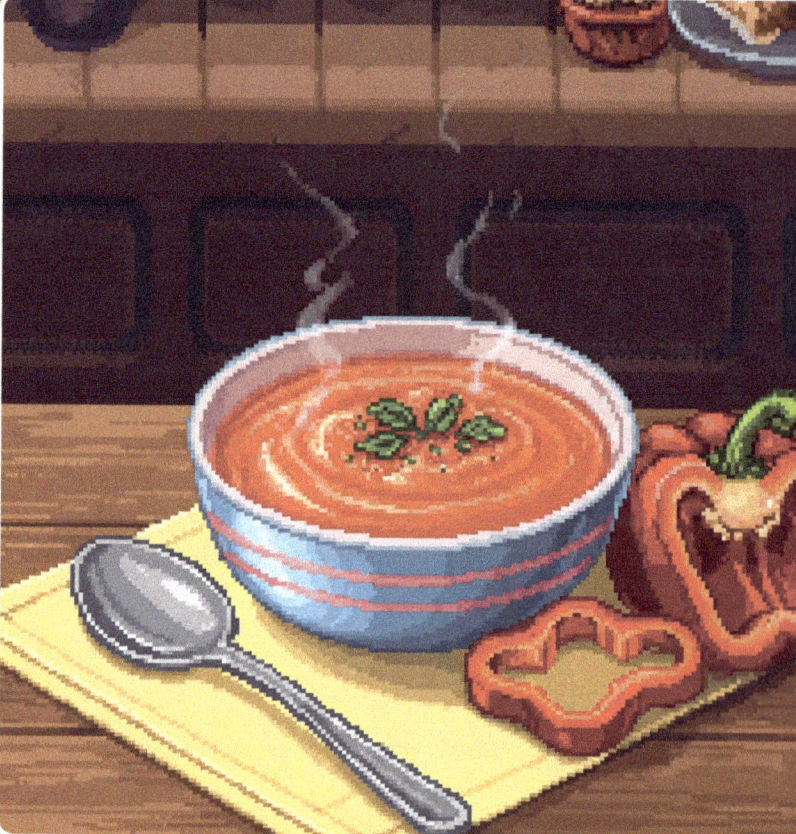

Cooking Directions

1 Set broiler to High and move a rack so it is 6" - 8" away from broiler. Keep oven door open. Place a sheet of tin foil on lower rack. When hot, place peppers on rack, above the foil sheet, and roast for 20 minutes rotating peppers every 5 minutes. When charred all over, remove peppers from oven. Place peppers in a heat safe bowl and cover tightly with plastic wrap. Turn off oven.

2 While the peppers are cooling, cut and measure all ingredients.

3 Once cool enough to handle, remove the skins and seeds from the peppers and roughly chop.

4 Place a 4 Qt. pot over Medium heat. When hot, add oil.

5 When oil is shimmering, add onion and cook until browned, 8 - 10 minutes. Add garlic and cook for 1 minute.

6 Add zucchini, peppers, tomatoes and spices. Cook for 2 - 3 minutes. Raise heat to High.

7 Add stock and bring to a boil. Reduce heat to Medium Low and cover. Cook for 20 minutes.

8 Add the coconut milk. Cook for 3 minutes more. Remove bay leaf from pot.

9 Using either an immersion blender or a heat safe blender/food processor, blend soup until smooth. Taste test, adjust seasoning as needed, and remove from heat. Serve Hot.

ADEPT

Sausage & Lentil Soup

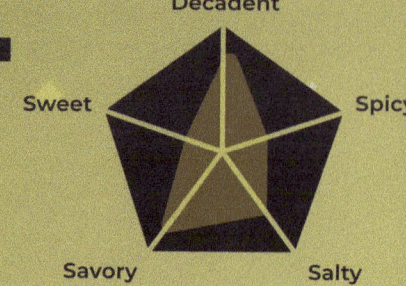

Decadent

Sweet

Spicy

Savory

Salty

This soup is a must-have when the days get short and the weather gets colder. The kale and lentils really stick to your ribs, and using hot sausage instead of sweet will really warm you up. Speaking of lentils, it's important to make sure you use green or brown lentils as they retain their shape and texture better than other varieties.

Ingredients

Green Lentils, Washed	¼ C
Water	1½ C
Italian Sausage, Sweet	1 Lb
Yellow Onion, Small Dice	1½ C
Celery, Small Dice	¾ C
Carrot, Small Dice	½ C
Chicken Stock	48 Fl Oz
Kale, Chopped	4 C
Garlic, Minced	1 Tbsp
Oregano, Dry	¾ tsp
Thyme, Dry	½ tsp
Basil, Dry	½ tsp
Salt	½ Tbsp
Black Pepper, Ground	¾ tsp
Bay Leaves	2 ea
Olive Oil	1 Tbsp

Prep Time	Cook Time	Servings
35 Min	35 Min	6 - 8 Bowls

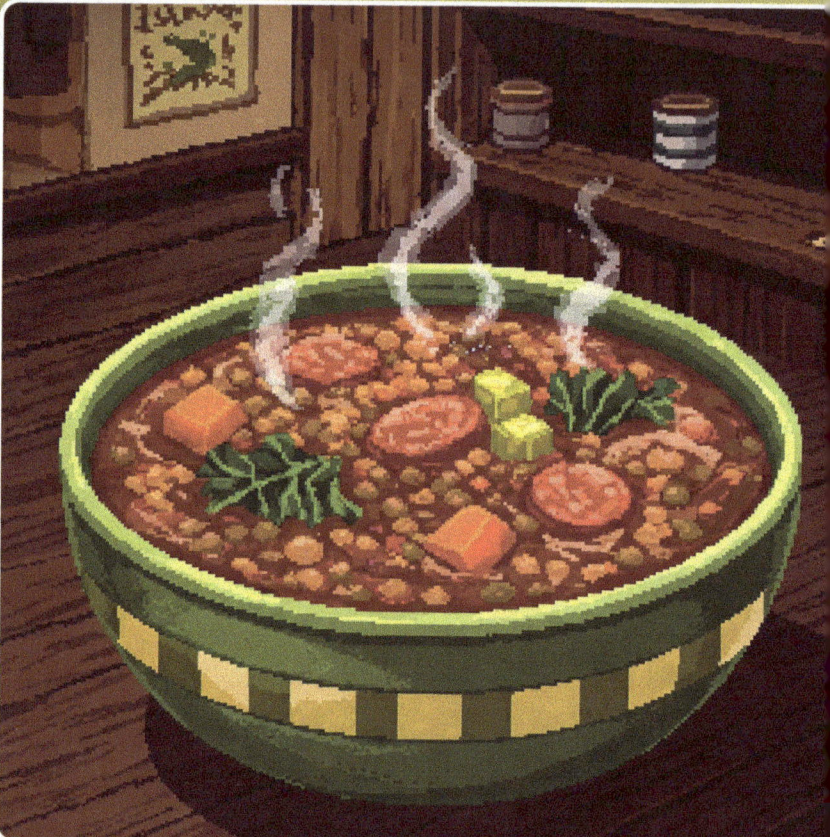

Recipe Tip

Test the lentils after the first cook to see how firm they are, and adjust the time they simmer in the soup accordingly. You want them to be slightly firm, but not grainy or chunky. They should come apart fairly easily as you bite into them when you finish cooking.

▼

Cooking Directions

Place the water in a 1 Qt. pot and place pot over High heat. When boiling, add lentils. Return to a boil then reduce the heat to Medium Low to hold a gentle simmer. Cook with lid tilted for 20 minutes. Drain from pot and set aside.

As the lentils are cooking, tear the sausage into clumps that are roughly 1" in size and roll into balls.

Place a 4-6 Qt. pot over Medium High heat. When hot, place sausage balls in pot and cook for 2 - 3 minutes, stir gently, and cook for 2 more minutes. Make sure to roll the balls around so that at least 2 'sides' of the ball get nicely browned. Remove from pot, retain grease in bottom of pot.

Lower heat to Medium and add the oil. When shimmering, add onion, celery, and carrot, cooking each until soft before adding the next, about 2 minutes each. Add 4 oz. of the stock and scrape the bottom of the pot well to remove any stuck on browned bits and spots (the fond).

Add garlic, cook for 1 minute. Add seasonings, lentils, kale, and return sausage to pot.

Raise heat to Medium High, add the stock. Bring to a boil, reduce the heat to Medium Low and cover. Simmer for 10 - 15 minutes, until the lentils are soft and the sausage balls are fully cooked (155 internal temperature.)

Taste test, adjust salt and pepper as needed, then remove pot from heat. Serve Hot.

Sides & Appetizers

ADEPT

Blistered Green Beans

Cooking the oil is a necessary step in all wok cookery, to develop a distinct smoky flavor that will be imparted on the food. However, when cooking the oil be careful that dark smoke is not produced. If this happens, remove from heat and discard oil, as the taste will be wrong. If at any point your oil is smoking blue, remove from heat and DO NOT add any food to the oil. Even in small quantities, blue smoke can produce a large flame when agitated, and is dangerous.

Decadent
Sweet
Spicy
Savory
Salty

Ingredients (Muffins)

Green Beans, Washed & Trimmed	12 oz
Garlic, Minced	2 tsp
Soy Sauce	2 Tbsp
Oil With High Smoke Point	1 Tbsp
Salt for Blanching	2 tsp
Water for Blanching & Shocking	
Ice for Shocking	
A Pinch of Salt & Pepper	

 Prep Time 10 Min

 Cook Time 5 - 7 Min

 Servings 4 Portions

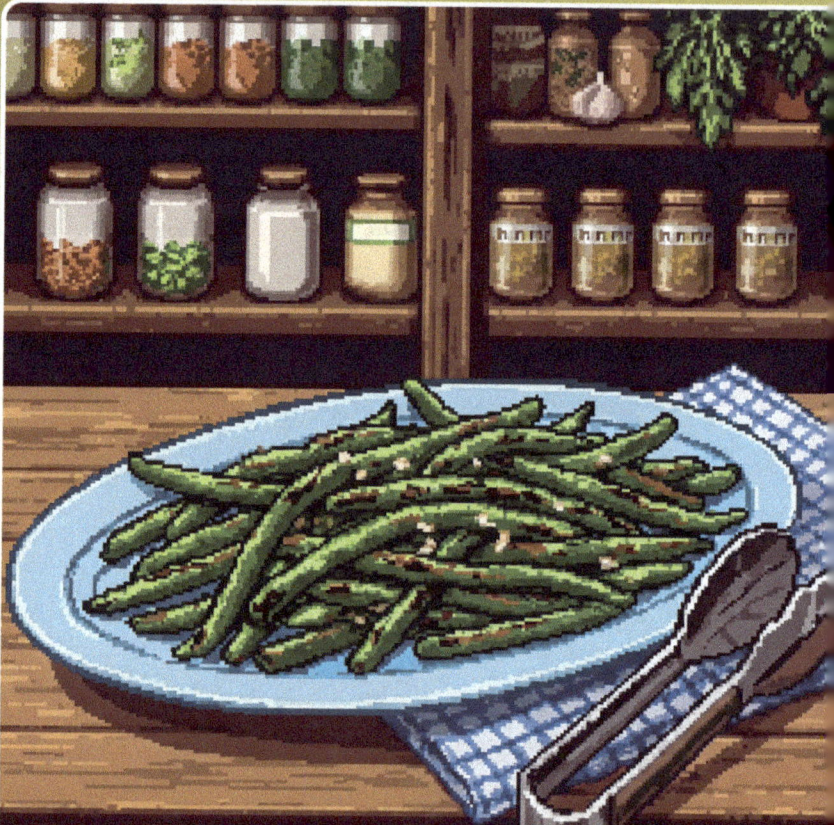

Recipe Tip

This recipe produces a fair amount of smoke, so proper ventilation is recommended when cooking. However, if there is too much smoke being produced, your heat is too high and should be reduced slightly until the smoking is lessened.

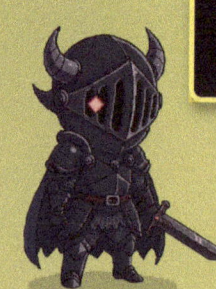

Cooking Directions

1. Fill a 4 Qt. pot halfway with water and place over High heat. When water is boiling, add 2 tsp. of salt. Place ice in a large bowl, fill with cold water leaving room for the green beans. Add green beans to boiling water and cook for 3 minutes.

2. Strain green beans from boiling water, then place in the bowl of ice water to shock and chill.

3. Once cool, strain the green beans and remove any ice from the beans. Dry thoroughly with a clean towel and set aside.

4. Place a wok or 12" - 14" skillet over High heat. When hot, add oil. Cook the oil until it is slightly smoking. NOT heavily smoking, and NEVER with blue smoke. If the smoke is too dense, or blue, remove pan from heat and wait about 5 minutes before starting over.

5. Add green beans and toss well. Cook for 5 - 7 minutes, tossing frequently, until black blisters start to form on the beans.

6. Reduce heat to Medium and remove the pan from the heat for 30 seconds. Add garlic, toss, and return pan to heat. Add soy sauce and cook for 30 - 45 seconds, tossing often.

7. Sprinkle a pinch of salt and pepper, toss and serve Hot.

Crispy Creamy Grit Cakes

These cakes make for excellent side items or passed hors d'oeuvres . Just like with crab cakes, simply increase or decrease the diameter of your cakes to suit your needs. As long as they are still 1" thick, they will take the same amount of time to shallow fry. Keep in mind you may need more of the breading and more eggs depending on the size of your cakes.

The grits can be made in advance, and held in the fridge for up to 24 hr. before use, just be sure to cover with plastic wrap or a lid if not using after 1 hour.

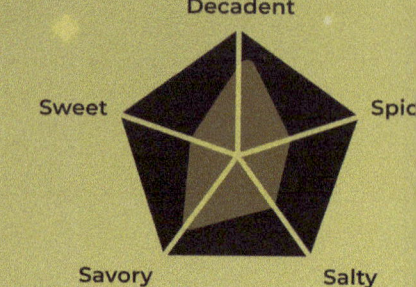

Decadent
Sweet
Spic
Savory
Salty

Ingredients (Muffins)

Dry Grits	½ C
Heavy Cream	8 Fl Oz
Chicken Or Vegetable Stock	8 Fl Oz
Poblano Or Bell Peppers	2 ea
Green Onion, Chopped	2 Tbsp
Parmesan Cheese, Grated	3 Tbsp
AP Flour	½ C
Panko Bread Crumbs	½ C
Salt	¼ tsp
Black Pepper, Ground	¼ tsp
Water	2 Tbsp
Large Eggs, Beaten	2 ea
Oil, For Shallow Frying	1 C

Prep Time
90 Min

Cook Time
15 Min

Servings
6 Cakes

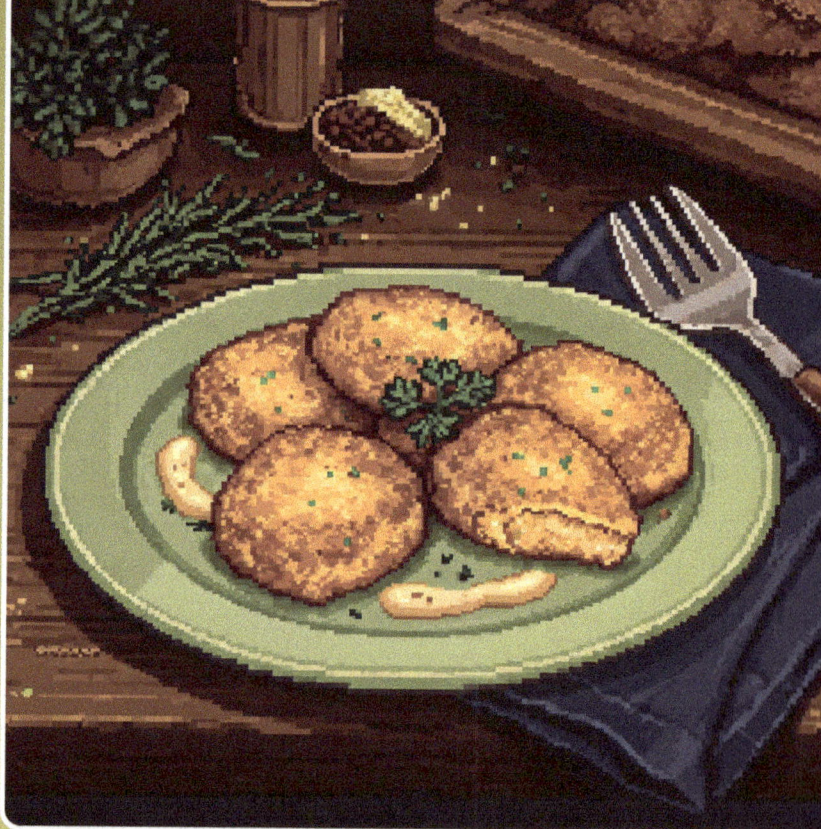

Cooking Directions

1 Set broiler to High heat. Adjust a rack so it is 6" - 8" away from broiler. When hot, place pepper on rack and broil for 15 - 20 minutes, turning peppers every 5 minutes. When fully charred remove peppers from oven and place in heat safe bowl. Turn off broiler. Tightly cover the bowl with plastic wrap and set aside.

2 While the peppers are cooling, place the heavy cream and 4 oz. of the stock in a 1 Qt. pot and place over Medium High heat. Bring to a boil, stirring often. In a separate bowl, combine the grits and remaining stock, whisking well. Pour the mixture into the boiling cream and stock, stirring continuously until well incorporated. Reduce heat to Low and cover.

3 Cook for 18 - 20 minutes, stirring often until thick and grits begin to pull away from the pot while stirring. While cooking the grits, remove the skin and seeds from pepper and cut into small dice.

4 When grits are done cooking add the scallions, parmesan, and roasted pepper (without their juice). Stir well.

5 Transfer to a heat safe container or bowl, spreading evenly so the mix is level. Cool for 45 - 60 minutes.

6 Place the flour in a bowl, or on a plate. In a separate bowl combine the panko, salt and pepper. In a third bowl, whisk the eggs and the 2 Tbsp. of water together.

>>>> CONTINUED >>>>

7   Once cooled, shape the grits into 6 equal sized cakes, about 1 inch thick. Dredge in the flour mixture, then place in egg mixture and coat evenly, then place in the panko mix. Press the breading gently into the cakes to coat evenly. Set cakes aside to rest out of fridge.

8   Heat oil in a large skillet over Medium heat until it reaches 350.

9   Place cakes carefully into skillet, making sure not to overcrowd, cooking in batches if needed. Fry for 4 - 5 minutes per side, until golden brown on both sides. Place on paper towels to absorb excess grease before serving. Serve Hot.

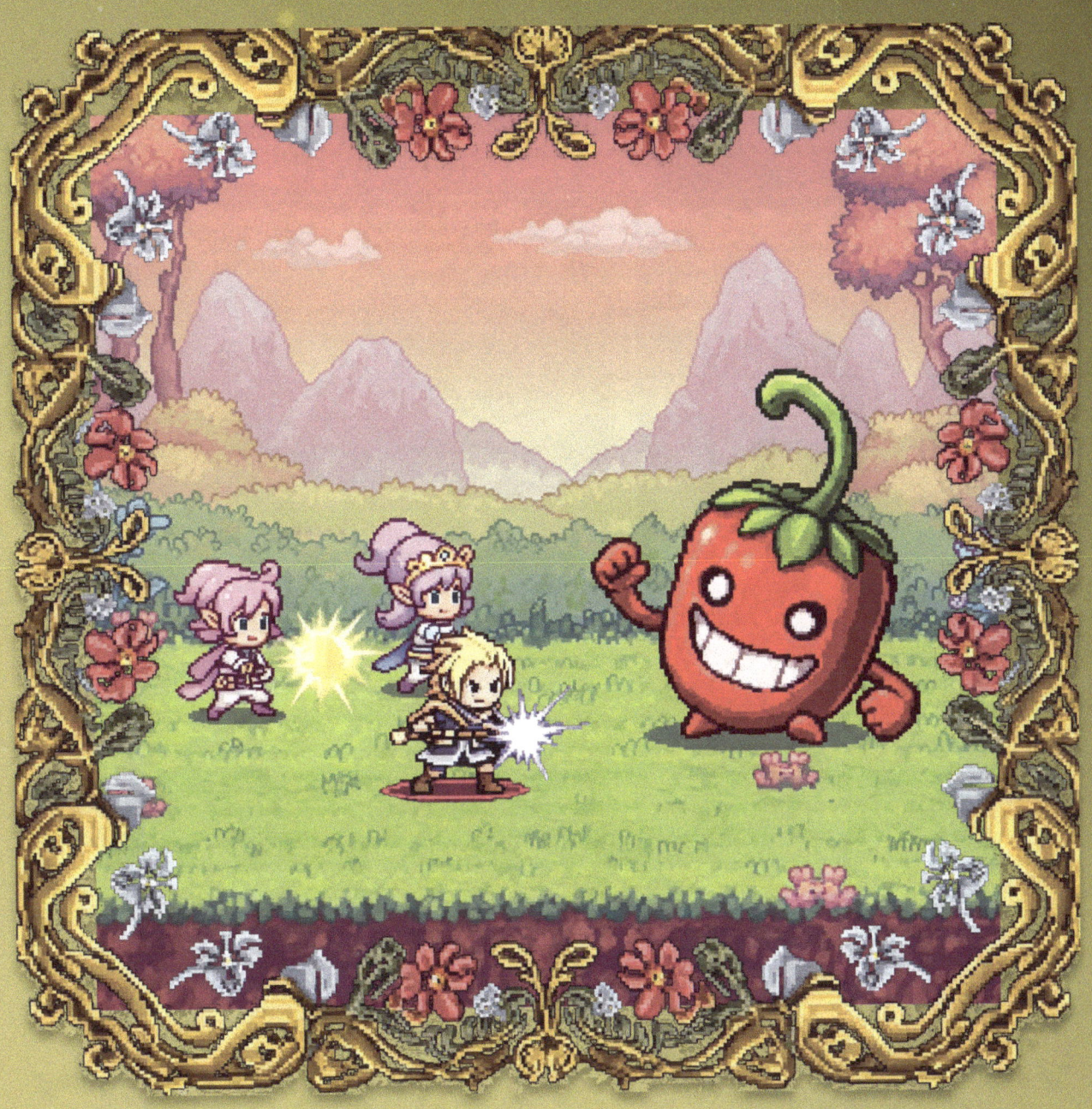

New England Crab Cakes

Decadent

Sweet — Spic

Savory — Salty

This recipe can be used to make crab cake hors d'oeuvres , side dishes, or as an entree. The only difference would be how much of the mixture you use to make the cakes. Just make sure to form patties that are uniformly 1½" thick, and the cooking time will remain the same. Served with remoulade, tartar sauce, or just a twist of lemon, these cakes are delicious.

Ingredients

Lump Crab Meat	1 Lb
Mayo (Pg 145)	½ C
Large Egg, Beaten	1 ea
Dijon Mustard	1 Tbsp
Bread Crumbs	⅔ C
Worcestershire Sauce	1 Tbsp
Hot Sauce	½ tsp
Neutral Oil	¼ C
Lemon Wedges	6 - 8 ea

Prep Time	**Cook Time**	**Servings**
12 - 15 Min	10 - 20 Min	8 Cakes

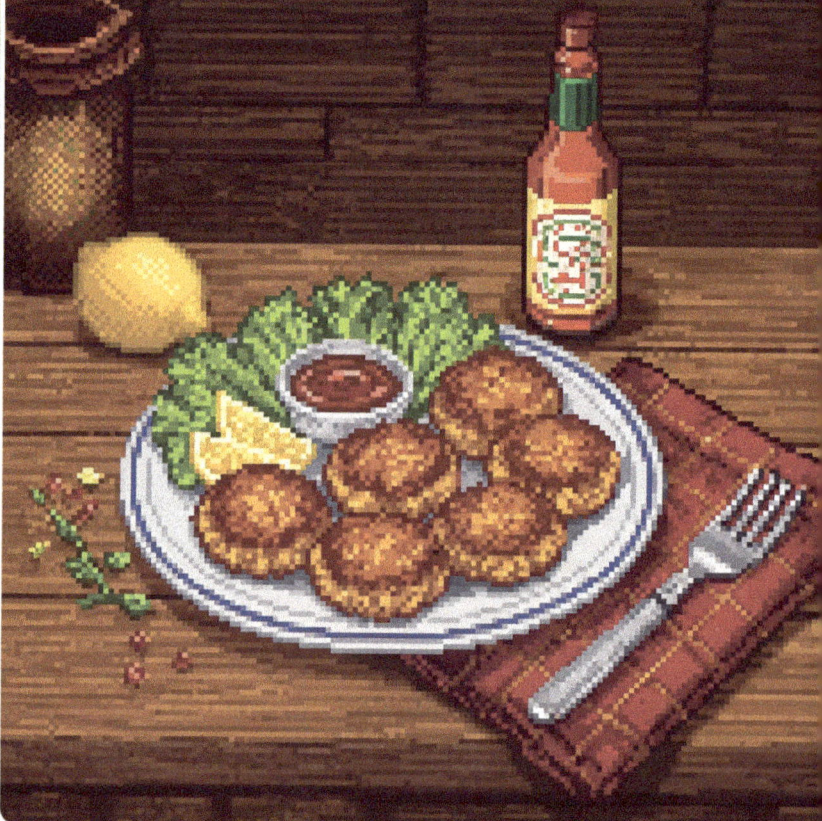

Recipe Tip

Instead of breadcrumbs, instead you may want to use saltines. Just substitute the bread crumbs for 20 saltine crackers, crushed or processed into a fine crumb. This gives the crab cakes a softer texture, and allows for a crunchier bite when seared properly. However, they are more prone to burning when you use saltines, so be careful of the heat of your pan if you choose this option.

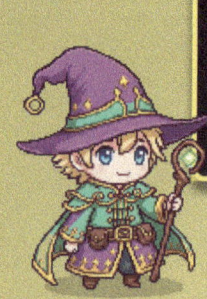

Cooking Directions

Before beginning, be sure to sift through the crab meat thoroughly and pick out any pieces of shell or cartilage, if using canned crab meat.

In a large bowl, whisk the egg, mayo, mustard, Worcestershire, and hot sauce until well blended and smooth.

In a separate bowl, fold the bread crumbs into the crab meat with a rubber spatula or wooden spoon. Add the mayo mixture to the crab meat and gently fold together.

Cover tightly with plastic wrap and refrigerate for at least 1 hour, no more than 24.

Using a measuring cup, scoop the mix into ⅓ C mounds. Lightly pack them into patties roughly 1½" thickness.

Place a large skillet (cast iron or non-stick) over Medium High heat. Add oil.

When oil is shimmering, place crab cakes gently in pan without overcrowding, working in batches if needed. Cook 3 - 4 minutes per side until browned and they reach an internal temperature of 155.

Transfer to a plate lined with paper towels to absorb excess oil before serving. Squeeze lemon wedges over cakes and serve Hot.

ADEPT

Sweet & Sour Green Beans

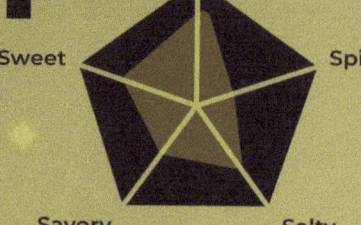

Decadent

Sweet · · Spicy

Savory · · Salty

This side dish is a tangy and savory addition to any plate, especially good with grilled pork or chicken. Be sure to let the sauce reduce in the pan, but not so much that it starts to burn. It should coat the vegetables in a glaze. Make sure to add the bacon at the very end to help ensure you have crunchy pieces throughout the dish.

Ingredients (Muffins)

Green beans, Washed & Trimmed	12 oz
White Onion, Julienne	½ C
Bacon, Cut Into 1" Pcs	3 oz
Button Mushrooms, Sliced	⅔ C
Rice Vinegar	1 Tbsp
Soy Sauce	2 tsp
White Sugar	1 ½ tsp
Ginger, Minced	½ tsp
Garlic, Minced	½ tsp
Salt	⅛ tsp
Black Pepper, Ground	⅛ tsp
Salt, For Blanching	2 tsp
Water for Blanching	
Ice Bath for Shocking	

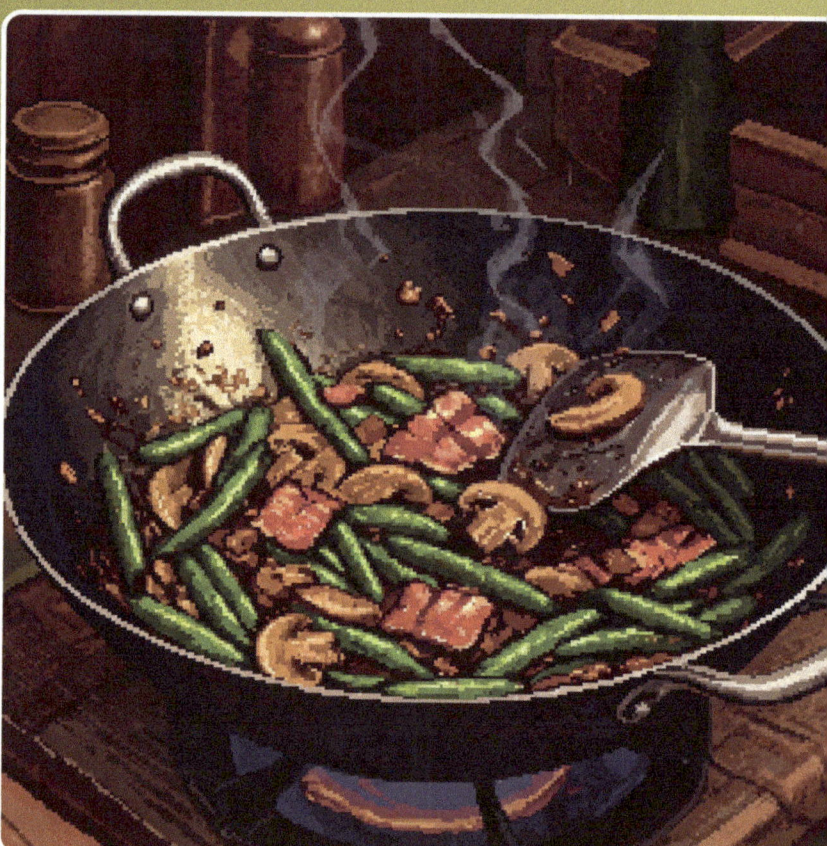

Prep Time
10 Min

Cook Time
25 - 30 Min

Servings
4 Portions

Recipe Tip

The bacon in this recipe can be substituted with any salty, flavorful meat you have on hand. Thin strips of ham, smoked turkey meat, or even Crispy Pork Belly! (Pg 213)

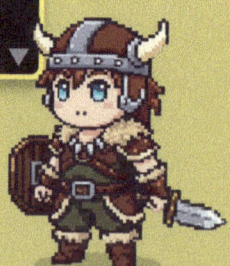

Cooking Directions

1 Fill a 4 Qt. pot with enough water to boil the green beans in so they have room to freely move. Place the pot over High heat. When the water is boiling add 2 tsp. of salt and place the green beans in the water. Boil for 3 min. While boiling, place ice cubes in a large bowl and fill with cold water. Combine the rice vinegar, sugar, salt, soy sauce pepper, ginger and garlic in a small bowl. Whisk well until the sugar is mostly dissolved.

2 Strain the green beans in a colander and transfer to the ice bath to stop the cooking process. Strain again, then remove from colander and dry thoroughly with a clean towel. Set aside.

3 Place a 12" - 14" skillet or wok over Medium heat. When hot, place the bacon pieces in the pan and cook until crispy, stirring often.

4 Remove bacon from pan and set aside. Keep the bacon grease in the pan.

5 Add the mushrooms to the pan and cook for 4 minutes, stirring occasionally.

6 Add the green beans to the pan, toss well and cook for 2 min.

7 Add the onions to the skillet and raise heat to Medium High. Cook for 2 minutes, tossing often.

8 Add the sauce to the pan, tossing thoroughly, letting it cook for about 30 seconds to reduce it and glaze the vegetables. Remove pan from heat and return bacon to pan, tossing all ingredients together. Serve Hot.

Mains

Baked Enchiladas

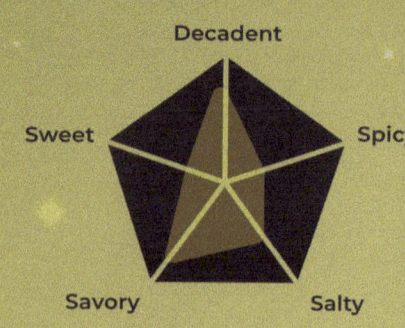

Decadent

Sweet · Spicy

Savory · Salty

This recipe has many steps, but don't be too intimidated, you've got this! Making your Ground Beef and the Enchilada sauce ahead of time will make your life much easier, and will provide you with excess ingredients for different dishes. Also, keep in mind that this recipe is delicious when using All Purpose Braised Pork (see Pg 197) or braised beef.

This recipe can be made ahead of time, up to 24 hr. in advance. Just assemble the casserole dish of enchiladas, cover with the sauce, and cover tightly before placing in the fridge. When ready to cook, cover them with the shredded cheese, cover the pan with tin foil, and bake for 40 - 45 min. at 350.

Ingredients

Restaurant Style Fluffy Beefy (Pg 117)	2 Lb
Colby Jack Cheese, Shredded	½ C
Enchilada Sauce (Pg 135)	24 Fl Oz
Bell Pepper, Diced	¾ C
White Onion, Diced	½ C
Chili Powder	2 tsp
Onion Powder	½ tsp
Cumin	½ tsp
Salt	½ tsp
Black Pepper	¼ tsp
Water	6 Fl Oz
Oil, For Sautéing	1 Tbsp
Oil, For Frying	1 C
White Corn Tortillas, 6" Wide	12 ea

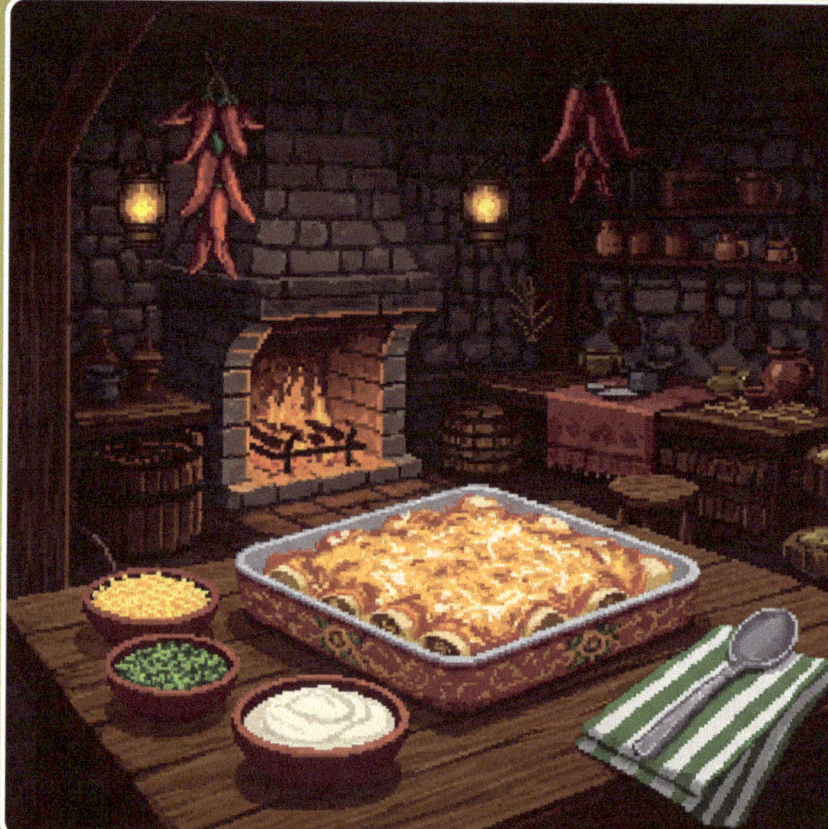

Prep Time	Cook Time	Servings
40 Min	30 Min	12 Enchiladas

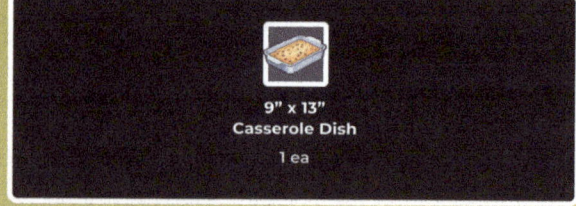

9" x 13"
Casserole Dish
1 ea

Cooking Directions

Place a small pot over Medium Low heat, add the enchilada sauce, and cover. Stir occasionally until the sauce is warmed through, then remove from heat. It doesn't need to be hot. Preheat oven to 350.

Place a large skillet over Medium High heat. When hot, add 1 Tbsp. of oil. When the oil is shimmering, add the peppers and onions. Tossing often, cook for 4 - 5 min. until they start to get soft. Place your ground beef into the pan and stir well to combine. Add your seasonings and water, stirring until the water has all been evaporated. Remove pan from heat.

Place a pot wide enough to fit the tortillas in over Medium heat and add 1 C of oil. Using a thermometer, bring the oil up to 200 and adjust the heat to hold it there.

Set up a station of the following, in a line if you can: A sheet pan to place your fried tortillas on, a bowl with about 1 ½ cups of enchilada sauce in it, a bowl full of the ground beef filling, a plate to roll your enchiladas on, and the 9" x 13" baking dish for your enchiladas.

Place a tortilla in the oil and fry for 3 sec. then flip with a pair of tongs, and fry for 3 more seconds. Carefully remove from the oil, let the excess drip off, and set it on the pan to rest. Do this with ½ of the tortillas.

> > > > CONTINUED > > > >

6   Take a slightly fried tortilla, once cooled enough to handle, and coat it on both sides with enchilada sauce. Place the tortilla on the plate, and use a large spoon to scoop 2 - 3 spoonfuls of the beef onto the tortilla. Gently roll the tortilla up and wrap it around the filling. Place it in the casserole dish. Repeat steps 5 and 6 until all the tortillas are filled. Make sure to place the enchiladas so they are touching, but aren't mashed together.

7   Once the pan is filled, pour the remaining enchilada sauce evenly over your enchiladas. Next, distribute the shredded cheese evenly over them. Cover tightly with tin foil.

8   Bake for 30 min. until the cheese is melted and the enchilada sauce is bubbling. Remove from oven and let rest, covered, for 5 min. before serving.

Recipe Tip

With the leftover ingredients, try out an enchilada omelet or breakfast scramble, or maybe make a batch of Hot Water Crust dough (Pg 165) and make some Central American inspired meat pies.

▼

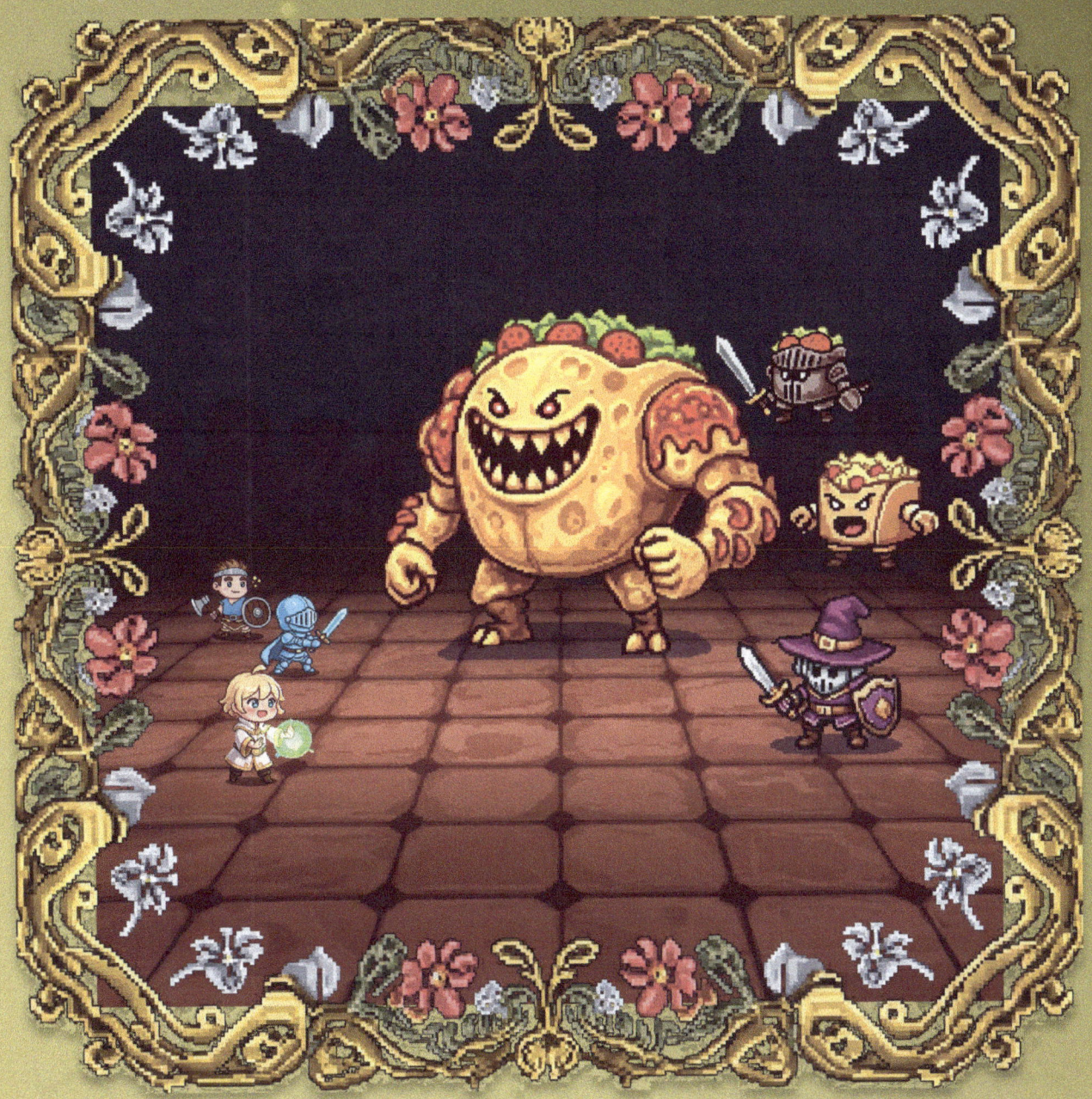

Baked Mac & Cheese

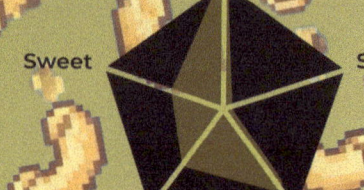

Decadent

Sweet

Spicy

Savory

Salty

This recipe is a favorite of all ages, and it's challenging both in practice and in theory. The largest potential hang up you should be wary of is not whisking enough when adding the cheese. Keeping the cheese moving will make sure that it blends into the sauce evenly, and won't form lumps.

Try this recipe out with various additions to the sauce. Some fresh peas, pieces of grilled chicken, or even seasoned pumpkin puree (like you would use for the Pumpkin Cream Sauce, see Pg 249) will elevate this already decadent dish.

Ingredients (Pasta & Sauce)

Macaroni Pasta, Uncooked	12 oz
Butter/Olive Oil	4 Tbsp
AP Flour	3 Tbsp
Salt, For Sauce	½ tsp
White (Or Black) Pepper	¼ tsp
Garlic, Minced	2 tsp
Nutmeg, Ground	¼ tsp
Milk	18 Fl Oz
Heavy Cream	10 Fl Oz
Extra Sharp Cheddar, Shredded	4 C
Salt, For Pasta Water	1 Tbsp

Ingredients (Bread Crumbs)

Panko	1 ½ C
Parsley, Dry	1 tsp
Butter, Melted/Olive Oil	2 Tbsp

Prep Time
15 Min

Cook Time
35 Min

Servings
9" x 13" Dish

**9" x 13"
Casserole Dish**

1 ea

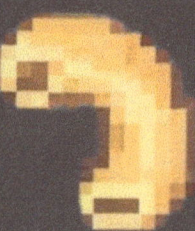

Cooking Directions

1 Preheat your oven to 350, making sure a rack is in the middle of the oven.

2 Fill a 6 Qt. pot ⅔ full with water and place over High heat. When boiling, add 1 Tbsp. of salt to the water and then cook pasta according to box directions, usually 10 min. When done cooking, reserve 2 Tbsp. of the pasta water before straining, then strain and set aside.

3 In a small bowl, combine the panko, parsley, and melted butter/oil. Stir together with a fork. Set aside.

4 While the pasta is cooking, get started on your sauce. Place a 12" - 14" skillet over Medium heat. When hot, add the 4 Tbsp. of butter/oil.

5 When the butter stops bubbling/the oil starts shimmering add the flour. Stirring constantly, cook for 2 min. to bring it to the Blanc Stage.

6 Add the garlic, salt, pepper, and nutmeg. Cook for 1 min. more.

7 Slowly add 8 oz. of the milk and whisk well, making sure to work out any lumps in your roux. Slowly add the remaining milk, then the heavy cream, and reserved pasta water. Whisk until the roux is completely combined.

8 Once bubbling, reduce the heat to Medium Low and cook or 5 - 7 min. until it thickens and coats the back of a spoon (nappe).

9 Add ½ of the cheese, stirring constantly, and mix until fully melted and combined. Remove from heat. Add the strained pasta to the sauce and stir carefully to coat all the noodles. Transfer ½ of the mix to a 9" x 13" casserole dish, sprinkle 1 C of the cheese over the pasta, then add the remaining pasta and sprinkle the remaining cheese over it. Top with your reserved bread crumbs.

10 Place in the oven on the middle rack and bake until the bread crumbs are golden brown and the cheese sauce is bubbling, 20 - 25 min. Remove from oven and let cool for 5 - 10 min. before serving.

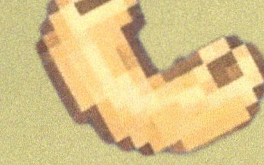

Recipe Tip

You can substitute the Panko for your own breadcrumbs by blending 4 slices of partially dried bread in a food processor. The homemade bread crumbs are an excellent addition, providing unique texture to the dish, but panko crumbs also work well.

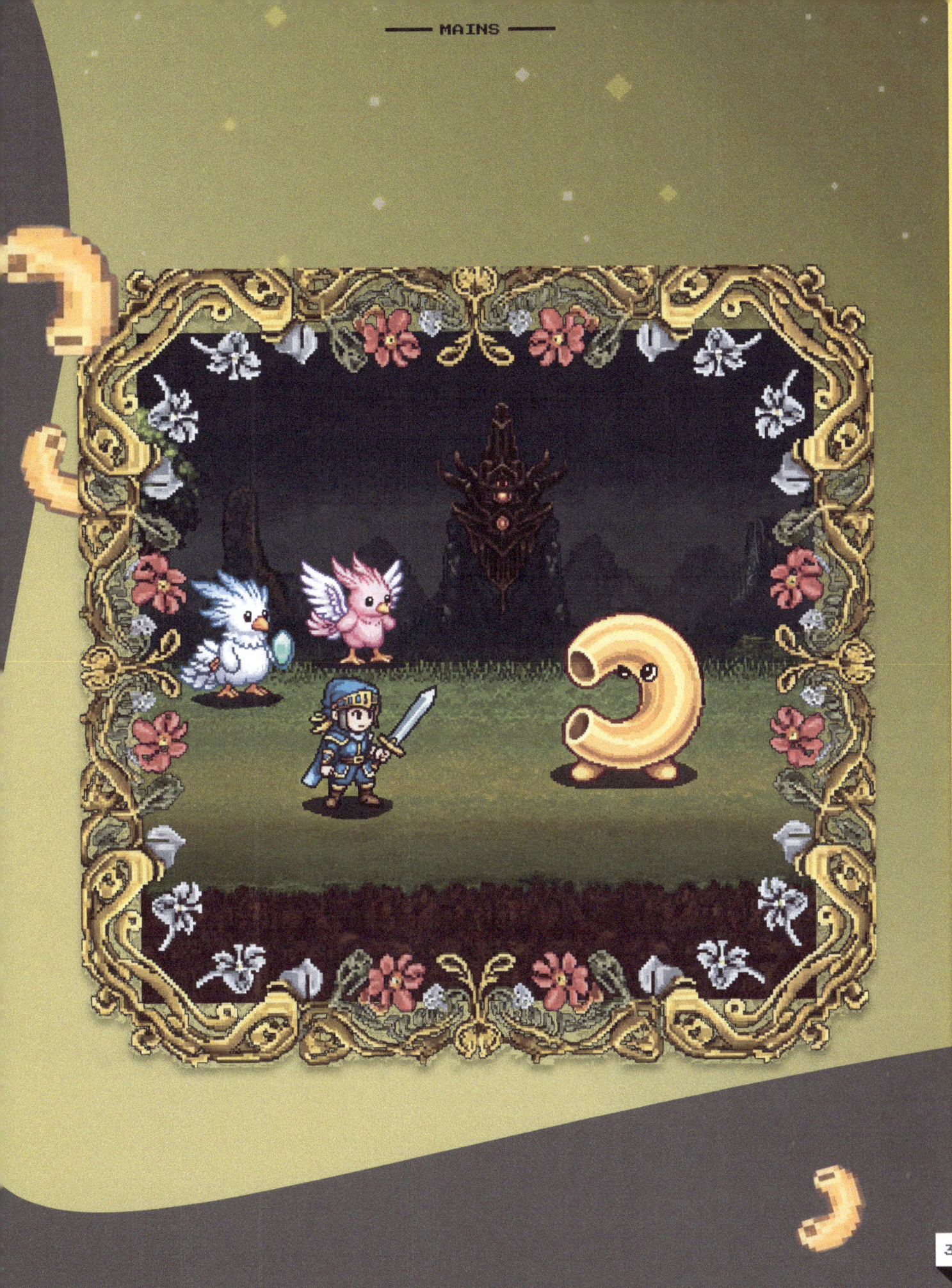

Chicken Cordon Bleu with Mustard Cream

This classic French dish is well known and for good reason! I've provided instructions for both stove top and oven cooking in case your largest skillet doesn't have a lid, or you are making a large batch of this recipe for a gathering. The delicate profile of this dish is what makes it so unique. It's simultaneously rich and light, the ham and Swiss working well with the mustard sauce.

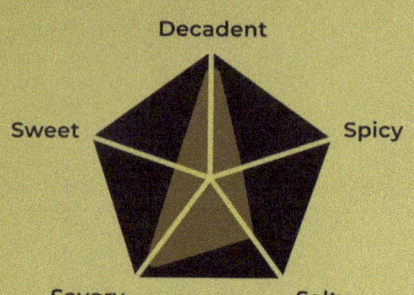

Decadent

Sweet

Spicy

Savory

Salty

Ingredients (Muffins)

Chicken Breasts, Boneless Skinless	4 ea
Swiss Cheese, Deli Slices	4 ea
Ham, Deli Slices	4 ea
White Wine (Chardonnay)	6 Fl Oz
Heavy Cream	8 Fl Oz
Dijon Mustard	2 Tbsp
Butter	6 Tbsp
Garlic, Minced	2 tsp
Salt	¼ tsp
Black Pepper, Ground	⅛ tsp
Paprika	2 tsp
AP Flour	3 Tbsp
Cornstarch	2 tsp

Prep Time	Cook Time	Servings
20 Min	35 Min	4 Portions

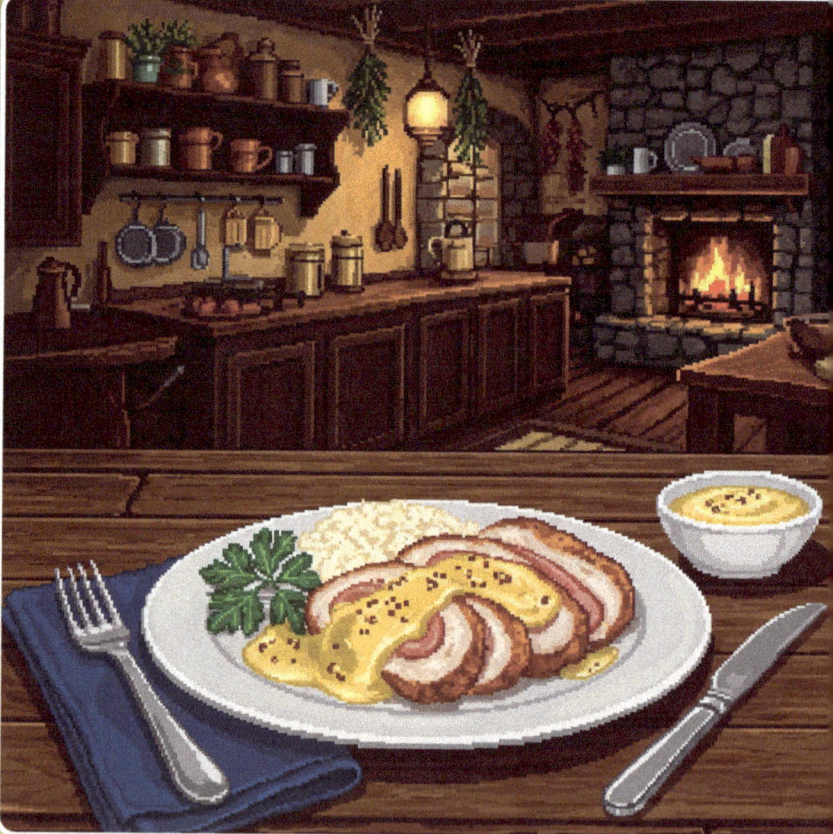

ADEPT

Cooking Directions
(Stove Top)

1   Starting at the side of the breast, cut it nearly in half, stopping just before the knife completely separates the halves and fold the top half over so the chicken breast now looks like a heart. This action is called butterflying. Do this to all 4 of the chicken breasts.

2   Evenly space them apart on the cutting board and cover the whole board with a piece of plastic wrap large enough to tuck both ends under the cutting board. Using a mallet or small frying pan, gently pound each piece 8 - 10 times, widening and thinning them.

3   Remove the plastic wrap, and lay down a slice of Swiss cheese, then a slice of ham, leaving about ½ an inch of chicken uncovered. Fold the chicken back together and press gently to help them hold the shape.

4   Combine the flour, paprika, salt, and pepper in a bowl large enough fit one of the chicken pieces. One at a time, carefully place each chicken piece in the flour mix and flip it over to evenly coat, gently shaking off excess flour before setting on a plate.

5   Place a 12" - 14" skillet (with lid preferred) over Medium High heat. Add the butter.

6   When the butter stops bubbling, place the pieces of chicken in the pan and cook for 2 - 3 min. per side so that both sides are well browned.

〉〉〉〉 CONTINUED 〉〉〉〉

7   Once browned, add the garlic and wine; bring to a simmer. Once you can no longer smell the alcohol coming off the wine, cover the pan and reduce heat to Low. Cook until the juices run clear and the center of the piece temps at 165, usually 20 min.

8   When chicken is done cooking, transfer onto a plate and tent with foil. Raise the heat for your pan to Medium High and scrape up any brown bits stuck to the pan (the fond).

9   Mix the cornstarch into the heavy cream. Once the wine is simmering, slowly add your heavy cream, stirring throughout. Bring to a simmer and add the mustard along with a pinch of salt and pepper to the pan. Stir to fully incorporate.

10 Simmer and reduce the sauce until it coats the back of a spoon thickly (nappe), 4 - 5 min.

11 Uncover the chicken, place one on each plate, and generously apply your Mustard Cream sauce. Serve Hot.

Cooking Directions (Oven)

1   Follow the previous steps 1 - 6. Preheat oven to 350 making sure there is a rack in the center of the oven. When done browning the chicken, remove the pan from the heat and transfer browned chicken pieces to a baking tray lined with foil.

⟩ ⟩ ⟩ ⟩ CONTINUED ⟩ ⟩ ⟩ ⟩

2   Cover the chicken with foil and place in the oven on the center rack. Cook for 25 - 30 min. until juices are running clear and the center of several pieces temp at 165.

3   Once the chicken is fully cooked, remove the tray from the oven and leave covered.

4   While the chicken is baking, take the pan you browned the chicken in and place it over Medium High heat. Let heat for about 30 sec. then add the wine, and scrape up any brown bits stuck to the bottom of the pan (the fond).

5   Bring to a simmer and follow the previous steps 9 - 11. Serve Hot.

Recipe Tip

You can use stone ground mustard instead of Dijon, if you prefer, just note that you may need to use less salt due to the fact that stone ground mustard is sharper, and usually has more sodium in it.

Chicken Tikka Masala

This dish is a healthy and delicious option for anyone who wants a hearty meal with plenty of leftovers. The vegetable medley is an optional ingredient if you prefer your curry to be a bit more filled out. The vegetables add a nice texture difference, and are a way to improve both the density and health of the dish.

Decadent

Sweet

Spicy

Savory

Salty

Ingredients

Chicken Breast, 1" Cubes	3 C
Garlic, Minced	2 tsp
Ginger, Minced	2 tsp
Yellow Onion, Small Dice	¾ C
Cayenne	½ tsp
Cumin	1 Tbsp
Cinnamon, Ground	½ tsp
Turmeric	½ tsp
Cardamom, Ground	½ tsp
Garam Masala	1 tsp
Paprika	2 tsp
Salt	1 tsp
White Sugar	1 Tbsp
Butter Or Ghee	3 Tbsp
Tomato Sauce, Canned	14 Fl Oz
Heavy Cream	8 Fl Oz
Frozen Vegetable Medley, Thawed	¾ C
Oven Baked Rice (Pg 89)	

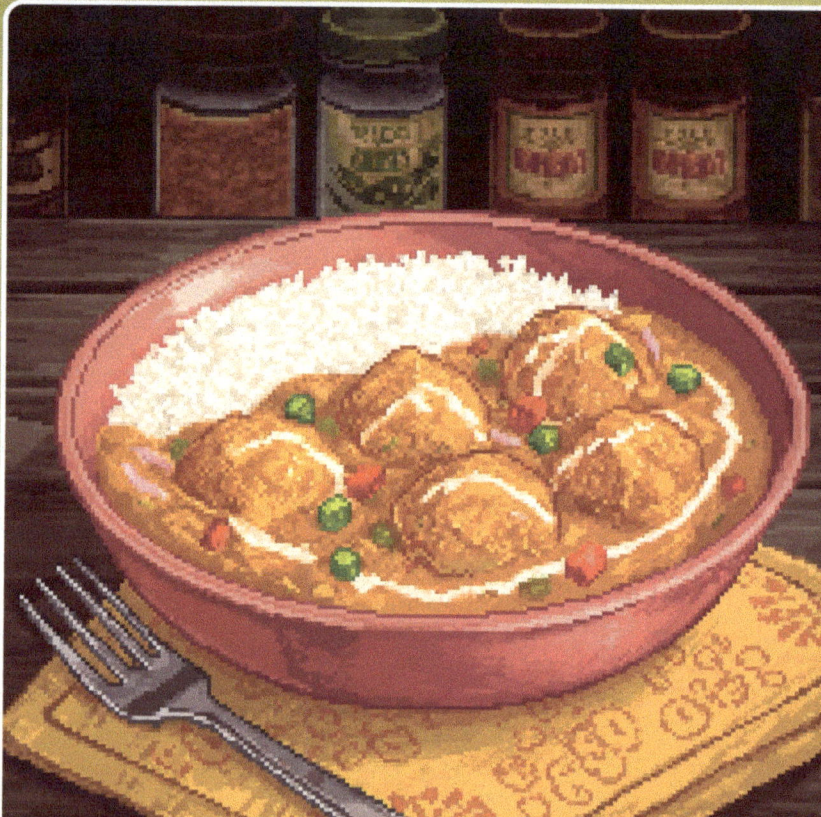

Prep Time
20 Min

Cook Time
40 - 50 Min

Servings
4 - 6 Portions

Recipe Tip

When you make the rice to be served with this dish, try adding some whole cardamom pods or other spices to give the rice a fragrant and earthy taste that'll compliment your curry nicely.

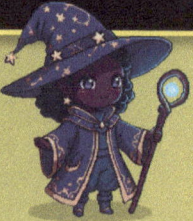

Cooking Directions

1. Place a large skillet (at least 3" deep) over Medium heat. Add 1½ Tbsp. of butter or ghee.

2. When butter stops bubbling, or ghee is shimmering, add the chicken pieces. Cook for 4 minutes, stirring halfway through. Remove chicken from pan and set aside.

3. Add the remaining butter or ghee. When the butter stops bubbling, or ghee is shimmering, add the onion. Cook until translucent, about 5 min.

4. Add garlic and ginger, cook until fragrant about 1 min. Next, add all the spices and stir well. Cook for 2 min.

5. Add tomato sauce, stir well and bring to a simmer. Reduce heat to Low and cook, uncovered, for 10 minutes.

6. Add the cream and the sugar, stir well, and raise heat back to Medium. Bring to a simmer. Cook uncovered, stirring often until thickened, 10 min.

7. Return the chicken and their juices to the sauce. Add the vegetable medley, if using, and stir well. Reduce the heat to Low and cover. Cook for 10 - 12 min. until chicken is fully cooked (internal temperature of 165).

8. Remove the lid and cook for 5 min. to reduce to nappe.

9. Taste test, adjusting the salt and sugar as desired. Serve Hot over ¾ - 1 C of Oven Baked Rice.

Creamy Shrimp Scampi

Decadent

Sweet

Spicy

Savory

Salty

This recipe is a quick meal that requires little preparation ahead of time. You can elevate the recipe slightly by using fresh herbs instead of dry ones, just be mindful that you need to use a 3:1 ratio of fresh herbs to dry for the same flavor effect. This increase in volume will necessitate using slightly more liquid ingredients to make sure you have the right amount of sauce for your shrimp and pasta. Remember, you aren't looking for the dish to be swimming in sauce, just enough to make sure that the pasta and shrimp are well coated.

Ingredients

Shrimp, Peeled & Deveined, 26 - 30 Ct	½ Lb
Spaghetti/Linguine	8 oz
White Wine (Pinot Grigio)	⅓ C
Heavy Cream	4 Fl Oz
Yellow Onion, Minced	2 Tbsp
Garlic, Minced	1 tsp
Lemon Juice	1 Tbsp
Parsley Dry	½ tsp
Basil, Dry	⅛ tsp
Oregano, Dry	⅛ tsp
Red Pepper Flakes	⅛ tsp
Black Pepper, Ground	⅛ tsp
Salt, For Sauce	⅛ tsp
Olive Oil	1½ Tbsp
Parmesan Cheese, Grated	2 Tbsp
Salt, For Pasta Water	2 Tbsp

Prep Time	Cook Time	Servings
5 - 10 Min	15 Min	3 - 4 Bowls

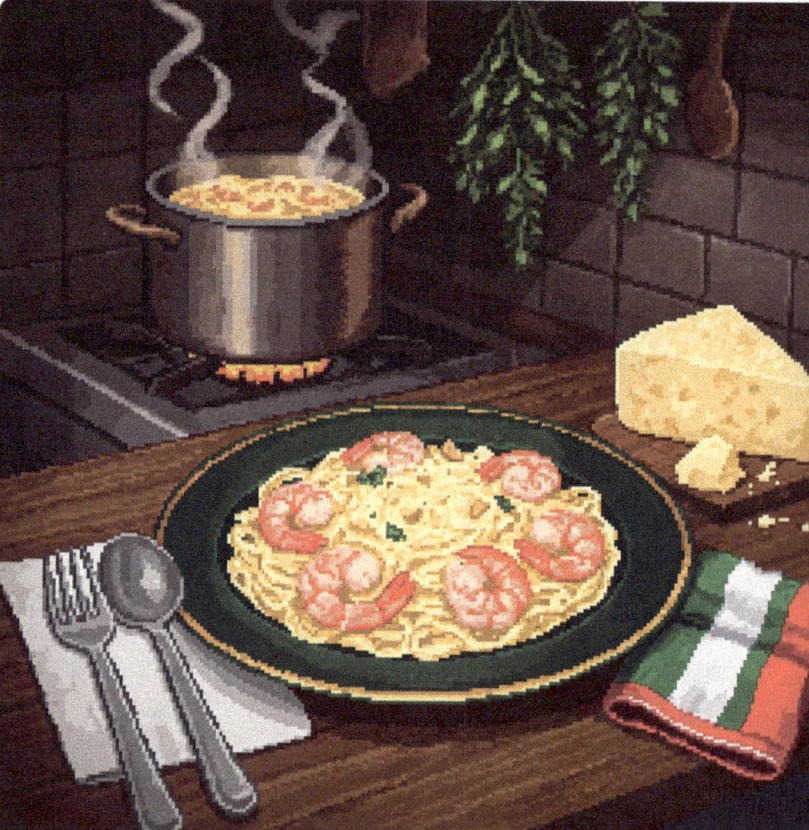

Cooking Directions

1   Fill a 6 Qt. pot ⅔ full with water and place over High heat. Place a 12" - 14" skillet over Medium High heat. Add the olive oil.

2   When the oil begins to shimmer, place the shrimp in the pan. Cook for 2 - 3 minutes per side until the shrimp are pink and springy. Remove from pan and set side.

3   Reduce the heat to Medium and add the onion to the pan. Stirring constantly, cook for 2 min. Then add the garlic and cook for 1 min. more.

4   Add the wine and bring to a simmer. Reduce the wine for 2 min. making sure that all the alcohol is cooked out. Next, add the remaining ingredients except the heavy cream and parmesan. Continue to cook for 2 more minutes, then reduce heat to Low.

5   When the water is boiling add 2 Tbsp. of salt to the water. Add the pasta and cook following the box instructions. If you are using your own homemade pasta, it will only take 3 - 4 min. for al dente.

6   When the pasta is nearly done cooking, with about 4 min. remaining, raise the heat to Medium High under your sauce pan and add the heavy cream. Bring it to a simmer, and cook until it coats the back of a spoon (nappé).

7   When the pasta is done, transfer 2 Tbsp. of the pasta water into the sauce along with the parmesan, stir well and then strain the pasta.

8   Return the shrimp to the pan, toss to coat, then transfer the pasta to the pan. Toss/stir well to coat fully. Remove the pan from heat. Serve immediately.

Herbed Chicken Hash

Decadent

Sweet

Spicy

Savory

Salty

This dish works well both as a quick dinner option and as a delightful brunch offering. Don't be deceived by the short list of directions; this dish requires finesse and proper timing. But you can do it!

This dish is elevated with the application of hot sauce or malted vinegar after cooking. Or try placing cheese on top during the last step of cooking or an Over Easy egg on top once in the bowl. Or all three!

Ingredients

Chicken Thighs, ½" Pcs	3 ea
Red Potatoes, Small Dice	2 C
Bell Pepper, Diced	½ C
Red Onion, Diced	½ C
Paprika	½ Tbsp
Garlic Powder	¼ tsp
Rosemary, Dry	⅛ tsp
Sage, Ground	¼ tsp
Parsley, Dry	⅛ tsp
Black Pepper, Ground	⅛ tsp
Salt	¼ tsp
Neutral Oil	3 Tbsp

Prep Time	Cook Time	Servings
15 Min	30 - 35 Min	4 Portions

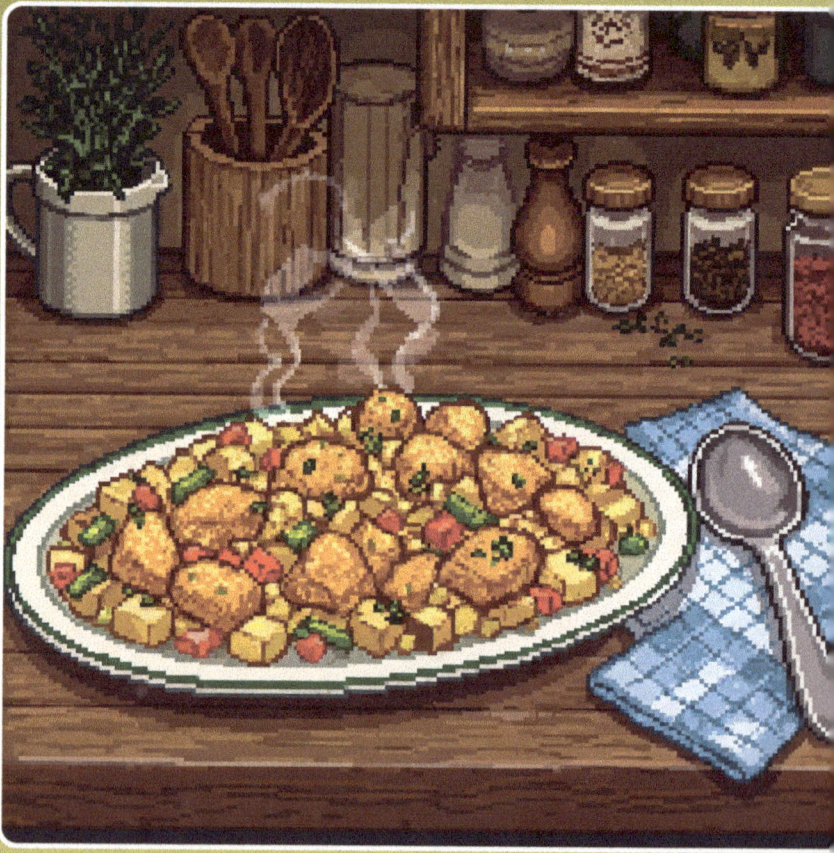

Recipe Tip

You can use fresh herbs instead of dry, however when you do consider altering the rule of a 3:1 ratio. Try a 2:1 ratio, otherwise it may give your hash an overwhelming flavor.

Cooking Directions

1 Set a large cast iron skillet over Medium heat. When hot, add 1 Tbsp. of oil. When shimmering, add the chicken pieces. Cook for 5 - 8 min. stirring occasionally until fully cooked. Remove from pan and set aside.

2 Add remaining oil to pan. When shimmering, add the potatoes and cook for 10 min. stirring occasionally, until browning begins.

3 Add the bell pepper, cook until soft. Next add the onion and the seasonings and stir well. Cook for 10 - 15 min. more, until potatoes are soft.

4 Return the chicken to the pan and stir well. Cook for 3 - 5 minutes, until all ingredients are heated evenly. Serve Hot.

Pumpkin Pasta with Candied Prosciutto and Walnuts

Decadent

Sweet

Spic

Savory

Salty

Having to make two recipes for one dish means you need to be on top of your Mis en place. Remember: having all your ingredients measured out and ready to use before you begin is the key to successful cooking.

The salty-sweetness of the candied nuts and prosciutto is a wonderful compliment to the creamy earthiness of the pumpkin sauce. Add more cayenne if you like a real kick, but keep in mind that the heat is not the focus of the dish, it is merely an accent to the flavors.

Ingredients (Muffins)

Macaroni Or Rigatoni, Uncooked	12 oz
Prosciutto Slices, Torn Into Lg Pcs	3 oz
Pumpkin Cream Sauce (Pg 249)	16 Fl Oz
Walnut Halves	½ C
Brown Sugar	2 Tbsp
Cayenne Pepper	⅛ tsp
Salt, For Pasta Water	2 T
Butter	½ Tbsp
Parmesan Cheese, Grated	2 Tbsp

Prep Time	Cook Time	Servings
15 Min	15 - 20 Min	4 Portions

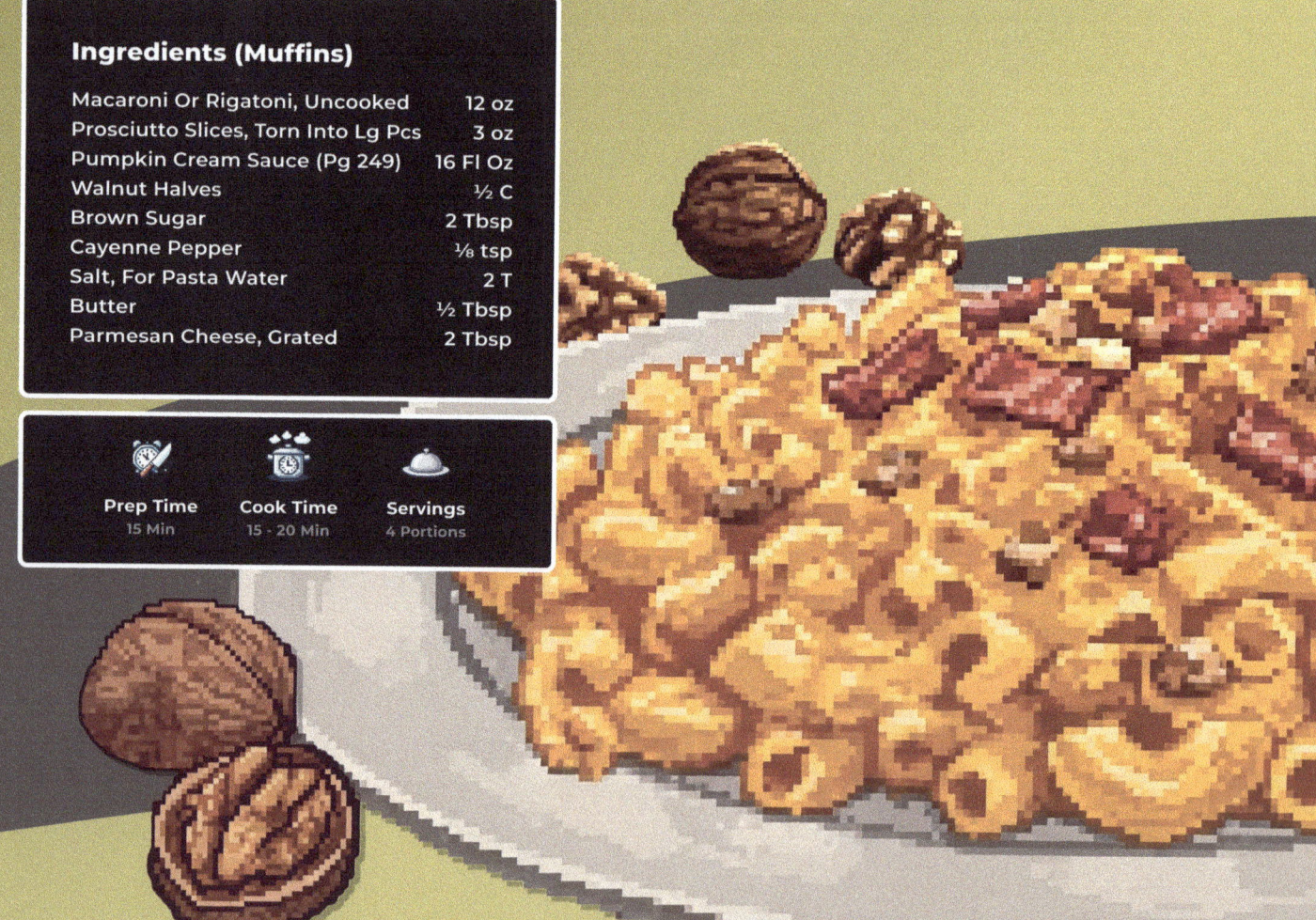

Cooking Directions

1 Place a nonstick 10" - 12" skillet over Medium heat. Line a baking sheet with parchment paper. When skillet is hot, add the butter.

2 When the butter stops bubbling, add the prosciutto pieces and cook for 1 - 2 min. Next, add the cayenne, sugar, and walnuts to the pan. Stirring constantly, cook until the sugar has melted, usually 5 - 7 min.

3 Once the walnuts and prosciutto are completely coated, immediately transfer them to the lined baking sheet and use a rubber spatula to separate them into small clumps. Working fast is essential at this stage, as the glaze will start hardening right away. Set aside and let cool.

4 Fill a 6 Qt. pot ⅔ of the way with water and place over High heat. Next, place a 12" - 14" skillet over Medium heat and make the Pumpkin Cream Sauce according to the recipe instructions while the water is heating up. If you made it a day in advance, gently heat it back up to simmering over Medium Low heat.

5 When the water is boiling, add 2 Tbsp. of salt to the pot. Then add your pasta and cook according to the box instructions, usually 10 min. or so. Think about your timing, and have the cream sauce made and being held over Low heat when your pasta is done cooking.

6 Before straining the pasta, add 1 - 2 Tbsp. of the pasta water to the sauce, whisking it in quickly. Strain the pasta well, then add to the pan. Sprinkle the parmesan over the pasta before stirring together; this helps your sauce stick to your pasta.

7 To serve, portion out the pasta into 4 separate bowls then top with ¼ of the candied nut and prosciutto clumps. Enjoy!

Roasted Pork Loin with Cinnamon Apples

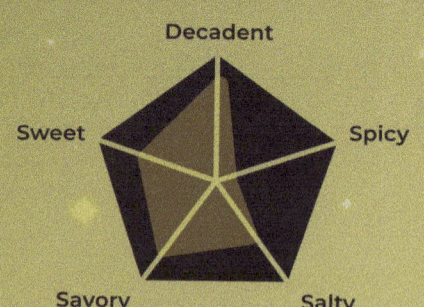

Decadent

Sweet

Spicy

Savory

Salty

Pork and Cinnamon Apples is a combination from most people's childhood memories, so making it for yourself now is a great way to bring some comfort. Try using a variety of spices and seasonings with both the pork and the apples to alter the dish. Maybe take things in a South Asian direction by adding elements of your preferred curry powder blends? Or use mace and paprika to give it an African influence? It's a versatile dish that won't disappoint.

Ingredients

2 - 2 ½ Lb Pork Loin	1 ea
Large, Firm Apples	4 ea
White Sugar	1 C
Cinnamon	1 Tbsp
Nutmeg	¼ tsp
Ginger, Ground	¼ tsp
Apple Cider Vinegar	1 Tbsp
Butter	2 Tbsp
Water	¼ C
Neutral Oil	2 Tbsp
Salt and Pepper For Pork	

Prep Time
25 Min

Cook Time
1 Hr 30 Min

Servings
8 Portions

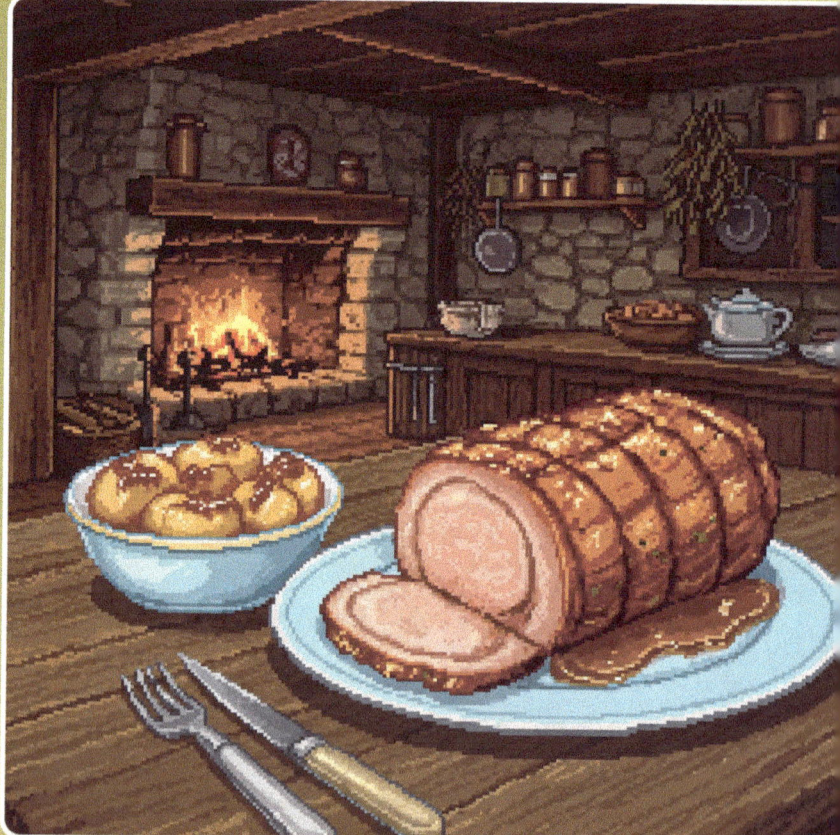

Cooking Directions

1   Preheat your oven to 350. Line a baking tray/roasting pan with foil and place a wire rack in the tray, if available.

2   Place a 12" - 14" skillet/pot over **High** heat. Add the oil and when it's shimmering, place the pork loin in the skillet/pot. Sear for 2 - 3 min. per side excluding the side with the fat cap on it. Remove pan from heat and transfer the pork to your prepared baking tray/roasting pan. Sprinkle generously with salt and pepper.

3   When preheated, place pork in oven and cook for 20-30 min. per pound. In this instance, for 1½ - 2 hr. Rotate the pan 180 degrees halfway through.

4   While pork is cooking, peel and core the apples. Cut the apples into pieces of desired size (I recommend a large dice) and set aside.

5   Place a 1 Qt. pot over Medium heat. When hot, add the butter. When butter stops bubbling, add your spices and stir to incorporate. Cook for 1 - 2 min. Raise heat to Medium High, add apples, sugar and water. Stir well to combine and keep stirring until sugar is dissolved.

6   Bring to a simmer and reduce the heat to Low. Cook, uncovered, for 10 min. until the apples are soft and the syrup is thickened to heavily coat the back of a spoon (nappe). Cover and hold on lowest heat setting until ready to use.

7   When the pork reaches an internal temperature of 140 remove from the oven. Let rest for 10 min. before transferring to a cutting board and slicing into 8 evenly thick pieces. The resting time is when 'Carry-Over Cooking' happens, and the internal temperature will continue to rise to reach the required 145, so it's important to not cut the pork until then. Top with apples when serving.

314

Steak Au Poivre

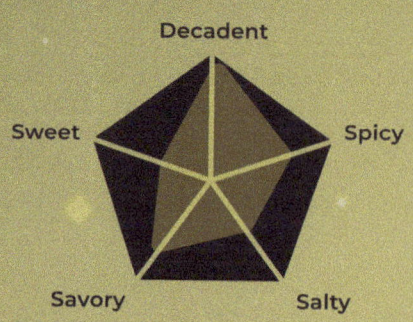

Decadent

Sweet

Spicy

Savory

Salty

This classic dish is not made very often any more, which is a real shame. It's timeless and delicious, and a simple way to elevate a home dining experience. Serve with roasted garlic mashed potatoes, couscous, or any starch that will help you enjoy the sauce as much as possible. Any vegetable side will pair with this dish, blistered green beans being my favorite.

When choosing which steaks you want for this dish, keep in mind that tougher cuts will need to be tenderized before cooking. While filets, strips, and rib-eyes are best served between Rare and Medium, cuts such as skirt steak or chuck eye benefit from cooking a bit longer, Medium to Medium-Well.

Ingredients

6 oz. Steaks (Filet or Strip)	2 ea
Brandy	4 Fl Oz
Heavy Cream	8 Fl Oz
Butter	2 Tbsp
Beef Stock	¼ C
Salt	½ tsp
Whole Peppercorns	2 Tbsp

Prep Time	Cook Time	Servings
10 Min	10 - 15 Min	2 Steaks

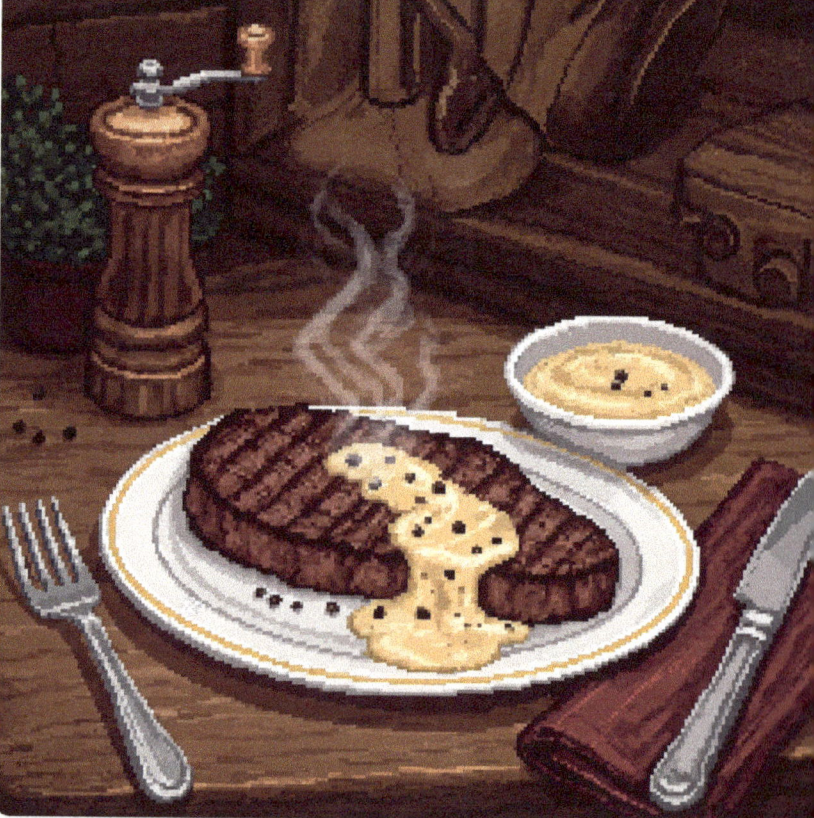

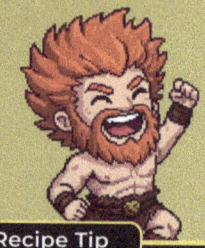

Recipe Tip

The larger your piece of beef, the more peppercorns and sauce you'll need. This recipe is for 6 oz. steaks, so use it as a baseline for figuring out how you need to scale the recipe for your cuts.

Cooking Directions

1 Preheat oven to 170. Place the peppercorns in a plastic bag and crush into small pieces with a pan or mallet. Once crushed, transfer them to a plate. Pat the steaks dry with a paper towel then press both sides into the crushed peppercorns. Reserve any extra pepper.

2 Place a 12" - 14" skillet over Medium High heat. Melt the butter in the pan; when the butter stops bubbling and smokes slightly place the steaks in the pan.

3 Cook to desired doneness. See the chart on Pg 386 for proper cooking temps.

4 Remove the steaks from the pan, set on plates, and place in oven to hold. Raise the heat on the stove to High, add the beef stock and scrape all the browned bits (the fond) off the bottom of the pan. Add the cognac away from the heat source, and carefully ignite with a long lighter after about 5 seconds. This part involves flame, so make sure there's nothing near you that might catch fire. Don't be afraid, so long as you maintain a firm hold on the pan and don't panic, it'll all be fine. When flames reduce or go out, return the pan to the heat.

5 Once all the flames dissipate, add the cream, salt, and remaining pepper. Lower the heat to Medium. Whisking frequently, reduce the sauce until it coats the back of a spoon (nappe).

6 Remove pan from heat. Remove the steaks from the oven. Careful, the plates may be hot. Cover the steaks evenly with the sauce and serve.

Steak Diane

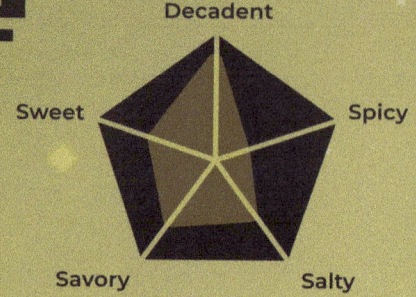

Decadent

Sweet

Spicy

Savory

Salty

This is another classic dish that's not made very often anymore. It's a simple but elegant dish that will elevate any at-home date night or special event. Serve with roasted potatoes, roasted vegetables, or on its own as part of a multiple course meal.

As with the 'Steak Au Poivre' recipe, you can use a variety of cuts of beef for this dish, the important thing is that the steaks are pounded thinly. Eye of Round steaks are a good alternative to Filet Mignon, as they are lean and easily tenderized.

Ingredients

6 oz. Steaks	4 ea
Mushroom, Sliced	⅓ C
Brandy	8 Fl Oz
Garlic, Minced	1 tsp
Butter	1 Tbsp
Neutral Oil	1 Tbsp
Cornstarch Slurry	1 Tbsp
Dijon Mustard	2 tsp
Salt & Pepper For Steaks	

Prep Time	Cook Time	Servings
10 - 15 Min	15 Min	4 Steaks

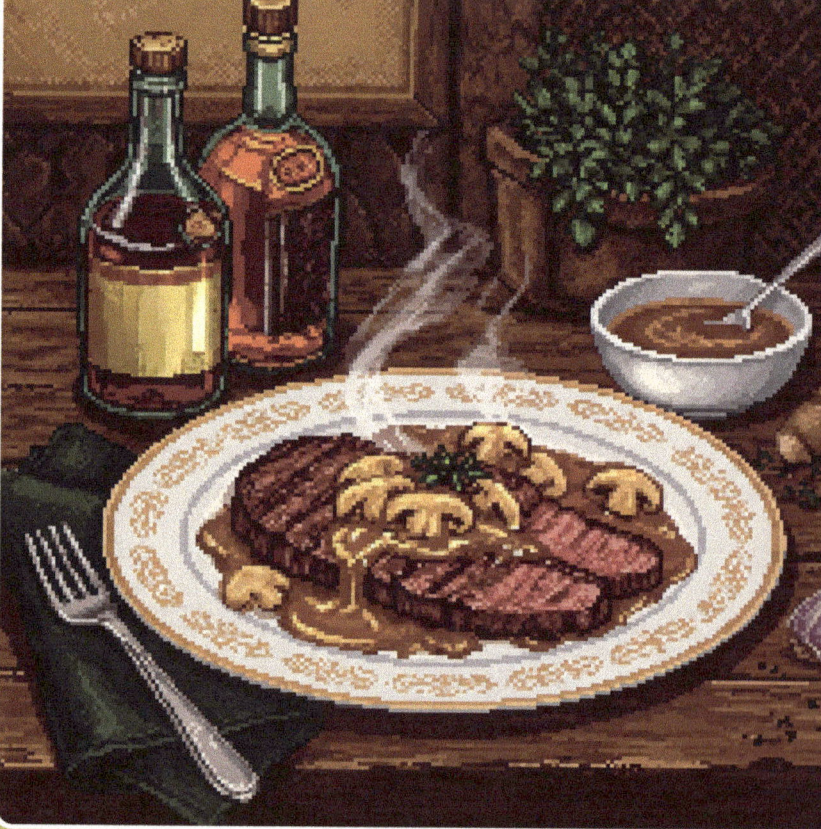

Recipe Tip

It's advised that you stay away from cuts like chuck and flank steak for this dish. The steaks are meant to be Medium Well; those cuts do benefit from being cooked to a higher level of doneness but they won't have the time needed to break down the fat and connective tissue in them.

Cooking Directions

1   Pound the steaks so that they are roughly ⅜" - ½" thick, as evenly as possible.

2   Heat a 12" - 14" skillet over Medium High heat, add the butter and oil. Salt and pepper the steaks generously.

3   When the butter mix stops bubbling and is slightly smoking place the steaks in the pan. Cook for 1 - 2 min. per side. Remove from pan and set aside.

4   Add the mushrooms to the pan and cook for 2 - 3 min. then add the garlic and cook for 1 min. more.

5   Remove the pan from the heat, and add the cognac/ brandy to the pan. Ignite the fumes with a long lighter carefully. There will be a fair amount of flames when you do this, but that's ok. So long as you don't panic and maintain a firm hold on the pan, it'll be alright.

6   When the flames reduce in size, return the pan to heat. When the fire is out, add the mustard and stir well.

7   Next, add the slurry slowly, stirring constantly, to thicken so it coats the back of a spoon (nappe).

8   Place the steaks back in the pan and turn off the heat. Let the steaks sit in the pan for 45 - 60 sec. to warm them up. Turn to coat both sides in the sauce and place on plates. Evenly distribute the sauce over the 4 steaks. Serve Hot.

Dressings
& Sauces

ADEPT

Cherry Bordelaise

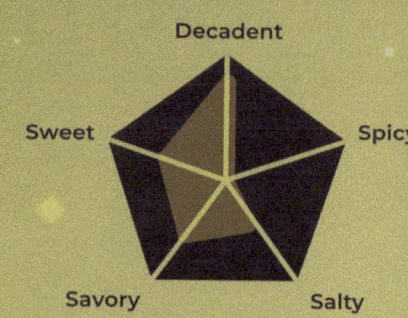

Decadent

Sweet

Spicy

Savory

Salty

This unctuous, slightly sweet, sauce is a great pairing for beef or poultry. Combining half of the wine and stock with the roux and letting that reduce is how you bring out those latent flavors in the wine and help them shine. Adding the butter at the very end (known as 'monter au beurre', literally 'mount with butter') gives the sauce a keen sheen and a lovely mouthfeel.

Mother Sauce: Demi-Glace

Ingredients

Dark Cherries, Pitted, Chopped	½ C
Stock (Beef Or Vegetable)	16 Fl Oz
Red wine	16 Fl Oz
Salt	¼ tsp
Black Pepper, Ground	⅛ tsp
Thyme, Dry	⅛ tsp
AP Flour	4 Tbsp
Butter	4 Tbsp
Butter, Room Temp (For Finishing)	½ Tbsp

Prep Time
10 Min

Cook Time
20 Min

Servings
24 oz

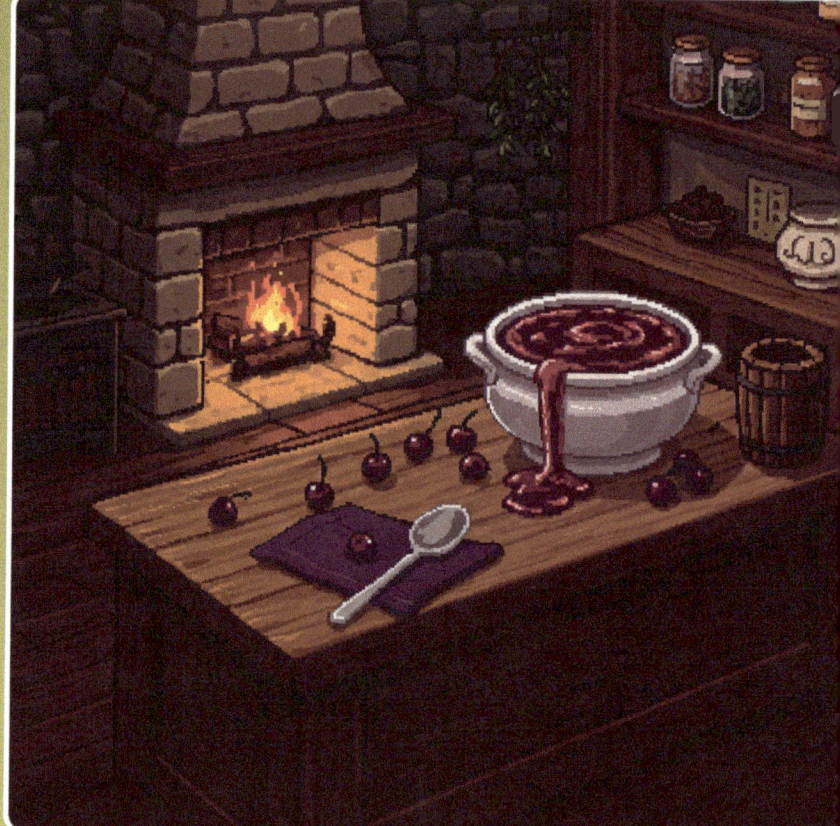

Cooking Directions

1 Place a 1 Qt. pot over Medium heat. When hot, add the butter.

2 When the butter stops bubbling add the cherries.
   Cook for 2 min. until the cherries are slightly soft.

3 Add the seasonings and flour; mix well. Stirring very frequently,
   cook for 6 - 8 min. to bring your roux to the Brun level.

4 Add ½ of the wine, stirring constantly to work out any
   lumps in the roux. Once the roux is smooth, add ½ of
   the stock and whisk well to fully incorporate the roux.
   Be sure to scrape up any fond.

5 Bring to a simmer and cook uncovered for 4 - 5 min.
   until the liquid in the pot has reduced by roughly
   half. It will be very thick, which is good.

6 Once reduced, add the remaining wine and stock slowly,
   whisking throughout. Continue whisking until completely
   incorporated. Bring back to a simmer, reduce the heat to
   Medium Low and cook for 3 - 4 min. stirring often. Reduce
   heat to lowest heat setting to hold the sauce, and add the
   ½ tbsp. of butter right before serving to finish the sauce.

7 Hold over lowest heat setting, covered, for up to 1 hr. If
   making for prep ahead of time, transfer to a heat safe
   container and cool completely before covering. Will
   hold in fridge for 4 days.

Recipe Tip

The type of wine you use has a huge impact on the flavors in
this sauce, so I recommend fruit-forward wines such as Merlot
or Pinot Noir. Malbec wouldn't be a bad choice, but you should
always make sure to taste your wine before cooking with it.

Puttanesca Sauce

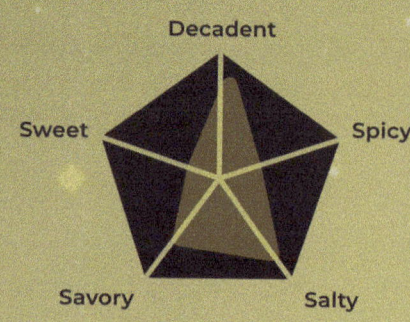

This classic sauce gives your pasta a good kick of flavor from the garlic and anchovies. The olives add a buttery texture and flavor that balances nicely with the red pepper flakes.

While traditional Puttanesca is made with fresh (or canned) tomatoes forced through a sieve, I find that using Pomodoro gives the recipe some much needed sweetness to help balance with the red pepper flakes. While an element of heat is important for this sauce, it's not the focus like with Fra Diavolo.

Mother Sauce: Tomato

Ingredients

Pomodoro Sauce (Pg 151)	2 C
Garlic, Minced	1½ tsp
Anchovy Fillets, Rinsed, Finely Chopped	4 - 6 ea
Capers, Drained	2 tsp
Castelvetrano Olives, Pitted, Chopped	½ C
Red Pepper Flakes	¼ tsp
Olive Oil	2 Tbsp

Prep Time	Cook Time	Servings
10 Min	12 - 15 Min	16 oz

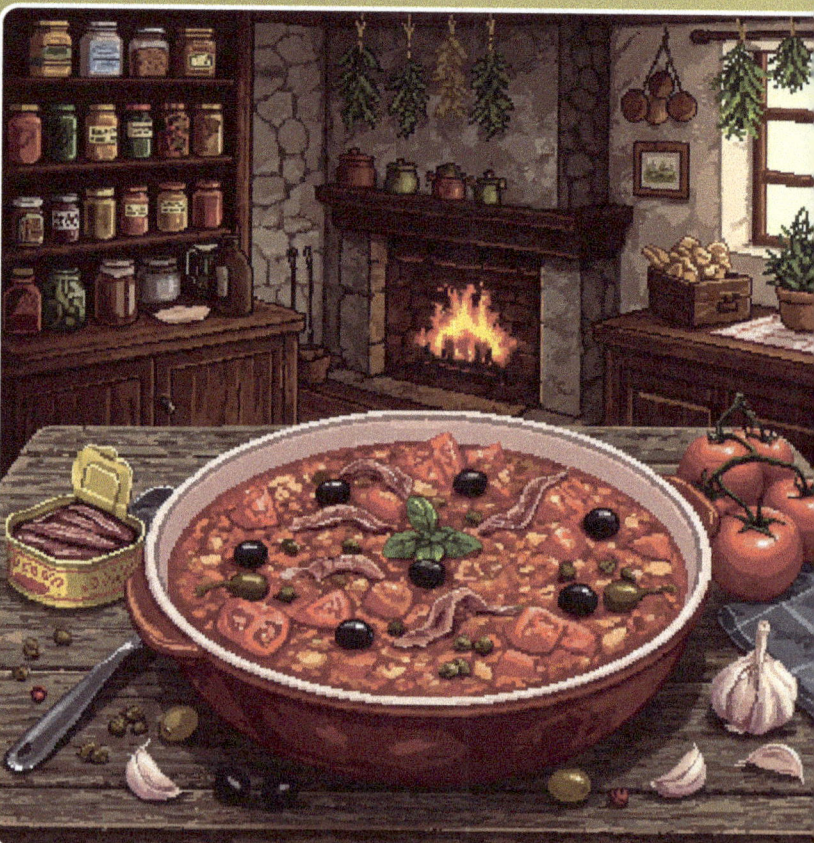

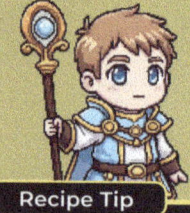

Recipe Tip

I prefer to use Castelvetrano olives when I make this sauce, but any type of green or black olive would work well. Use the olives you like best, just be careful of the sodium content!

Cooking Directions

1 Place a 12" - 14" skillet over Medium High heat. When hot, add oil.

2 When oil is shimmering, add the olives and cook for 1 min. Add the garlic, anchovies, and red pepper flakes. Cook for 1 more minute, until fragrant.

3 Add the Pomodoro to the pan carefully; it may splatter. Stir and bring to a simmer. Reduce the heat to Medium Low, cover, and cook for 10 - 12 min.

4 Use immediately, or store in airtight container and refrigerate. Keeps for 4 days in the refrigerator.

Desserts & Baking

Blueberry Muffins

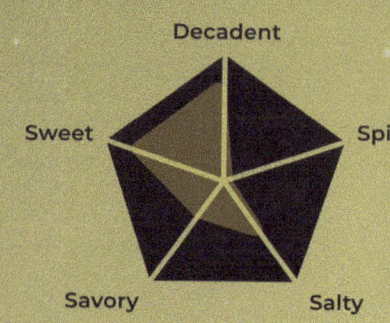

Decadent

Sweet

Spic

Savory

Salty

These muffins have an amazing rise to them, and the sour cream makes them extra fluffy and soft. Any kind of fresh fruit can be used, not just blueberries. Try them with chopped up strawberries, mango, or raspberries. And of course, adding chocolate chips (white or dark) would make for a delightful accompaniment for your fruit pieces. Just cut the fruit amount in half and replace that with the chips.

Ingredients (Muffins)

AP Flour	2¼ C
White Sugar	1 C
Large Eggs	2 ea
Butter, Melted	8 Tbsp
Baking Powder	2 tsp
Baking Soda	½ tsp
Vanilla Extract	1 tsp
Salt	½ tsp
Water	¼ C
Sour Cream	3 Tbsp
Blueberries, Fresh	1 C
Zest Of ½ A Lemon	

Ingredients (Crumble)

Butter, Melted	3 Tbsp
Brown Sugar	½ C
AP Flour	½ C

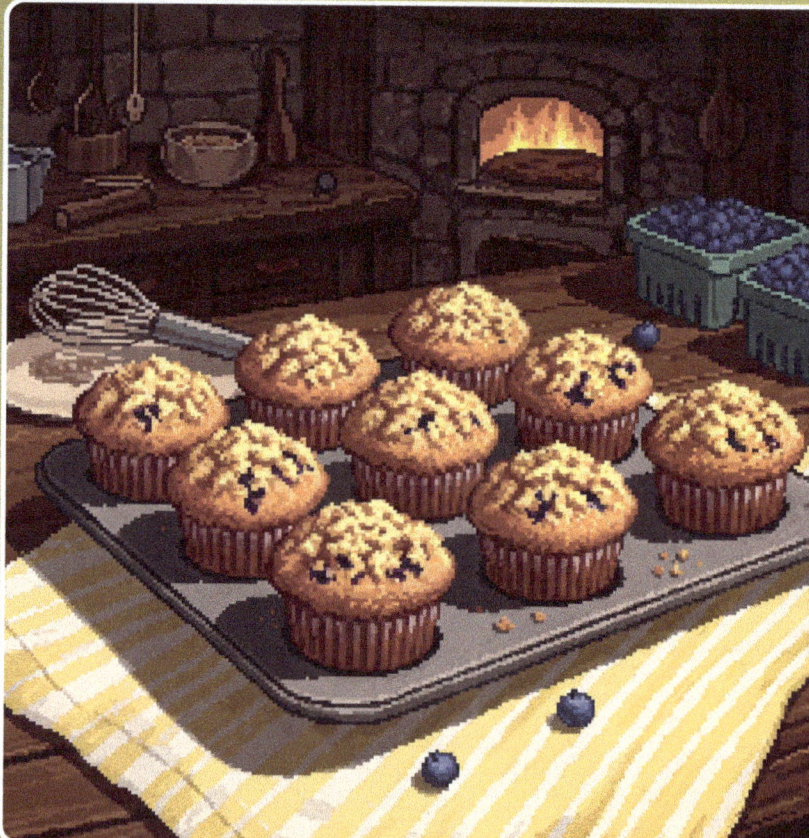

Prep Time	Cook Time	Servings
20 Min	30 - 35 Min	12 Regular or 6 XL Muffins

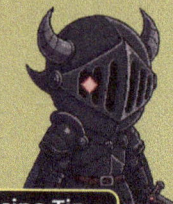

Recipe Tip

This recipe was adapted from one for sourdough muffins. If you have your own sourdough starter that you enjoy using to bake, simply remove the ¼ cup of water and reduce the flour amount to 2 cups, and add in ½ cup of your sourdough starter.

Cooking Directions

1 Preheat the oven to 350. Grease your muffin tins,
   or line them with paper inserts.

2 Combine all crumble ingredients in a small bowl. Mix
   with a fork until the flour and sugar have combined
   and formed balls of various sizes, with as little excess
   flour and sugar loose in the bowl as possible. Set aside.

3 In a large bowl, sift the flour, baking soda and powder,
   and salt together. Add the zest, mix with a fork, and then
   add the blueberries. Toss to coat and set bowl aside.

4 In a medium bowl, combine the sugar, sour cream,
   water, vanilla, eggs and melted butter. Whisk
   vigorously until smooth.

5 Pour the wet ingredients into the dry and stir
   with a rubber spatula or wooden spoon until just
   combined. If batter is too stiff, add 1 - 2 Tbsp. of
   water, and if too runny add 1 - 2 Tbsp. of flour.

6 Divide the batter evenly into your muffin tins
   and sprinkle with the crumble. Gently press
   the crumble topping into the top of the batter.

7 Bake for 30 - 35, until a toothpick inserted into the center
   of a muffin comes out clean. Let muffins cool in the tin
   for about 10 min. before transferring to a cooling rack.

8 Good for 3 days covered at room temperature, good
   frozen for 3 months in a freezer bag.

Homemade Naan Bread

Decadent

Sweet   Spicy

Savory   Salty

Working quickly with finesse is the key to making this recipe. Letting the dough sit too long on the counter will cause it to dry out too much for cooking. Having a hot surface is important to quickly cook the bread, but not so hot that it causes major burning on your dough.

Try mixing in chopped up cilantro, minced onion or garlic, or even spice blends to give this naan your own unique flavor. Soon enough, you'll have ideal pairings for when you make curries at home.

Ingredients

Self-Rising Flour	1¾ C
Salt	½ tsp
Greek Yogurt, Plain	1 C
Butter, Melted	1 Tbsp

Prep Time
10 Min

Cook Time
30 - 40 Min

Servings
6 - 8 Pieces

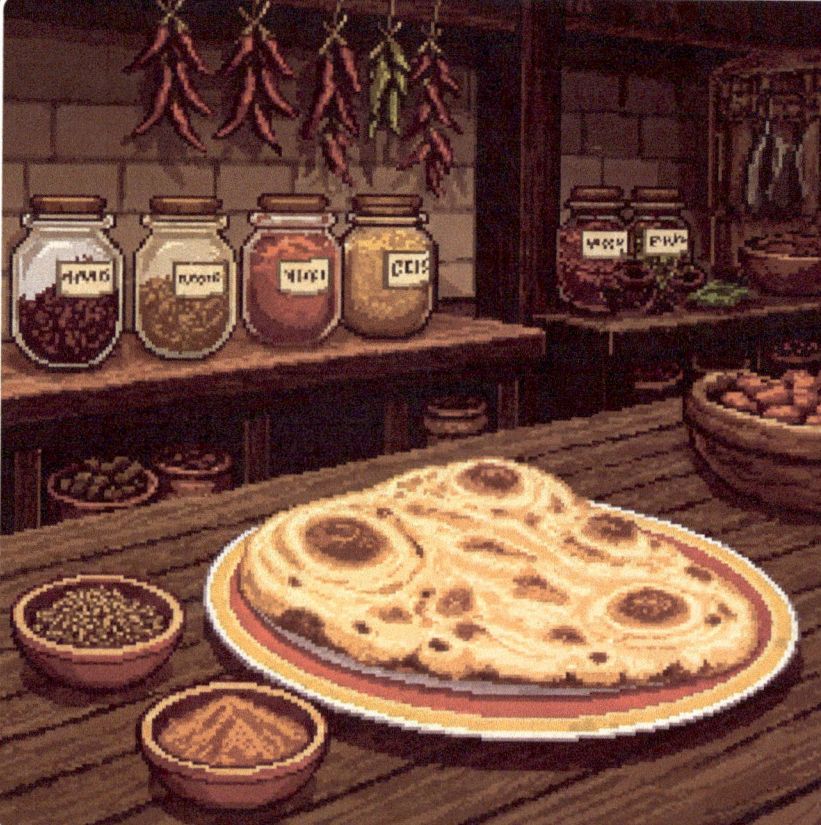

Cooking Directions

1   Preheat oven to 170.

2   Sift the flour and salt into a large mixing bowl. Add the yogurt and mix together until thoroughly combined. If using a stand mixer, keep the speed low and slow to prevent messes.

3   Remove the dough from the bowl and form into an even ball.

4   Place dough ball on a floured surface. Flatten the ball into a rough rectangle about 1" - 1¼" thick.

5   Divide the dough into 6-8 even pieces, and form them into your desired shape, making sure they are roughly ¼" - ⅜" thick. Keep other dough pieces covered until formed.

6   Place a 10" - 14" non-stick skillet over Medium heat. When hot, place a piece of dough in the skillet, more if they will fit, but don't overcrowd or have the dough pieces touching.

7   Cook for 3 min. then flip and cook for 2 min. more. Remove from the pan and brush with melted butter before placing on a baking tray and covering with foil. Repeat for all your dough pieces.

8   Hold the finished bread pieces in the oven as you are cooking the others.

LVLUPCookBook Channel

EXPERT

One Final Trial

You have moved beyond mere competency, and you're now excelling at your cooking. Novice and Apprentice level recipes come naturally to you, as well they should. Adept recipes are likewise easier than they used to be.

These Expert recipes and challenges will push you, and will show you that there is still knowledge for you to attain. But you're not afraid.

This is the final leg of your journey, and you will finally see those last few challenges completed on your Skill Tree.

Once that is done, revel in your accomplishment, enjoy your own cleverness and skill. Then, don't be afraid to choose a new Class for yourself; find new ways to grow and Level Up!

LEVEL 30

Achievements Unlocked

Doughn't Forget
- You've made different types of dough and used them in various dishes

Multi Tasker
- You're now capable of making 3 different recipes in tandem

Meal Planning Master
- Your grocery lists and meal plans are inventive and unique

Peacemaker
- You've grown proficient in pairing dishes so they complement one another

Mother May I?
- You're familiar with The Mother Sauces and various derivations

Flame On!
- The power of flambé is now yours

The Roux-d Less Travelled
- You can now make any kind of Roux you need for a recipe

Hitting The Sauce
- You can craft any sauce, for any recipe

Sides & Appetizers

Classic Gyoza (Potstickers)

Gyoza are a traditional Japanese food that I absolutely love. They are a little labor intensive, so I recommend making a large batch all at once and freezing plenty for later enjoyment. If doing so, just remove the frozen dumplings from the bag and cook following the recipe directions. Note that frozen dumplings may take an extra minute or two to cook fully.

Folding the dumplings is by far the most difficult aspect of this dish. With practice, it'll become second nature in no time. However, to save time, you can also purchase a dumpling press online. They are cheap, easy to use, and I find it's beyond helpful if you enjoy making large amounts and varieties of dumplings (like I do!).

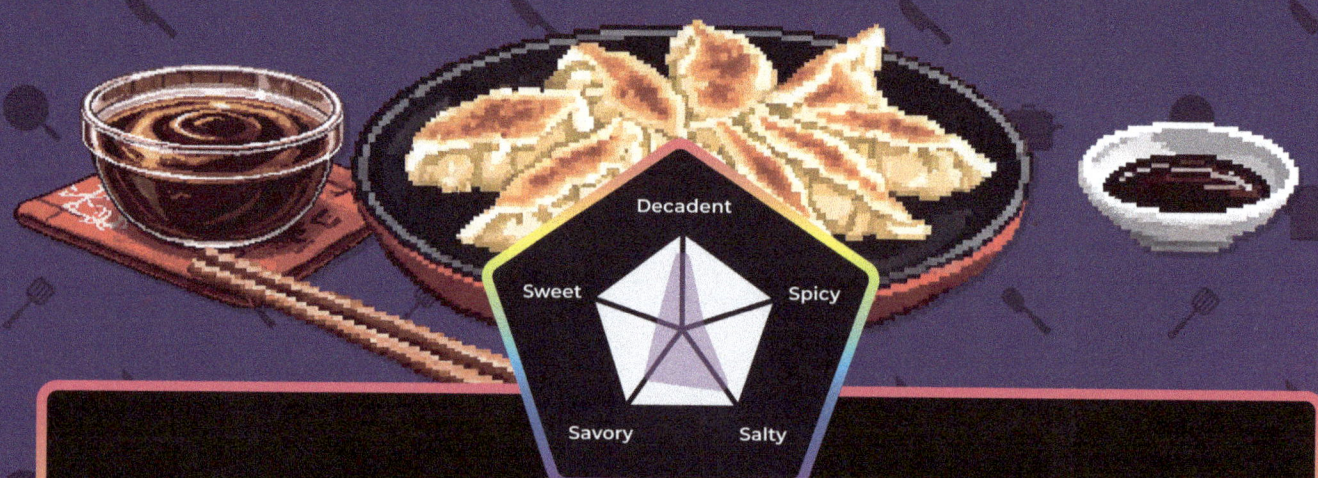

	Decadent	
Sweet		Spicy
Savory		Salty

Ingredients (Filling)

Prep Time	Cook Time	Servings
45 Min	10 Min	18 - 20 Gyoza

Pork Belly, Finely Minced	¼ Lb	White Sugar	½ tsp
Pork Loin, Minced	¼ Lb	Chicken Stock	½ tsp
Scallions, Finely Minced	¼ C	Black Pepper, Ground	½ tsp
Chives, Minced	2 Tbsp	Sesame Oil	½ Tbsp
Celery, Minced	2 Tbsp	Mirin/Shaoxing Wine/Sake	½ Tbsp
Napa Cabbage, Minced	¼ C	Round Dumpling Wrappers,	20 ea
Salt	¾ tsp	Thawed	
Ginger, Minced	1 tsp	Water For Wrapping	

Ingredients (Dipping Sauce)

Soy Sauce	4 Tbsp	Sesame Oil	1 tsp
Rice Vinegar	4 Tbsp	Ginger, Minced	1 tsp

Ingredients (Cooking)

Neutral Oil, Divided	2 Tbsp	Water	⅓ C

Folding Directions

Special Equipment

Half-Moon
Dumpling Press
1 ea

10" - 12" Lid
1 ea

1   Set out the dumpling wrappers to thaw, I advise placing them in the fridge the night before.

2   Combine all ingredients in a large bowl, mixing well to fully combine.

3   Moisten the edges of the wrapper with a small amount of water. Place 1 heaping Tbsp. in the center of the wrapper.

4   Pinch one end shut and begin to make pleats to seal. To do this, fold the wrapper sides together, slightly overlapping, and pinch to seal, repeating this all along the length of the dumpling. It will require 5 - 6 pleats to seal properly. Make sure to gently push the filling in with a free finger as you work so it's evenly distributed. When you reach the end, gently pinch the two ends together to seal.

5   Repeat until all dumplings are folded into crescents and sealed. Set aside. If freezing some dumplings, place them on a baking sheet lined with parchment paper and transfer to freezer. Let rest for 2 hr. until frozen through. Transfer to a freezer bag and store for up to 3 months.

Cooking Directions

1 Measure out ⅓ cup of water and place in a microwave safe bowl. Combine the dipping sauce ingredients in a small dish and stir well. Let rest 10 min. before use. Will hold in fridge for 7 days.

2 Place a 10" - 12" non-stick skillet over Medium High heat. Add the oil.

3 When the oil is shimmering, place your dumplings down in a circle, arranging them close together, but not touching. Cook for 2 - 3 min. until the bottoms of the dumplings are browned.

4 Sprinkle 1 - 2 tsp. of oil on the dumplings. Heat your water in the microwave for 10 - 15 seconds and then pour the water into the skillet. Be careful, as it will rapidly boil and splatter. Cover the pan and cook for 6-7 min. until the water has nearly all evaporated.

5 When almost all the water is gone, remove the lid and allow the rest of the water to evaporate. Use a thermometer to make sure your dumplings are 155 internal temperature.

6 Carefully remove from pan and set on a plate with the browned and crispy side showing. Serve Immediately.

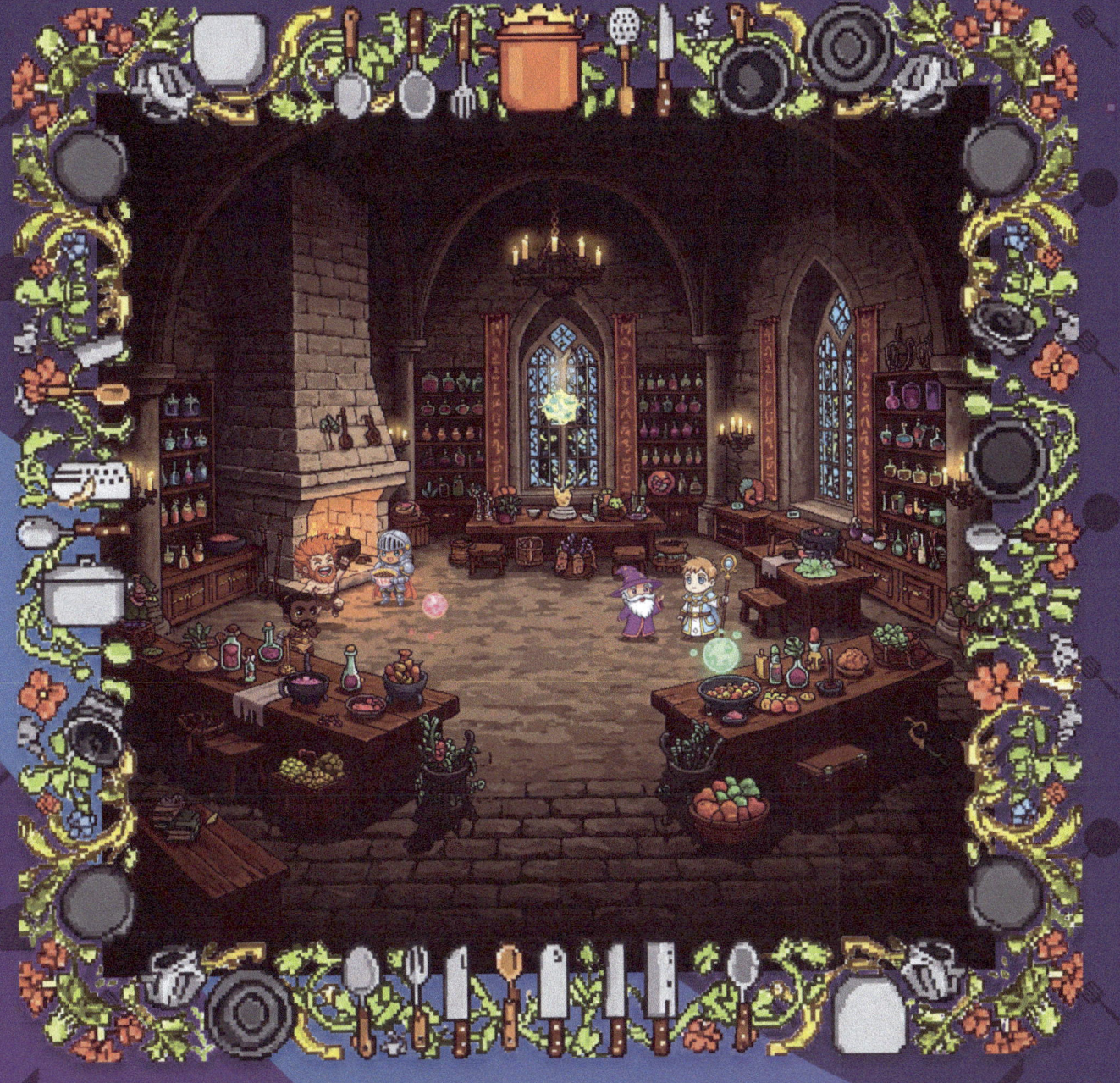

Recipe Tip

The dipping sauce recipe I give is very basic, but pairs perfectly with the filling of these dumplings. Experiment with different ingredients and flavors to find your unique favorite. If you omit the ginger from the ingredient list, the sauce will keep indefinitely in the fridge. So, you can make the base in a larger quantity and then portion it out for your experiments.

Mushroom Risotto

This classic dish is a delightful addition to any plate, and makes for a perfect side with roasted chicken, grilled pork, or a vegetarian meal. This method of cooking risotto yields a creamier and softer result than by cooking it like normal rice. Do not wash the Arborio rice before use: the starches that coat the grains are essential for developing the proper texture and consistency.

Don't be deceived by the short list of instructions; this recipe is tricky to pull off correctly. It requires the cook to understand their stove top well. Too much heat, and the stock/broth will evaporate without absorbing. Too little heat, and the rice won't absorb the liquid efficiently, leading to longer cooking times.

It's possible to prep ahead of time by cooking the risotto, according to the recipe, until just before it is al dente. However, this is also tricky to pull off correctly, and I advise not attempting this method until you are quite familiar with the recipe, and the process of cooking risotto this way.

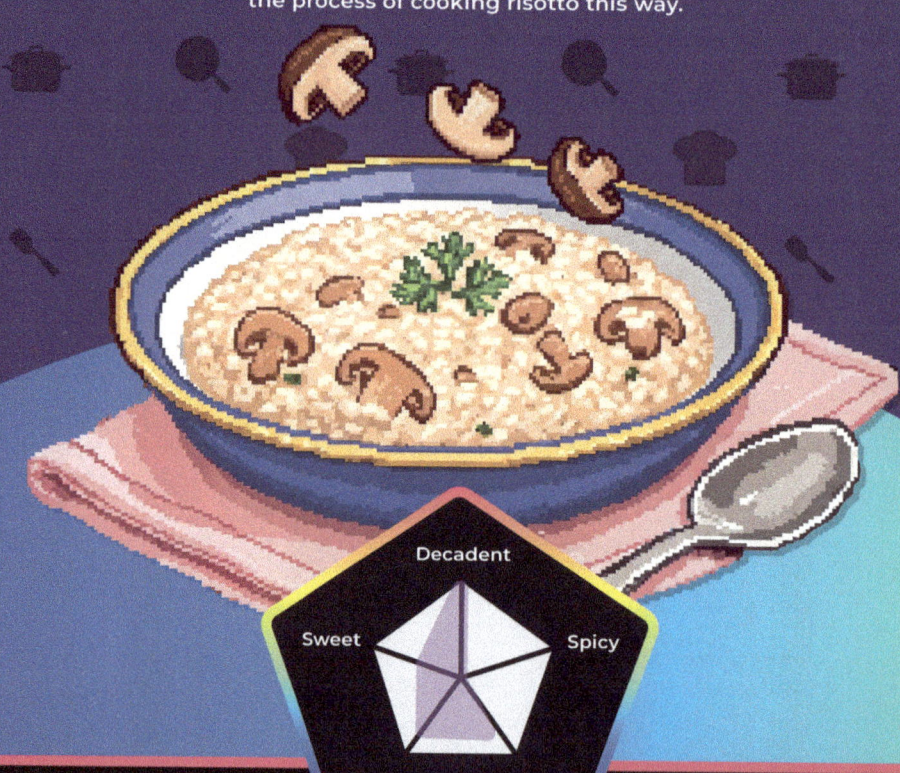

Decadent

Sweet · Spicy

Savory · Salty

Ingredients		Prep Time 10 Min	Cook Time 25 - 30 Min	Servings 6 Portions
Arborio Rice	1 C	Salt		¼ tsp
Stock/Broth (Any Kind)	1 Qt	Black Pepper, Ground		⅛ tsp
Heavy Cream	½ C	Parmesan, Grated		¼ C
Cremini Mushrooms, Diced	½ C	Olive Oil		1½ Tbsp

Cooking Directions

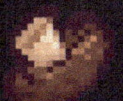

1. Place the stock/broth in a microwave safe container, and heat on Medium setting for 45 - 60 sec. The liquid only needs to be room temp/warm, not hot. Set aside.

2. Place a 12" - 14" skillet over Medium heat. Add the olive oil.

3. When shimmering, add the mushrooms. Stirring often, cook until they start to become tender, 1 - 2 min.

4. Add the risotto and stir well. Cook in the pan until the rice starts to brown slightly and smells nutty, 2 - 3 min.

5. Begin adding the stock/broth, 4 - 6 Fl. Oz. at a time, stirring well as you do. You want to bring the liquid to a simmer, and stir the rice well. Cook it in this fashion until the liquid is nearly all absorbed, then add another 4 - 6 Fl. Oz. If the stock/broth is evaporating too quickly, reduce the heat slightly. Repeat until all the stock/broth has been cooked into the rice, and the rice is al dente when tasted with a spoon. Be sure to test for texture once you've added about 3 cups of the liquid.

6. Add the salt and pepper with your final addition of stock/broth, stir well. When nearly all the liquid has been absorbed, add your heavy cream and parmesan to the pan. Cook until the heavy cream has reduced and the rice is thoroughly coated in the cream-parmesan mixture.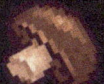

7. Test the taste, adjust salt and pepper as desired. Serve Hot, will hold over Low heat on the stove top, covered, for up to 40 min.

Mains

Butter Chicken

This recipe is labor intensive, but well worth the effort. It also lends itself to cooking with lamb, paneer, or extra-firm tofu. If using lamb, a more tender cut such as a loin chop would be ideal, but shoulder or leg will also work. Keep in mind that cuts like the shoulder, leg, or blade chops require more cooking time, so it's advised that they be braised ahead of time and gently folded into the curry at the end.

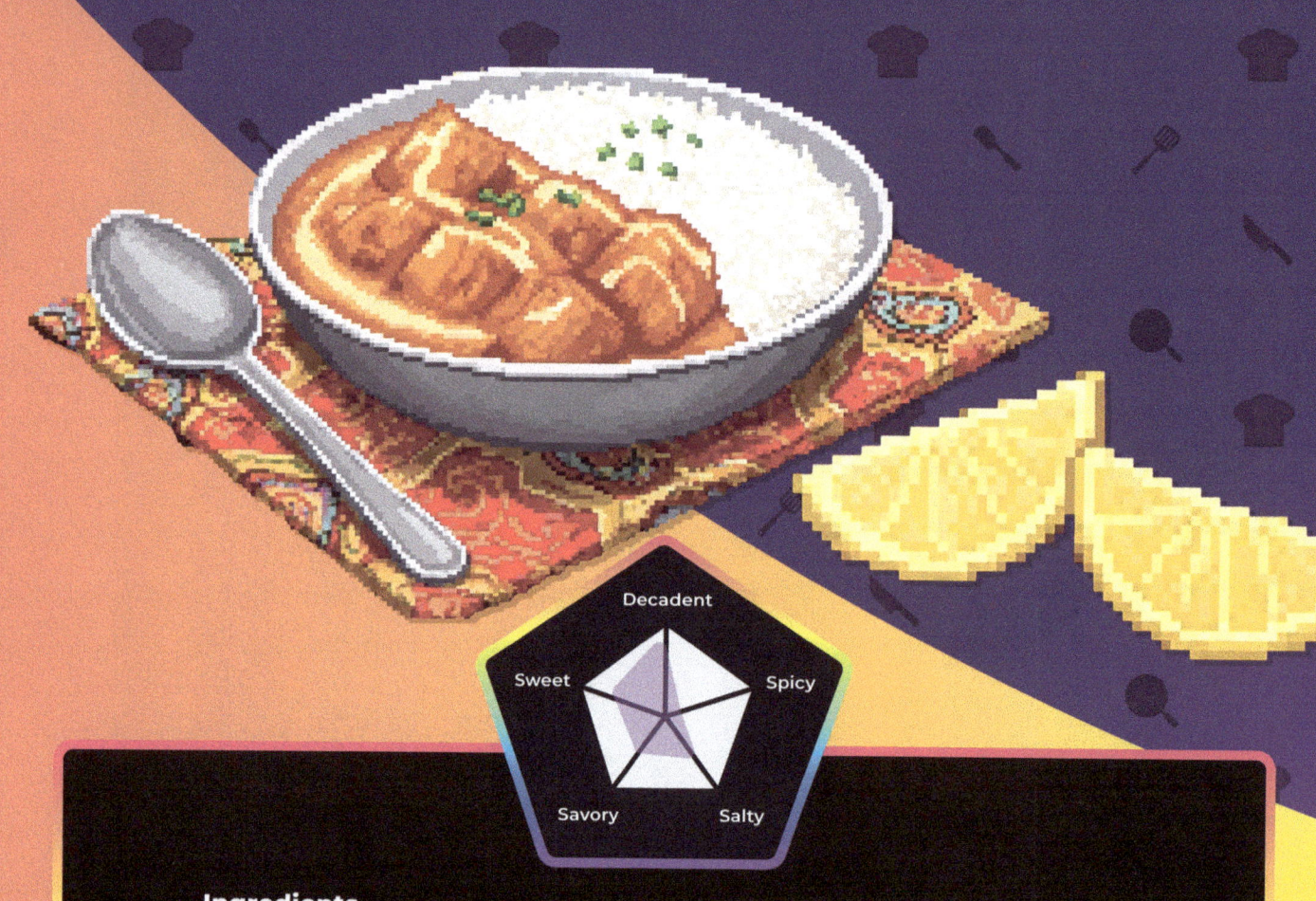

Decadent

Sweet

Spicy

Savory

Salty

Ingredients

Prep Time	Cook Time	Servings
1 Hr	40 Min	4 - 6 Portions

Chicken Breast, 1" Cubes	1 ½ C	Garam Masala, Divided	1 Tbsp
Cayenne	⅛ tsp	Onion, Diced	1½ C
Lemon Juice	1 Tbsp	Tomato Paste	1 C
Paprika	¾ tsp	Green Chiles, Diced	¼ C
Yogurt, Plain	⅓ C	Chili Powder	2 tsp
Neutral Oil, Divided	2 Tbsp	Sugar	1 tsp
Turmeric	⅛ tsp	Butter or Ghee, Divided	3½ Tbsp
Ginger, Minced, Divided	1 Tbsp	Cashews, Raw	28 ea
Garlic, Minced, Divided	1 Tbsp	Water	1 C
Cumin, Divided	1 tsp	Stock (Any Kind)	¼ C
Coriander, Ground, Divided	2½ tsp	Heavy Cream, Warmed	⅓ C
		Oven Baked Rice (Pg 89)	

Cooking Directions (Preparation)

Special Equipment

Cheesecloth or
Fine Mesh Sieve
1 ea

Heat Safe Blender/
Food Processor
(Required)
1 ea

1   Combine chicken pieces, lemon juice, paprika, cayenne and ¼ tsp. salt in a bowl and mix together. Refrigerate and let rest for 20 minutes.

2   Add yogurt, 1 Tbsp. oil, turmeric, ½ Tbsp. ginger, ½ Tbsp. garlic, 1 tsp. coriander, ½ tsp. cumin, and 1 tsp. garam masala to the bowl, mix well. Marinate for 30 min. minimum, 6 hours maximum.

3   Place a 10" - 12" skillet over Medium heat. Add ½ Tbsp. oil. When the oil is shimmering, add the onion and cook until light brown, stirring often, about 10 minutes. Remove from pan and set aside. Remove pan from heat and turn off stove eye.

4   Place a small pot on High heat. Add water and bring to a boil. When boiling, add cashews and reduce heat to Medium Low. Cover and simmer for 10 min. Place the tomato paste and onion in a blender. When cashews are done, measure out ½ C of the water and add to blender. Strain the cashews and add them to the blender. Blend to a puree. Pull chicken out of fridge to warm up.

Cooking Directions

5. Strain the puree through a sieve or cheesecloth and set aside. Discard the strained parts.

6. Place the same pan in which you cooked the onions over Medium heat. Add 3 Tbsp. of butter/ghee. When hot, add the remaining ginger, garlic and the green chiles. Cook until fragrant, 1 minute.

7. Add the spices to the pan, stir well and cook for 1 minute. Add the strained puree to the pan and mix well. Bring to a simmer, then reduce heat to Medium Low and cook until it coats the back of a spoon (nappé).

8. While sauce thickens, place the skillet you cooked the onion in over Medium High heat. Add ½ Tbsp. of oil. When shimmering, add the chicken. Sear well for 5 - 8 minutes, stirring occasionally. When seared, and the sauce is thickened, add the chicken to the sauce. Deglaze the chicken pan with ¼ C of Stock, making sure to scrape up all the fond. Add this to the sauce.

9. Bring the sauce to a simmer, and cook for 5 min. covered, then 5 min. uncovered. Be sure to check that the chicken is fully cooked, 165 internal temperature.

10. Add the salt and sugar, stirring gently. Remove the pan from the heat and add the warmed up heavy cream and ½ Tbsp. of butter or ghee. Stir well. Serve Hot with ¾ C rice.

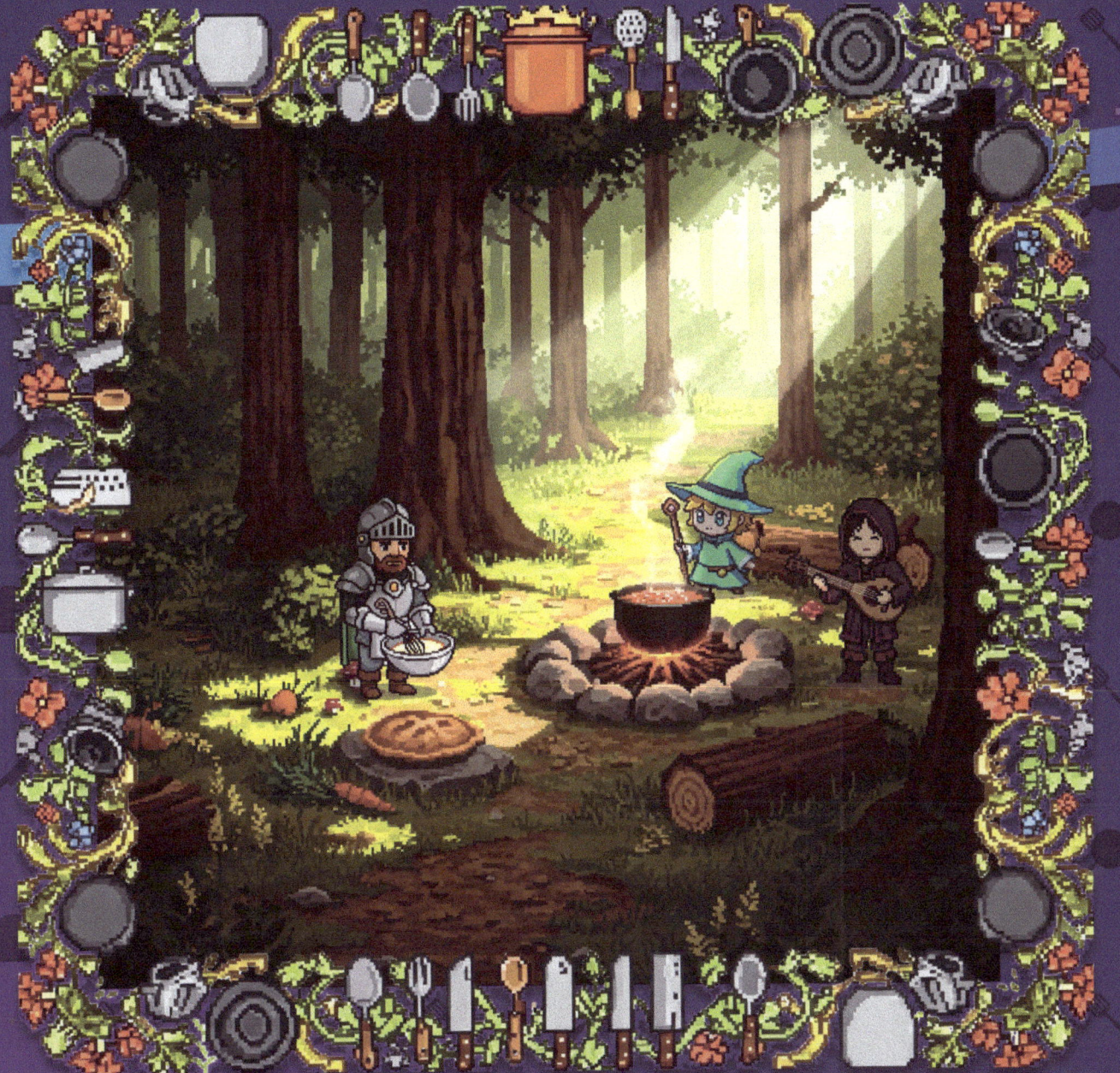

Recipe Tip

This recipe is on the sweeter side by it's nature, but that doesn't mean it wouldn't pair well with spicier side options. Try putting minced hot chiles in the rice when baking, or maybe making some spicy potatoes to put the sauce over instead of rice.

Thank You!

Chicken & Sausage Gumbo

This recipe takes a fair bit of time and concentration, but it's more than worth the effort involved. This dish is a staple in my kitchen, and I eat it at least once a month. Shredding your own chicken is the ideal way to prepare for this meal, but there isn't always time for that. If that's the case, I recommend purchasing a rotisserie chicken from the store and shredding the meat you need from that. Not only does it save time for this recipe, it also provides the meat needed for making your own chicken salad or homemade Chicken and Dumplin's.

Shredding the chicken up to 2 days in advance and making the roux in advance will certainly cut down on the prep time when you go to make the dish. Also, you can purchase the celery and dice the whole head during prep time and freeze the excess pieces in a freezer bag. They'll keep for up to 2 months, and will be ready for use whenever you need diced celery. If you've got the time and want to feel like a true Creole chef, doing it all at once is a rewarding experience.

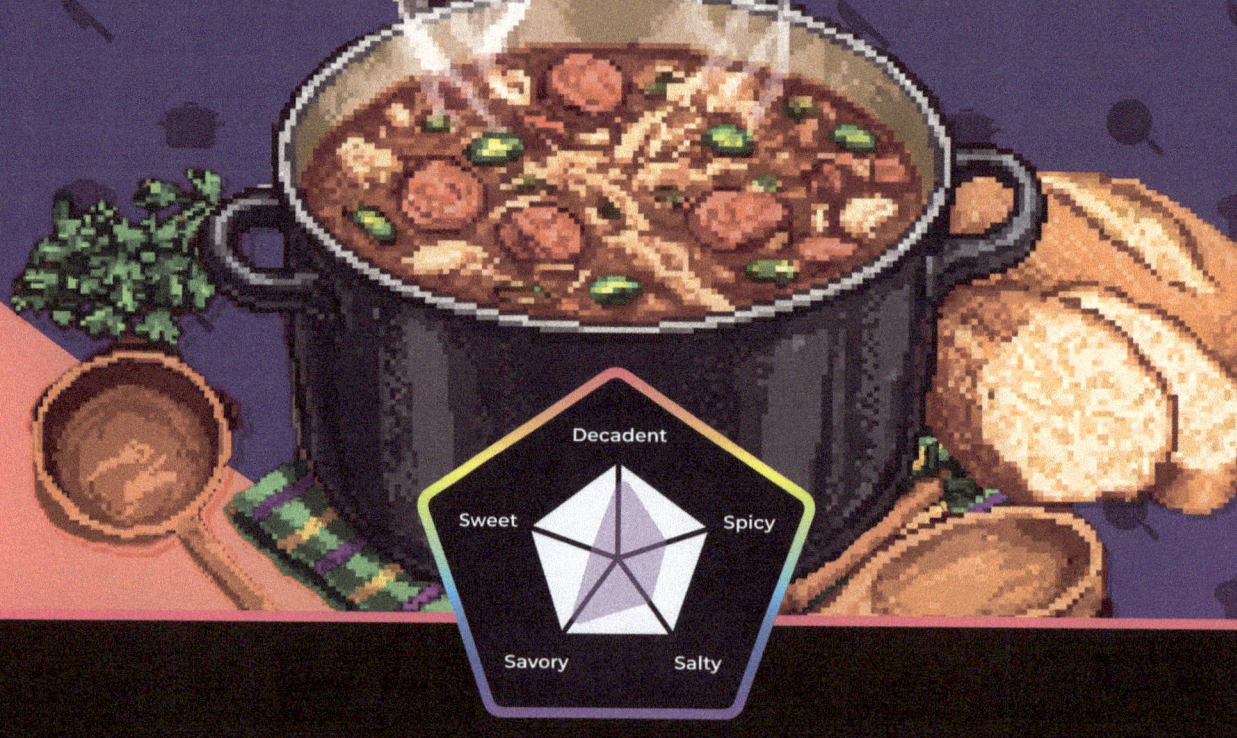

Decadent

Sweet — Spicy

Savory — Salty

Ingredients

		Prep Time	Cook Time	Servings
		40 Min	3 Hr	4 - 6 Bowls

Ingredients				
Chicken Breast, Shredded	1½ C	Paprika		1 tsp
Sausage, Sliced (Andouille)	1½ C	Thyme, Dry		½ tsp
Red Beans, Rehydrated OR	1 C	Parsley, Dry		1 tsp
15 oz. Can Red Beans	1 ea	Black Pepper, Ground		⅛ tsp
Tomato, Diced, W/ Juice	1 C	Bay Leaf		2 ea
White Onion, Diced	⅔ C	Worcestershire Sauce		¾ Tbsp
Green Bell Pepper, Diced	⅓ C	Black Roux		6 - 7 oz
Celery, Diced	⅓ C	Neutral Oil		2 Tbsp
Chicken Stock	2 Qt	Oven Baked Rice (Pg 89)		
Garlic, Minced	½ Tbsp			
Hot Sauce	1½ tsp			

Cooking Directions

1   Place a large pot over Medium heat. When hot, place
    sausage in pot, cut side down. Cook for 1 - 2 minutes
    on each side until browned. Remove sausage from pot
    and set aside. Add the oil. When oil is shimmering add
    the onion, bell pepper, and celery, cooking each until
    soft before adding the next. When done, add the garlic
    and cook for 1 min.

    *If making the roux during cooking, after the
    vegetables are done is the time to add the flour.
    Stirring nearly constantly, cook the flour for 7 - 9 min.
    to bring it to the Bien Colorè level, it should be the
    color of milk chocolate.

2   Add the premade roux and stir well, to make sure it's
    totally melted down. When the roux is ready, add
    8 Fl. Oz. of your stock/broth and stir thoroughly,
    making sure to work out any lumps in the roux. Then
    add your Worcestershire sauce and cook for
    30 seconds.

3   Add the tomatoes (with their juice), all seasonings, and
    the sausage. Stir well and cook for 1 min. Then add the
    chicken, the rehydrated beans, and your remaining stock.

〉〉〉〉 CONTINUED 〉〉〉〉

4   Raise the heat to High, stirring often, and bring to a boil. Add your hot sauce, then reduce the heat to Low/Medium Low and cover. Cook for 2½ hours, until the beans are soft. If using canned beans, you need to add them in the last 20 - 25 min. to avoid overcooking them.

5   Remove lid and raise heat to Medium. Simmer uncovered for 10 - 15 min. to thicken. Taste test and adjust salt, pepper, and hot sauce as desired. Serve hot over ¾ - 1 C of Oven Baked Rice.

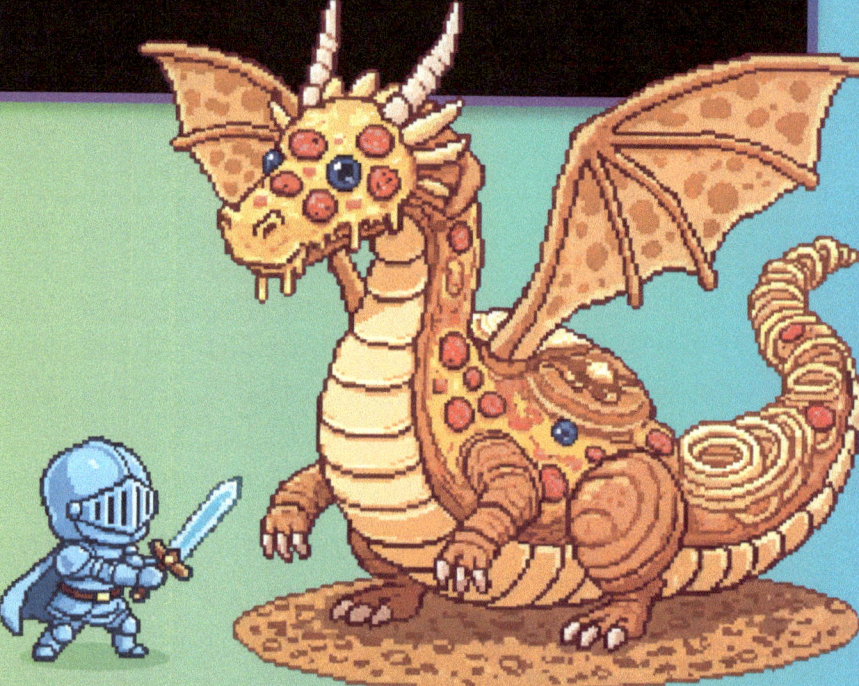

Recipe Tip

The use of green bell pepper, specifically, is required. The green bell pepper, white onion, and celery form what is known as "The Trinity", and it's the unique marker for almost all Cajun and Creole recipes. Without those three specific ingredients, the dishes just won't taste quite right.

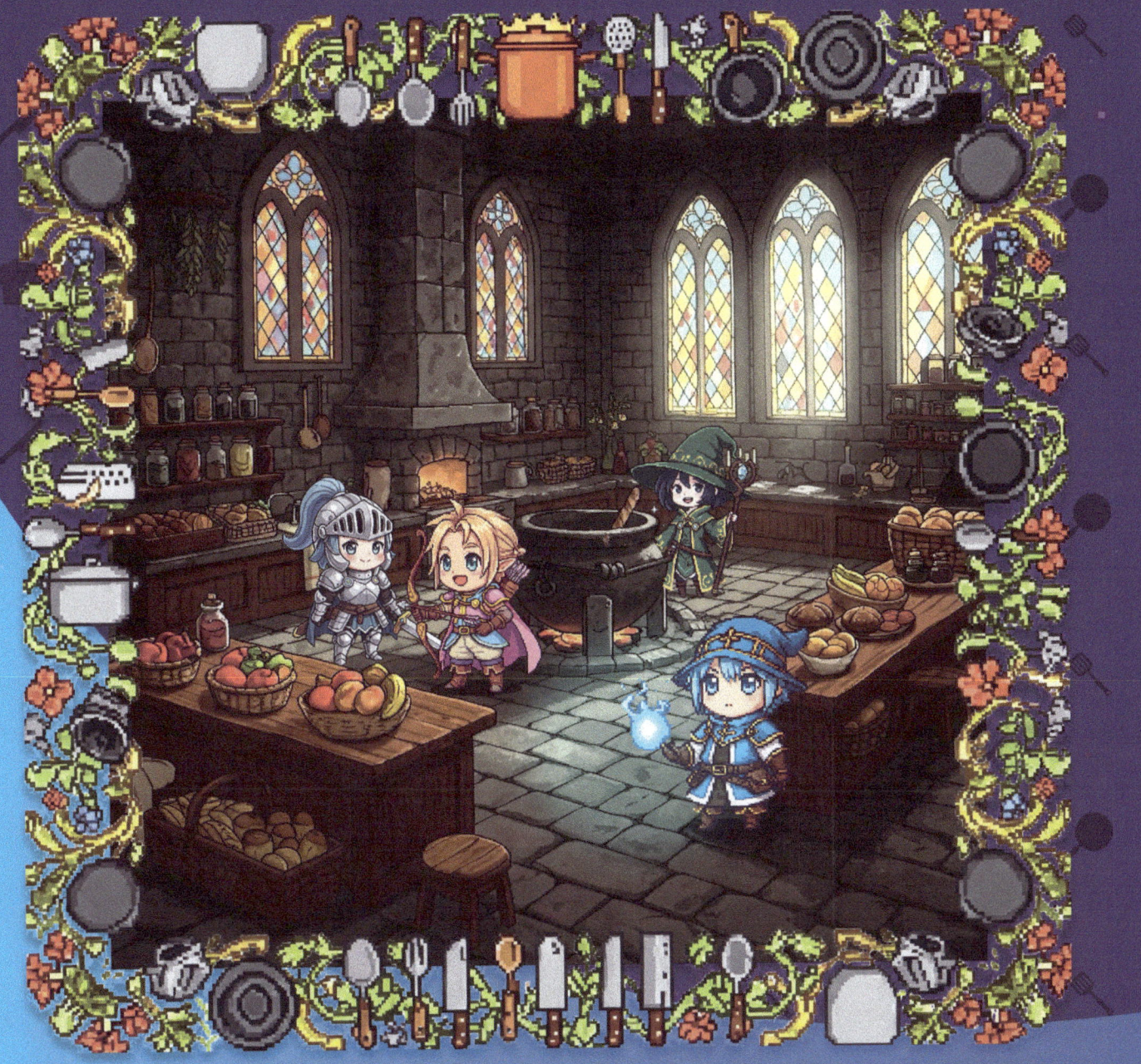

Chicken Tikka Saag

Tikka Saag has always been my favorite dish to order when eating at an Indian restaurant, and was one of the first recipes I learned how to make myself. I prefer milder curry blends, myself. If you are into very spicy foods, just increase the amount of cayenne you use. Be careful though, as cayenne continues to grow in strength not only as it cooks, but also during the cooling process for leftovers.

This recipe also works well with lamb, paneer, or extra-firm tofu. If using lamb, loin chops would be the best suited to keep cooking times down. If you want to use leg or shoulder make sure you prepare ahead of time by braising the meat and making sure it's soft enough for you to enjoy before making the sauce. Otherwise it'll take hours of cooking, and you run the risk of burning the sauce and overcooking the spinach.

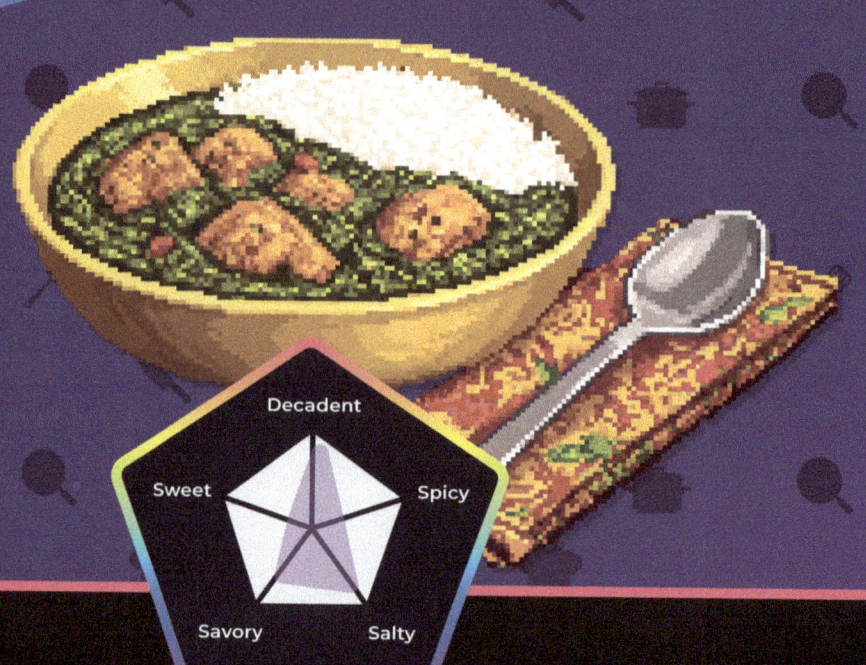

Ingredients

Prep Time	Cook Time	Servings
10 Min	35 - 40 Min	3 - 4 Portions

Chicken Breast, 1" Cubes	1½ C	Chili Powder	¼ tsp
Tomatoes, Diced, W/ Juice	1½ C	Turmeric	1 tsp
Onion, Small Dice	¾ C	Cumin	1 tsp
Spinach, Washed & Chopped	½ Lb	Yogurt, Plain	¾ C
Garlic, Minced	1 tsp	Neutral Oil Or Ghee, Divided	1½ Tbsp
Ginger, Minced	2 tsp	Salt	¼ tsp
Coriander, Ground	1½ tsp	Black Pepper, Ground	¼ tsp
Cardamom, Ground	½ tsp	Water Or Stock	¼ C
Garam Masala	1½ tsp	Oven Baked Rice (Pg 89)	
Cayenne	¼ tsp		

Cooking Directions

1. Place a 12" - 14" skillet over Medium High heat. When hot, add 1 Tbsp. of oil/ghee.

2. When shimmering, add the chicken pieces. Sear pieces for 2 - 3 min. per side, turning to get two sides of each piece. Remove from pan and set aside.

3. Add ½ Tbsp. of oil/ghee, lower the heat to Medium and add the onions. Cook for 5 min. until lightly browned.

4. Add the spices, garlic, and ginger. Stir well and cook for 1 - 2 min. until fragrant.

5. Add the tomatoes, with their juice, and cook for 10 min. until they are soft and mixture is thickened.

6. Add spinach and cook until it sticks to the pan, stirring often. Add the water/stock.

7. Return the chicken to the pan. Bring to a simmer and cover. Cook for 7 - 10 min. until chicken reaches 165 internal temperature.

8. Uncover the pan, lower the heat to Medium Low, add the yogurt and stir well. Continue cooking until the sauce reaches your desired thickness.

9. Serve hot with ¾ - 1 C of Oven Baked Rice.

Homestyle Fried Chicken

This recipe is courtesy of my lovely wife Julia. She grew up making fried chicken like this with her grandmother, and was kind enough to permit me to share her family recipe with all of you. It takes a fair bit of time, and while it may seem intimidating, this recipe becomes simple once you get into the groove. Before you know it, your family and friends will be requesting this recipe whenever a gathering is happening. Mac and Cheese, Oven Baked Rice, Coleslaw, Old Fashioned Greens, or Blistered Green Beans are all excellent options as sides with this dish.

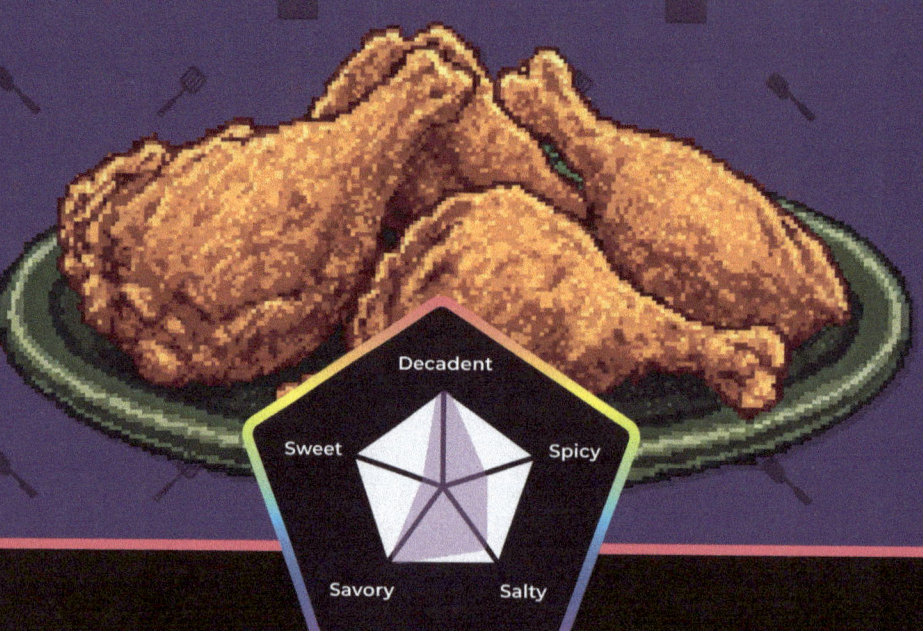

Decadent

Sweet   Spicy

Savory   Salty

Ingredients (Marinade)

Prep Time	Cook Time	Servings
20 Min	25 Min or 45 Min	4 - 6 Portions

Buttermilk	1 Pt	Cayenne	¼ tsp
Salt	½ Tbsp	Paprika	½ tsp
Onion Powder	½ Tbsp	Chicken (Tenders/Various Pcs)	2 Lb
Garlic Powder	½ Tbsp	Large Egg, Beaten	1 ea
Cumin	½ tsp		

Ingredients (Breading)

AP Flour	2 C	Black Pepper, Ground	1 tsp
Cumin	1 Tbsp	Ginger Powder	1 tsp
Sage, Ground	½ Tbsp	Mustard Powder	1 tsp
Rosemary, Dry	1 Tbsp	Chinese Five Spice Powder	1 tsp
Garlic Powder	½ Tbsp	Oil For frying, See Recipe	
Onion Powder	½ Tbsp	for Amounts	
Paprika	½ Tbsp		

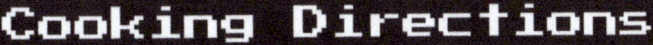

Cooking Directions

Special Equipment

Large Brown Paper Bag,
One inside the other
2 ea

1   Combine all ingredients for marinade in a large bowl,
    whisk well.

2   Place chicken in the bowl and mix well to coat. Make sure
    that as much of the chicken is submerged as possible.
    Cover and let rest in the fridge for 6 - 8 hours.

3   Combine all ingredients for breading in a large bowl.
    Set aside.

4   Remove the chicken from the bag and place in a
    colander in sink. Retain excess marinade if you
    wish to double bread your chicken.

5   After 1 - 2 minutes of dripping, transfer ¼ C of breading
    mix to the double bag. If cooking tenders, place 2 - 3
    tenders in at a time. For bone in pieces, place 1 - 2
    pieces in bag so they fit easily and can move around.

> > > > CONTINUED > > > >

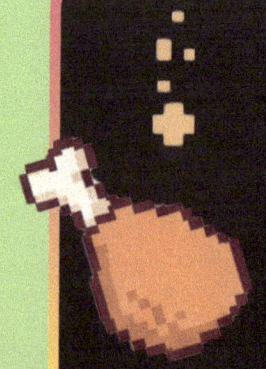

6   Hold bag so the top is sealed in your fist and shake vigorously for 5 - 10 seconds. Remove chicken from bag and place on a lined baking sheet or plate. Repeat for all pieces of chicken. If double breading, pour some of your marinade into a bowl, and place the chicken a few pieces at a time into it. Then remove, shake the excess marinade off, then put back into the bag and shake.

7   Set chicken aside and let rest on counter during this step. If Shallow Frying, you'll need your largest and deepest skillet, pouring in oil so it's 1½" - 2" deep. If deep frying, you'll need a counter top fryer or a large and deep pot with 6" - 7" of oil in it. Place your vessel over a Medium/Medium High heat and bring oil to 350 temperature. It's strongly advised you use a thermometer to make sure your oil is at the right temperature and note how quickly or slowly your stove top heats up the oil, adjusting your heat setting as needed.

8   When oil is holding at 350 carefully place as many pieces of chicken as will fit without touching or overcrowding the pan or basket.

Cooking Times

For Tenders   If Shallow Frying: Cook for 3 min. then turn over and cook for 3 min. more.

If Deep Frying: Cook for 5 - 6 minutes, agitating often. Use a thermometer to make sure the chicken is at 165 internal temperature

>>>> CONTINUED >>>>

For Bone-In Chicken

If Shallow Frying: Cook for 20 - 25 min. rotating the chicken every 5 minutes. Note that wings will take less time than legs or thighs, which in turn take less time than a breast piece. Don't be afraid to use your thermometer to chart your progress and make sure all chicken pieces reach an internal temperature of 165. Make sure to insert the thermometer near to the bone to get an accurate reading.

If Deep Frying: Submerge chicken in oil and fry according to piece. For Thighs and Legs: 18 - 20 min. For Breasts: 12 - 15 min.
For Wings: 12 - 15 min. agitating often and making sure they reach 165 internal temperature.

9   While frying, preheat your oven to 185. Line a baking tray with foil and place a wire rack in it. The rack isn't necessary, but it's ideal.

10   When chicken is fully cooked, remove from oil and place on the tray/rack. Hold the finished chicken in the oven while cooking the rest. Give the oil time to come back up to 350 in between batches.

11   Serve Hot and be careful: you'll probably fall in love at first bite.

Mushroom & Leek Tavern Pies

These pies are a tavern staple of British tradition, and as soon as you bite into the crunchy crust and the gooey, cheesy filling you'll understand why. The leeks provide a delicate unctuousness that balances the tang of the cheese and the earthiness of the mushrooms that makes for a wonderful bite. Making the pies in a XL Muffin tin makes a pie that's large enough to be the entrée of a meal by itself, while making them in a regular sized muffin tin will make for excellent hors d'oeuvers for a family gathering or holiday party. Just be careful, because once you serve these up everyone who eats one will want the recipe for them.

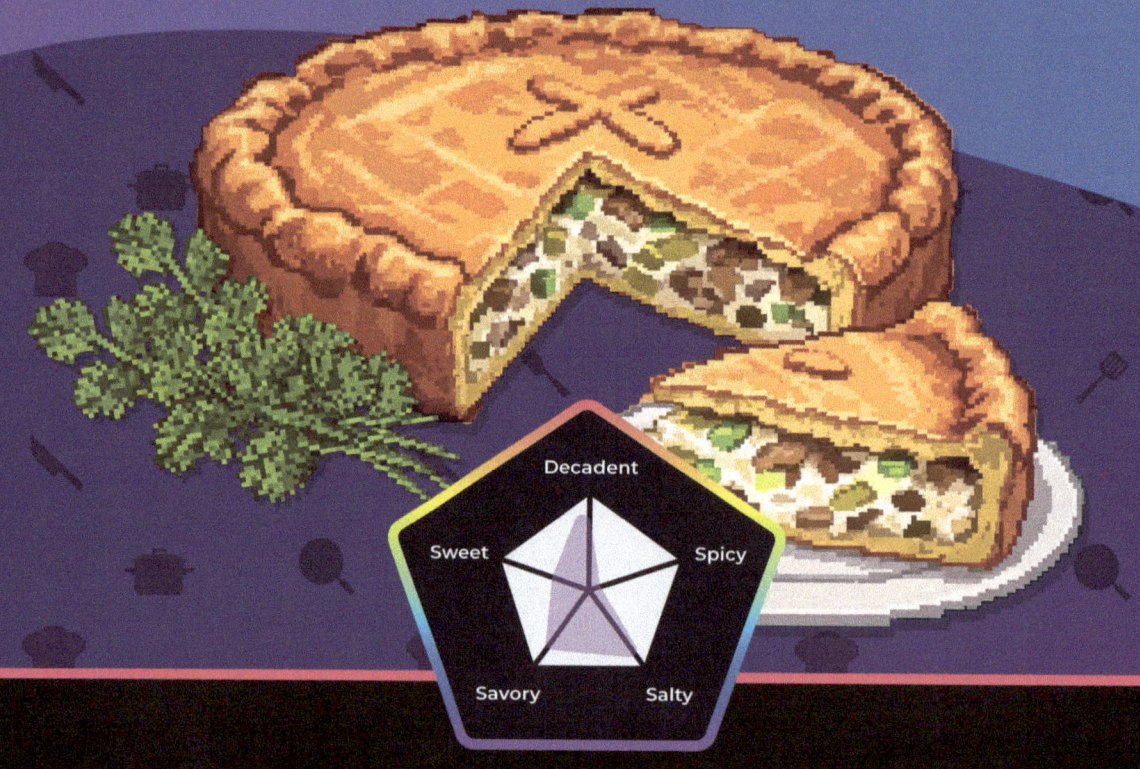

Ingredients

Prep Time	Cook Time	Servings
20 Min	30 Min	6 XL Muffin Size or 12 Reg. Muffin Size Pies

Button Mushrooms, Quartered	12 oz	Black Pepper, Ground	¼ tsp
Cremini Mushrooms, Quartered	12 oz	Fresh Parsley, Finely Chopped	4 Tbsp
Heavy Cream	4 Fl Oz	Nutmeg, Ground	⅛ tsp
Whole Milk	8 Fl Oz	Butter	2 Tbsp
Sharp White Cheddar, Shredded	1 C	AP Flour	1 Tbsp
Salt	½ tsp	Large Egg, Beaten	1 ea
Leeks, Washed, Thin Half-Moons	2 ea	Hot Water Crust Dough (Pg 165)	16 oz

Cooking Directions

Special Equipment

XL Muffin Tin, with 6 Muffin Cups or
Regular Sized, 12 Cup Muffin Tin
1 ea

1   Preheat oven to 425 making sure that a rack is in the middle of the oven.

2   Place a 4 Qt. pot over Medium heat. When hot, add the butter.

3   When the butter stops bubbling, add the leeks and cook for 2 - 3 min. until soft.

4   Add the mushrooms and stir well. Cook for 2 min.

5   Add the flour and stir to coat. Cook for 1 min, stirring throughout.

6   Pour in ½ of the milk and stir constantly until there are no lumps in the roux. Slowly add the remaining milk, then the cream, stirring constantly.

7   Still stirring, bring the mixture to a simmer. When simmering, add the parsley, salt, pepper, and nutmeg. Cook for 30 seconds, then add the cheese slowly, stirring as you do.

>>>> CONTINUED >>>>

8 Cook for 2 min. stirring constantly to make sure the cheese melts evenly. Cover and remove the pot from the heat.

9 Make your hot water crust dough according to the recipe and roll it out into a sheet ⅛" thick.

10 Measure your muffin cups and cut the dough into circles large enough so that they'll line the cups with a ¼ - ½" rim around each one, and then press the dough into the cups to line them. Next reincorporate the dough together, roll out to ⅛" thickness again and cut out the tops for each cup.

11 Divide the filling evenly into each cup, filling nearly to the top. Place your tops on each one and press the dough together, pinching all around to seal them. Cut 2 slits in the top of each pie to vent, brush each with the beaten egg, and sprinkle with salt.

12 Bake on the middle rack for 15 - 20 min. until the dough is golden brown. Remove from the oven and let rest in the tins for 10 min. before removing and placing on a plate or rack. Serve Hot. Wrap left over pies in foil and refrigerate. They will hold in fridge for 5 - 7 days, and can be wrapped in plastic then foil to be frozen for up to 3 months

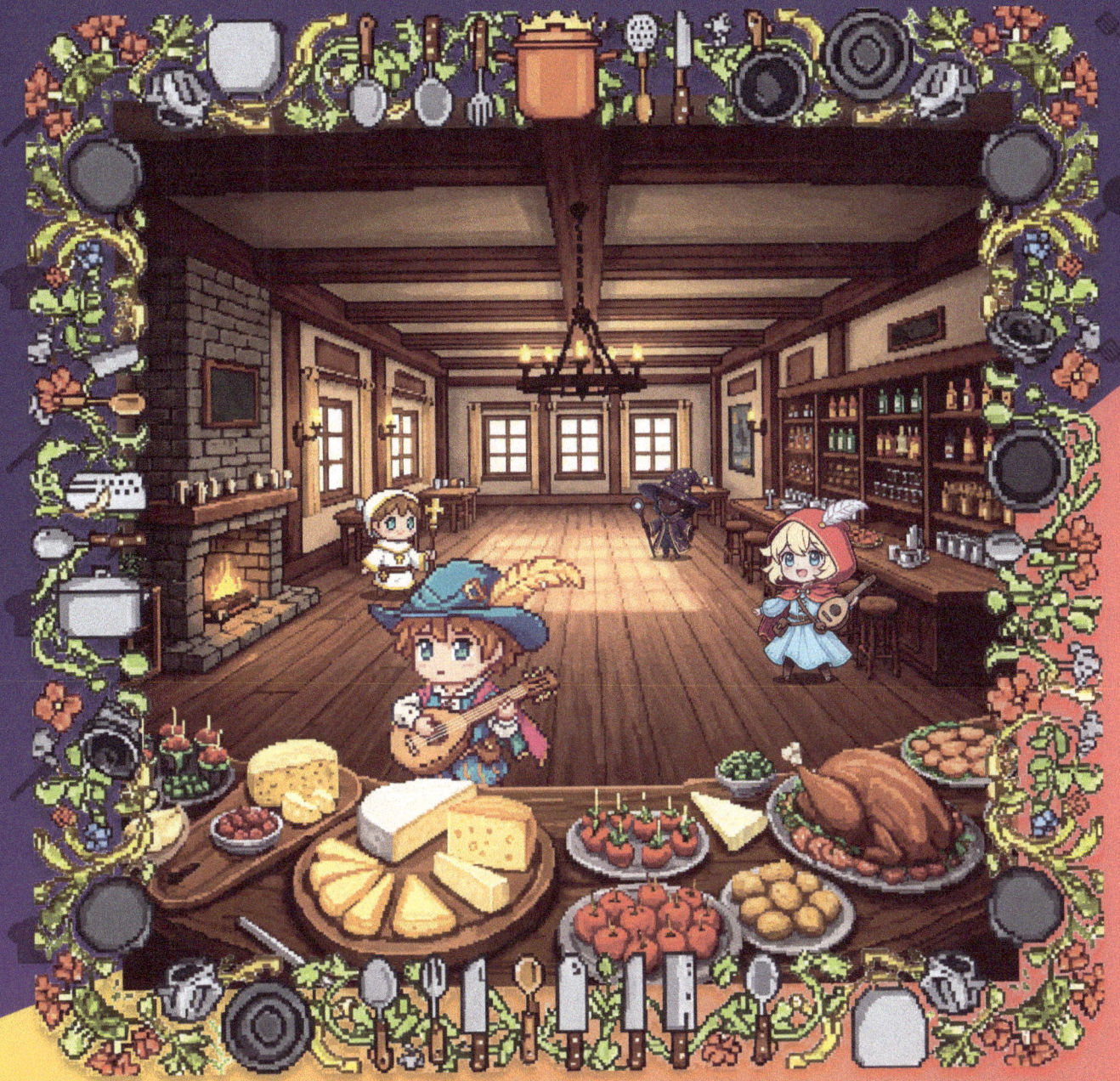

Recipe Tip

Don't be afraid to try out various kinds of mushrooms with these pies! Oyster, maitake, lion's mane, and more! All are good options, with many more besides. Be adventurous!

Quiche Aux Carnitas

This recipe is a great way to use leftover braised pork, and can be adapted to utilize a wide variety of proteins. This recipe is difficult and in-depth, requiring both proper planning and lengthy preparation. But the result is a soft, fluffy dish with distinct and robust flavor. Take this recipe, learn it well, and then use it to experiment and create your own unique, delightful combinations of flavors! Making the pie crust yourself takes time, but the Experience Points you get from making this dish from scratch are well worth the effort.

You can do some prep work ahead of time by making and pre-baking the pie crust, preparing the meat and vegetable mixture, and storing both in the fridge. This way, when dinner time comes, you only have to assemble the quiche and bake at 400. This method helps make this dish a good weekend prep idea for your meal plans.

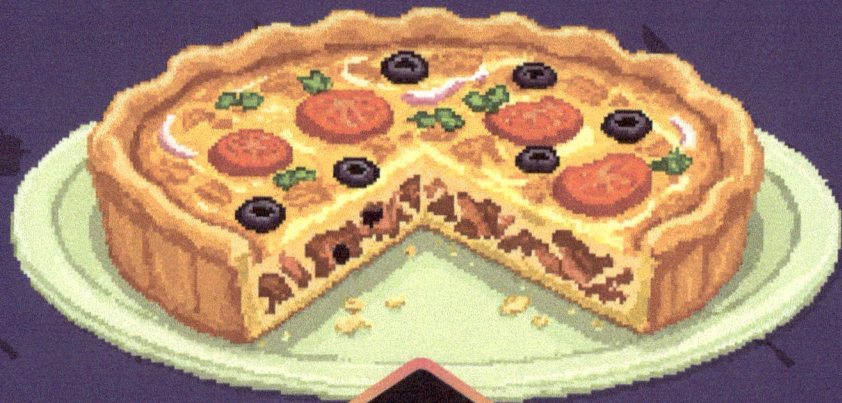

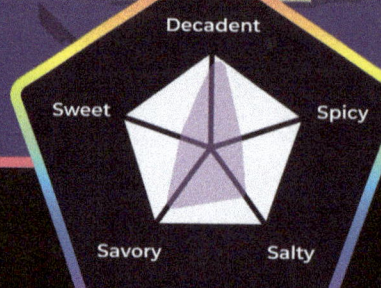

Ingredients

		Prep Time 1 Hr 20 Min	Cook Time 30 - 35 Min	Servings 9" Quiche
AP Braised Pork, Shredded (Pg 197)	1 C	Cumin		¼ tsp
Large Eggs	4 ea	Cinnamon		⅛ tsp
Tomato, Diced	¼ C	Paprika		½ tsp
Black Olives, Sliced	¼ C	Coriander		¼ tsp
White Onion, Diced	¼ C	Chili Powder		½ tsp
Monterey Jack Cheese, Shredded	1 C	Oregano, Dry		¼ tsp
		Salt		½ tsp
Milk	8 Fl Oz	Butter, Melted		1 Tbsp
Garlic, Minced	2 tsp	Olive Oil		1 tsp
Black Pepper	¼ tsp	Butter Crust Dough (Pg 159)		8 oz

Cooking Directions (Preparation)

Special Equipment

9" Pie Dish (Glass or Metal) 1 ea	Uncooked Rice or Beans for Pre Baking the Pie Crust 1 ea

1   Make your pie dough. Roll the pie dough out to a sheet that is ⅛" thick. Place dough in the 9" pie dish and trim the dough to ½" beyond the edge of the dish. Press the dough gently into the dish to completely line it, and then crimp the excess dough on the edge of the pie dish.

2   Place the pie dish in the fridge and let rest for 30 min. Preheat your oven to 425.

3   While the pie crust is chilling, cut and measure all other ingredients.

4   When the pie crust has finished chilling, remove from fridge and line the crust with foil or parchment paper. Fill the lined pie dish with dry beans, uncooked rice, or baking beads. Place in oven and bake for 15 - 20 min. Remove the weights and foil/parchment paper and bake for another 3 - 4 min. Remove from oven and let cool to room temperature on a wire rack. Reduce oven temp to 375.

>>>> BAKING DIRECTIONS >>>>

Cooking Directions
(Baking)

1   While the pie crust cools, place a 10" - 12" sauce pan over Medium High heat and remove the eggs from the fridge. Add the oil.

2   When the oil is shimmering, add the garlic, onions, tomatoes, and black olives. Stirring often, cook until the onions begin to soften, 2 - 3 min. Remove from pan, and turn off stove eye.

3   Transfer the cooked vegetables to a large bowl. Add the shredded pork, ½ of the cheese, and seasonings (except the salt). Stir well to combine, then transfer the mix into the pie dish and spread so it is evenly distributed. Top the mixture with the remaining cheese.

4   Melt the butter in the microwave on Low, using 10 sec. bursts; make sure the butter is melted, but not hot. In the same bowl you already used, whisk the eggs well. Then add your milk, salt, and melted butter, and whisk to combine.

5   Pour the egg mixture over your ingredients in the pie dish, and gently shake the pie dish so the egg distributes evenly. Cover the edges of the pie crust loosely with foil, and place the pie dish on a baking tray.

6   Bake in the oven until a knife inserted in the center of the quiche comes out clean, 30 - 35 min. Remove from oven and let cool for 10 min. before cutting and serving.

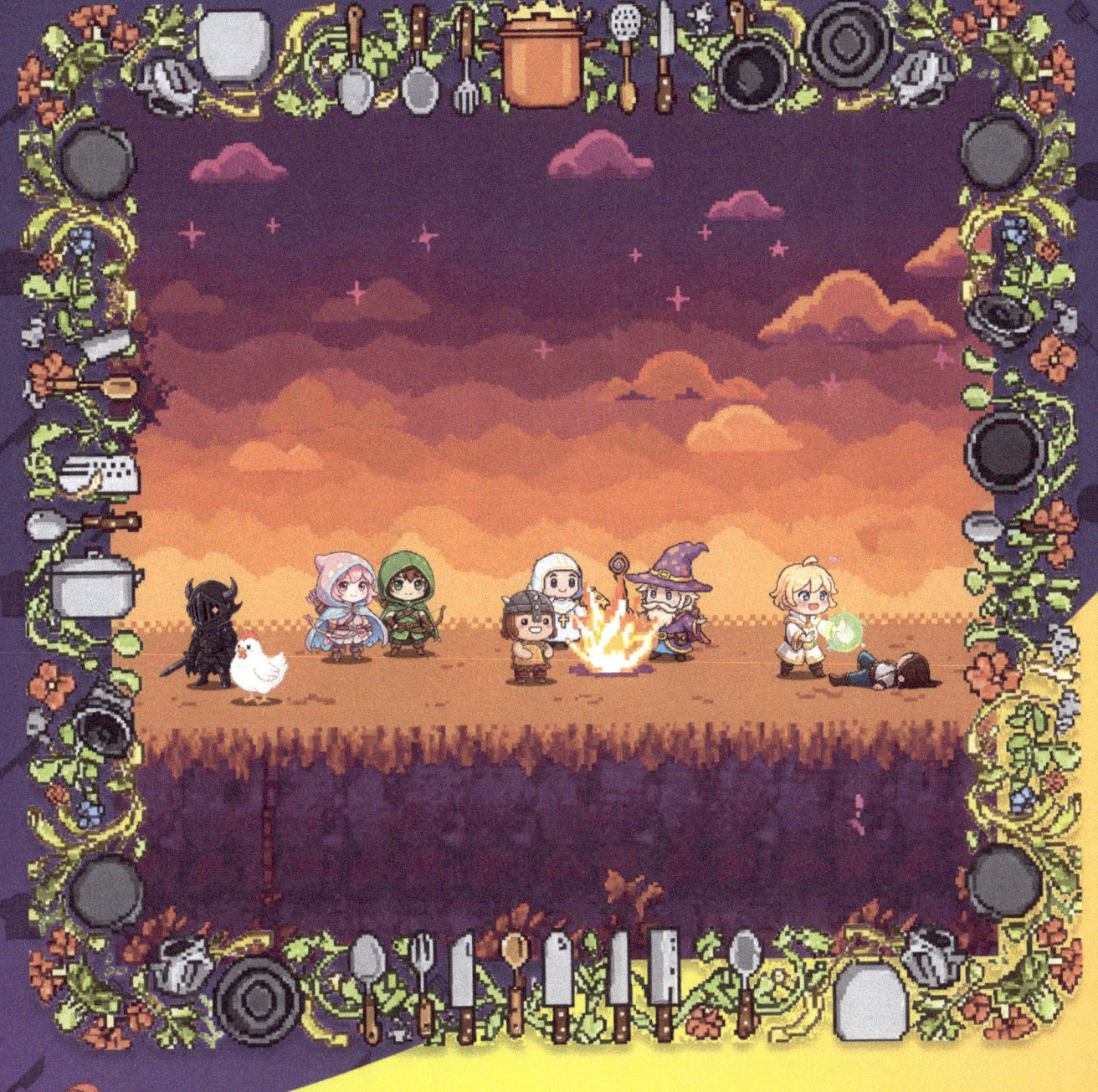

Recipe Tip

Once you've got the hang of making this recipe, try out different presentation methods. Make little quiche appetizers with a muffin tin, or try it out in XL muffin tins for single serving entrees. Get creative, and utilize everything you've learned to make this dish shine!

Shrimp Étouffée

This Creole dish is on the lighter side, and is a great way to enjoy a summer evening. It's traditionally made with crawfish tails, but I find shrimp are not only more readily available, but also more delicate in their flavor. Using homemade seafood stock is the way to go if you really want this dish to shine, but chicken or even vegetable works just fine. This dish is one that benefits from sitting in the fridge overnight before serving. This is great news for making leftovers, and it'll really help elevate the already delightful flavors. Just be sure to properly cool the sauce before covering in the fridge. When serving the next day, reheat gently and add water 1 Tbsp. at a time if it seems too thick.

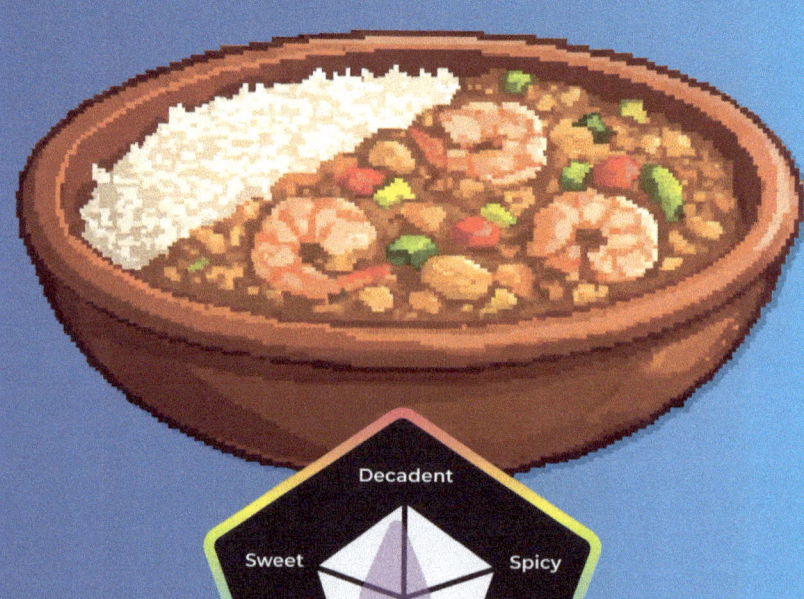

Decadent
Sweet
Spicy
Savory
Salty

Ingredients

		Prep Time 15 Min	Cook Time 1 Hr 40 Min	Servings 4 Portions

Shrimp, Peeled, Deveined, 16 - 20 Ct	1 Lb	Cayenne	⅛ tsp
White Onion, Small Dice	1 C	Salt	¼ tsp
Green Bell Pepper, Small Dice	½ C	Paprika	¼ tsp
Celery, Small Dice	½ C	Thyme, Dry	¼ tsp
Scallions, Thinly Sliced	⅓ C	Roux Blond	6 oz
Garlic, Minced	1½ Tbsp	Chicken/Seafood Stock	1 Pt
Parsley, Fresh, Minced	1 Tbsp	Butter/Oil	1 Tbsp
Lemon Juice	1 tsp	Oven Baked Rice (Pg 89)	
Black Pepper, Ground	½ tsp		

Cooking Directions

1 Place a 4 Qt. pot over Medium Low heat and place butter/oil in it. When the butter stops bubbling or the oil is shimmering, add the onions, bell pepper, and celery, cooking each until soft before adding the next. Add your garlic and salt, cook for 1 min. more. If using premade roux, now is the time ro put it in the pot and incorporate it. If not using premade roux, add your flour and stir well to incorporate. Stirring very often, cook the flour for 4 - 5 min. so it reaches the Blond level.

2 Add the scallions and all your seasonings, stirring well.

3 Raise the heat to Medium and add 1 C of the stock. Stir well, working out any lumps in the roux. Add the remaining stock and whisk to fully incorporate the roux. Bring to a simmer and cover.

4 Cook until the Etoufee forms a thick gravy that coats the back of a spoon (nappe). Remove the lid, add your shrimp and stir well. Bring back to a simmer, cover and cook for 5 - 7 min. until the shrimp are plump and bright pink. Taste test and adjust seasoning as desired.

5 Serve Hot over ¾ - 1 C of Creole Rice.

Shrimp in Sauce Creole

This is a staple of Creole cuisine, and the sauce pairs with any delicate flavored protein. Chicken is common, as well as crawfish, and if you are into it, give extra-firm tofu a try with this decadent sauce. Using homemade stock is preferred, either chicken or seafood, and using fresh tomatoes over canned will bring out a more herbaceous flavor profile in the dish. However, canned tomatoes work well and the flavor they produce might be more to your liking.

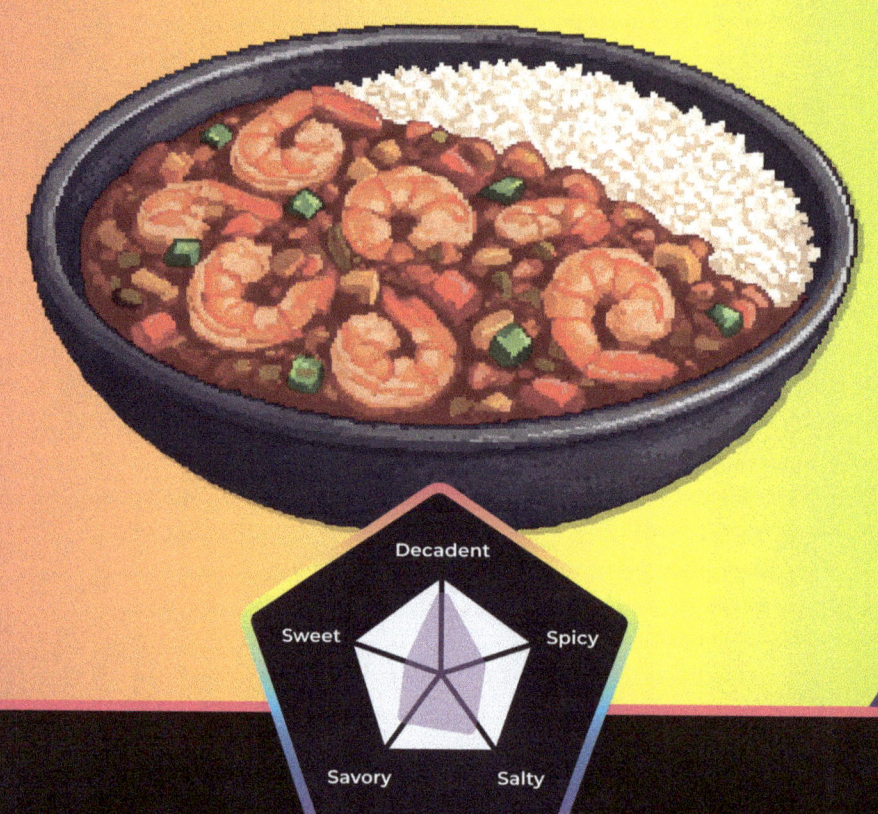

EXPERT

Decadent
Sweet
Spicy
Savory
Salty

Ingredients

		Prep Time 20 Min	Cook Time 1 Hr	Servings 6 Portions
Shrimp, Peeled, Deveined, 21-30 Ct	2 Lb	Hot Sauce		2 tsp
		Salt		1 tsp
White Onion, Small Dice	1½ C	Black Pepper, Ground		½ tsp
Green Bell Pepper, Small Dice	¾ C	Paprika		½ tsp
Celery, Small Dice	¾ C	Thyme, Dry		¼ tsp
Tomatoes, Diced W/ Juices OR	2 C	White Sugar		1 tsp
14.5 oz. Can Diced Tomatoes	1 ea	Cayenne		⅛ tsp
Scallions, Sliced	½ C	Tomato Paste		6 Tbsp
Garlic, Minced	1½ Tbsp	Chicken/Seafood Stock		1 Pt
Bay Leaf	1 ea	Butter/Oil		4 Tbsp
Parsley, Minced	2 Tbsp	AP Flour		2 Tbsp
Worcestershire Sauce	2 tsp	Oven Baked Rice (Pg 89)		

Cooking Directions

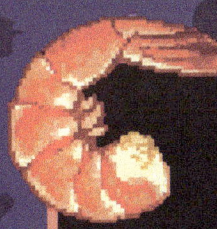

1   Place a 4 Qt. pot over Medium heat. Add the butter/
    oil to the pot. When the butter stops bubbling or the
    oil starts to shimmer add the onion, bell pepper, and
    celery cooking each until soft before adding the next.
    Add the garlic and salt, and cook for 1 min. more.

2   Add the remaining dry seasonings and stir frequently,
    cooking for 5 min. more. Add the tomato paste, stir
    well to combine, and cook or 2 min. until it starts to
    smell sweet.

3   Add the flour and cook, stirring constantly, for 1 min.
    Add the Worcestershire and cook for 30 seconds, then
    add the tomatoes, stock, and hot sauce.

4   Raise the heat to High and bring the mixture to a hard
    simmer. Reduce the heat to Medium Low and cover,
    cooking for 15 min. stirring occasionally to keep the
    sauce from sticking to the bottom of the pot.

5   Remove the lid and raise the heat to bring the mix
    back to a soft simmer and cook uncovered for 10 min.
    stirring often. Then, add your shrimp and cook for 5 - 7
    min. more until the shrimp firm and bright pink.

6   Taste test and adjust the seasoning as desired.
    Remove the pot from heat. Serve hot over ¾ C of
    Oven Baked Rice.

Desserts & Baking

French Bread

I am particularly proud of this recipe, as I have never been much of a baker. There's a reason I went to school for Culinary Arts, after all. However, after I went to New Orleans for my honeymoon, I fell in love with Creole and Cajun cuisine, especially the Po' Boy Sandwich. When I got back home, I made it my mission to be able to make crunchy, fluffy bread at home for my sandwiches. This recipe took months of testing and refining, but I did it.

Having a stand mixer is not necessary for this recipe to work. In fact, it helps only slightly as this recipe is a bit wetter than most bread dough, and a stand mixer won't be able to develop the gluten very well. Kneading is a bit of a workout, as the rice flour is a bit thicker and grainier than wheat flour. When kneading, apply the 'windowpane test'. This is a test to see how far along your gluten has developed. Simply pull the dough up and stretch it between several fingers and look at it in good lighting. If the dough stretches easily and you are able to faintly see through it, you are good to move on to the next step.

One item that I highly recommend to anyone looking to make their own baguette style loaves is a French bread pan. These are not expensive and can be found easily online. The pan helps the dough hold its shape during the second proofing and during baking. I purchased one after my first attempt at developing this recipe and it changed the game completely.

These loaves are perfect for making any kind of sandwich, and are also delicious as an addition to a charcuterie board, or as a side with any meal. When the bread grows stale, cut it up into cubes to make homemade croutons, or slice it into rounds and make some French Onion Soup (see recipe). The only trouble is that the bread is usually all eaten up before this can happen.

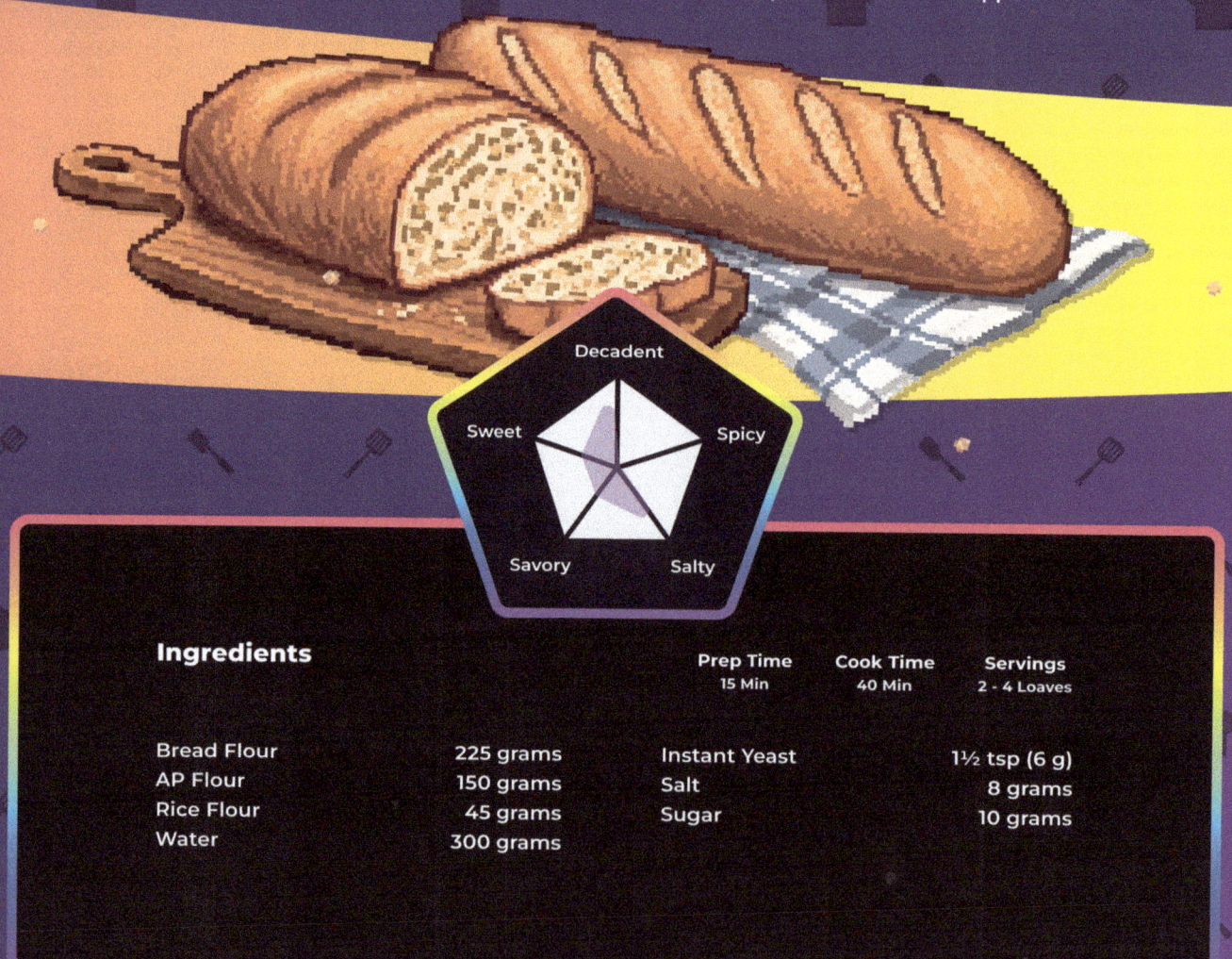

Decadent

Sweet · Spicy

Savory · Salty

Ingredients

			Prep Time	Cook Time	Servings
			15 Min	40 Min	2 - 4 Loaves

Ingredient	Amount	Ingredient	Amount
Bread Flour	225 grams	Instant Yeast	1½ tsp (6 g)
AP Flour	150 grams	Salt	8 grams
Rice Flour	45 grams	Sugar	10 grams
Water	300 grams		

Cooking Directions

Special Equipment

2 Slot French Bread Loaf Pan
1 ea

Scale that measures in Grams
1 ea

Stand Mixer (Not required)
1 ea

Bench Knife or Other Scraping Tool
1 ea

Large Plastic Oven Bag
1 ea

1   Measure and weigh out all ingredients, in separate bowls and containers. Keep the bread flour out for dusting.

2   Sift the flours together. Transfer them to a large mixing bowl and add the yeast, sugar, and salt. Mix together to combine.

3   Add the water and mix with a rubber spatula to form a shaggy dough. If using a stand mixer, mix on 1 at first, and work your way up to 4, scraping the sides as the mixer runs to incorporate all ingredients.

4   If not using a stand mixer, transfer the dough to a floured surface, coat your hands in flour, and knead vigorously for 8 min. If the dough begins to get sticky, sprinkle a small amount of flour on the counter and your hands to keep working it. If using a stand mixer, knead in the bowl for 2 min. on a 4, then transfer to the floured surface and knead vigorously by hand for 6 min. While kneading, be sure to scrape up any dough that sticks to the counter quickly to reincorporate into the dough ball.

> > > > CONTINUED > > > >

5   Spray a large bowl with cooking spray and place the dough in the bowl, cover tightly with plastic wrap. Bulk rise at room temperature (75 degrees) for 70 min. At the 50 min. mark, stretch and fold your dough. This process is where you lightly grease your hands, and work your fingers under ½ of the dough ball. Gently grip and pull it up, stretching it out. Then, fold it over onto itself and gently press the dough back together. Rotate the bowl 90 degrees, and repeat. Do this 4 total times, and return the plastic wrap to cover and finish rising.

6   Dump the dough out from the bowl onto a floured surface and divide it evenly into 2 pieces. Pre-shape the dough pieces into roughly the same size and shape, and let rest on the counter for 20 min.

7   Roll a dough piece out into a 13"W x 6"L rectangle. Get rid of any air bubbles, roll up the dough and seal by pinching along the seam. Then, roll out slightly to increase the length by about ½". Repeat with other dough piece.

8   Place on a baking sheet (in a French bread pan, if you have it) and then place the sheet into a proofing bag. I recommend using the large plastic roasting bags they sell at grocery stores. Place the sheet in the bag and tightly seal to prevent air flow, keeping the bag as far away from the dough as possible so it can rise. To do this, I find it helpful to blow some air into the bag before tying off to inflate it a bit.

> > > > CONTINUED > > > >

9   Proof at room temperature for 45 - 60 min. until the dough has doubled in size. Be sure to check on it and make sure to proceed to the next step as soon as it has doubled in size. Over-proofing is a sure way to mess up your bread. While proofing, preheat your oven to 425, make sure there is one rack in the center of the oven, and place an oven safe dish or metal bowl full of water on the lower or upper rack.

10 Remove from proofing bag, brush dough with water and cut 2 - 3 small strips on a bias using a very sharp knife.

11 Be careful of the steam when opening the oven door. Bake for 10 min. then reduce the heat to 375 and rotate the pan 180 degrees. Bake for 25 min. more, opening the oven door just a crack in the last 5 min.

12 Remove from oven and transfer to a wire rack to cool completely. The crust should be light brown and quite crispy.

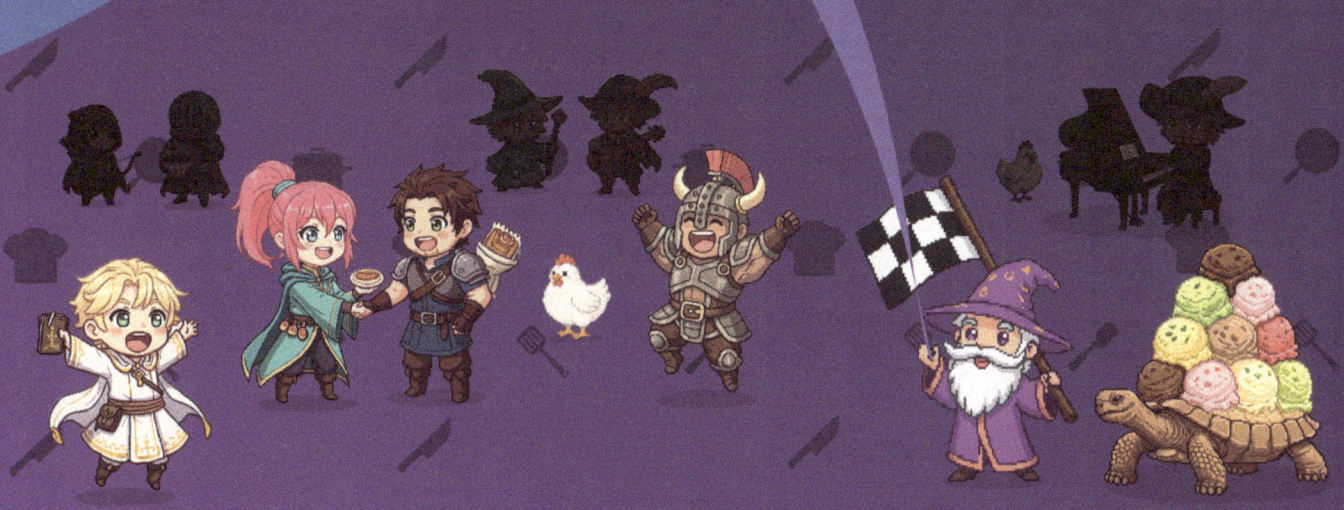

LEVEL 40

Achievements Unlocked

Around The World
- You're able to tweak recipes to alter their flavor and cultural profiles

Strategist
- You're familiar with making multiple courses for meals, and pairing them successfully

Crowd Pleaser
- You're now capable of feeding large groups of people, making multiple recipes in tandem

Switch Hitter
- You're proficient in utilizing multiple cooking methods in one recipe

Fu...sion Ha!
- You understand how to bring two distinct cuisines together in one dish

Sword Master
- You're familiar with and competent in all forms of knife cuts

Batter Up!
- You can now make battered and fried proteins like a pro!

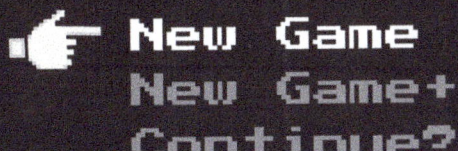
New Game
New Game+
Continue?

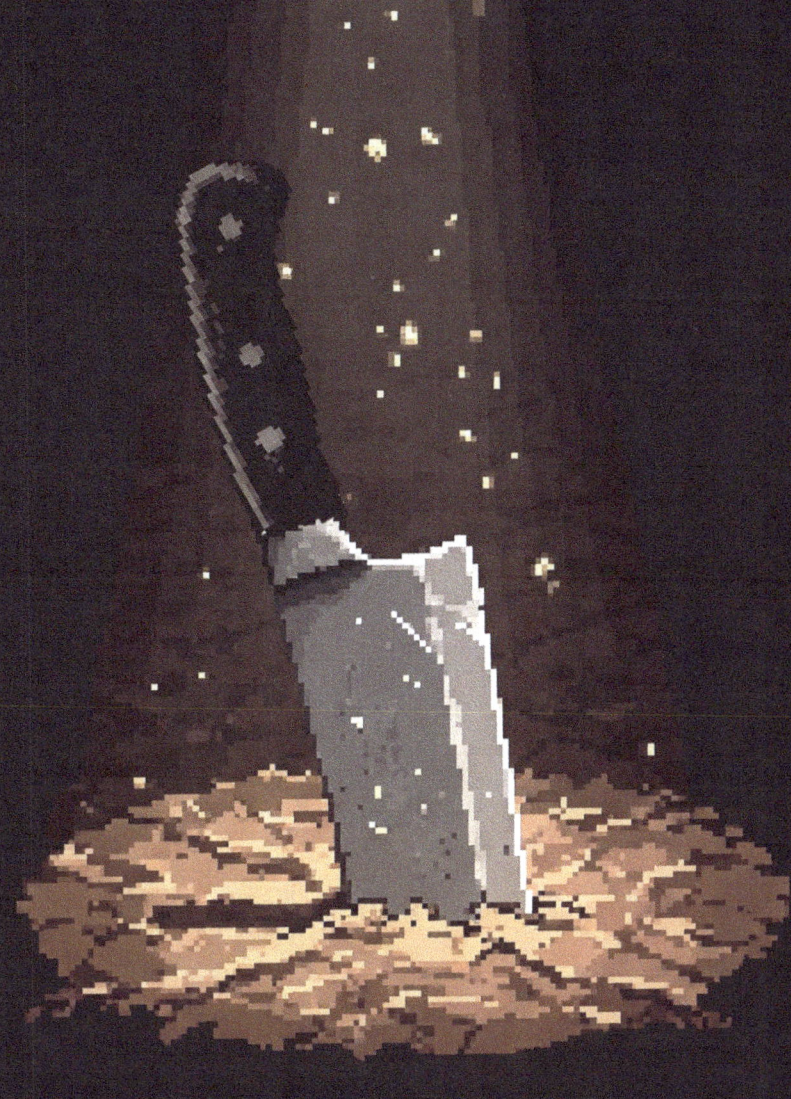

Published by: GWN Publishing
www.GWNPublishing.com
Illustration and Cover Design: Sterling Vanderhoof
ISBN: 978-1-965971-14-7

Recipe Index

Terms and Definitions

There are enough specialized techniques, terms, and names to fill a Library of Alexandria sized lexicon when it comes to cooking. However, in the main, there are some core and peripheral entries that are used by almost everyone, from a Novice to an Expert. I've provided a list of the entries I come across and utilize most, both in my private and professional pursuits, so you too can have firm footing when starting your journey.

Knife Cuts

Brunoise (Small Dice) (broo-NWAHZ)	• To cut a food into cubes that are ⅛" x ⅛" x ⅛"
Macédoine (Dice) (mass-uh-DWAHN)	• To cut food into cubes that are ¼" x ¼" x ¼"
Parmentier (Large Dice) (par-MON-tee-ay)	• To cut food into cubes that are ½" x ½" x ½"
Cube	• To cut food into pieces that are ¾" or thicker on all sides
Rough Chop	• To cut food into small pieces of a non-uniform size and shape
Mince	• To cut food into very small pieces of a non-uniform size and shape
Julienne	• To cut food into strips which are ¼" x ¼" x 1½"-2"
Chiffonade (Shred) (SHIF-o-nod)	• To cut lettuce or other leaves into very fine strips, accomplished by rolling the leaf up before slicing

Recipe Terms

AP Flour	• The shorthand for 'All Purpose", this is flour that has no leavening agents added to it, and is the most common flour used for culinary pursuits
Bake	• To cook in an enclosed space using temperatures between 200 and 375 degrees
Baste	• To apply liquids gathered at the bottom of a pan or tray during the cooking process to the surface of an item. Aids in moisture retention and flavor development
Blanch	• To partially cook a food item, usually by submerging it in boiling water
Boil	• To cook food by fully submerging in liquid that is at 212 degrees
Braise	• To cook by submerging food ¼ - ½ of the way in liquid between 145 and 190 degrees
Broil	• To cook with intense heat, with the heat source being 6"-12" above the food item
Cold Smoke	• To infuse flavor into a food item by placing it in an enclosed space and filling the space with smoke and warm air between 65 and 85 degrees
Cure	• To apply sugar, salt, and herbs to a food item to draw out moisture and infuse flavor. Used commonly as a method of preparation for long term storage
Divided	• In the context of a recipe, an ingredient value is given in its total amount and the amounts needed at different points in the cooking process are outlined in the directions.
Emulsify	• To combine an oil and an acid thoroughly in order to keep the molecules in suspension (mayo, vinaigrettes, etc.)
En Papillote (Ahn pa-pee-yote)	• To cook food wrapped tightly in parchment paper, tin foil, corn husk, or banana leaf by steaming or baking
Glaze	• To coat a food item in a sauce or syrup and apply heat to remove moisture from the coating
Grill	• To cook on a grate or griddle with intense heat, with the heat source being 6"-12" below the food item
Nappe (nap-pay)	• To reduce/thicken a sauce or liquid to the point where it coats the back of a spoon or similar smooth surface
Poach	• To cook by submerging food ½ - ¾ of the way in liquid between 145 and 175 degrees
Reduce	• To apply heat to a liquid in order to evaporate water and concentrate flavor and density
Roast	• To cook in an enclosed space using temperatures between 380 and 500 degrees
Roux (ROO)	• A mixture of equal parts flour and oil/melted butter that is heated and cooked to varying levels for different thickening effects (see section on Roux)
Sauté (saw-TAY)	• To cook in a skillet over high heat, lots of movement, little oil
Sear	• To use high heat to heavily darken the outside of a protein or vegetable, not to fully cook
Shock	• To place a hot food item in an ice water bath to rapidly cool and stop the cooking process
Simmer	• To hold a liquid between 165 and 200 degrees to facilitate flavor development or moisture evaporation; a soft boil
Slurry	• A mixture that is equal parts water and finely diced food matter, cornstarch or otherwise
Smoke	• To cook a food item by placing in an enclosed space and filling the space with smoke and hot air between 180 and 300 degrees
Steam	• To cook food in an enclosed space with the heat source being the hot, moist air that fills the space. Steam runs between 212 and 225 degrees

Helpful Conversions & Abbreviations

Below is a chart with the most common conversions used in a kitchen, along with another that has explanations of their abbreviations. This chart is a handy reference, and I strongly urge cooks of all levels to read it over thoroughly and work to memorize it. It may seem intimidating, but as you continue on your cooking journey you'll find yourself recalling this information easily and quickly.

Units	Abbreviations
Teaspoon	Tsp. / t
Tablespoon	Tbsp. / T
Cup(s)	C
Fluid Ounce(s)	Fl. Oz.
Ounce(s)	Oz.
Pound(s)	Lb.
Pint(s)	Pt. / P
Quart(s)	Qt. / Q
Gallon(s)	Gal. / G

Units	Measurements	Volume
Pinch	$\frac{1}{32}$ tsp.	
Dash	$\frac{1}{16}$ tsp.	
Teaspoon		⅙ Oz. Fluid and Dry
Tablespoon	3 tsp.	½ Oz. Fluid and Dry
Cup	16 Tbsp.	8 oz. Fluid and Dry
Ounce	2 Tbsp.	
Pound	16 Oz.	
Pint	2 C	16 Fl. Oz.
Quart	4 C, 2 Pt.	32 Fl. Oz.
Gallon	16 C, 8 Pt., 4 Qt.	128 Fl. Oz.

Keep in mind that the volumes given are just that, volume. The weights are obvious for Ounces and Pounds, but a pound of almost any given ingredient will have a very different measurement from 16 ounces by volume. This is why recipes are always given in units of volumetric measurement, unless stated as weight. While a cup is 8 ounces in volume, a cup of diced onions will not weigh 8 oz. All the recipes in my book are given in Imperial volumetric terms, with weight being specified for the ingredients that require it.

Safe Cooking Temperatures

The Food Item	Safe Internal Temperatures
Vegetables, Store Bought Processed Foods	135 Degrees
Whole Fish/Shellfish/Seafood	145 Degrees
Whole Pork	145 Degrees
Whole Lamb (Steaks, Chops, Roasts)	Rare: 120-125 Degrees
	-Medium Rare: 130-135
	-Medium: 140-145
	-Medium Well: 150-155
	-Well Done: 160
Whole Beef (Steaks, Chops, Roasts)	Rare: 120-125 Degrees
	-Medium Rare: 130-135
	-Medium: 140-145
	-Medium Well: 150-155
	-Well Done: 160
Ground Meat & Seafood	155 Degrees
Injected/ Marinated Meats & Seafood	155 Degrees
Poultry (Chicken, Duck, Turkey)	165 Degrees
Stuffed Meat, and the Stuffing inside it	165 Degrees
Leftovers & Dishes made using Leftovers	165 Degrees

*It is only safe to reheat properly cooled food twice. This means that after cooking, you properly cool the food. When you reheat it, make sure it reaches 165 internal temperature. Then properly cool it again. The second time it is reheated to 165 internal temperature is the last time it is safe to serve and eat. Any more and you risk Food Poisoning.

About the Author

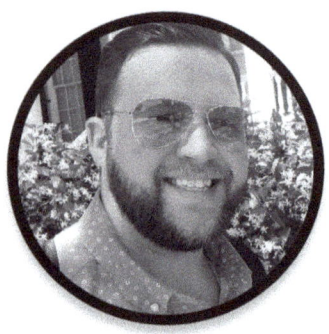

Cameron McCluskie

I am Cameron McCluskie, a professional chef and avid lover of all things food and drink. I have spent my entire adult life (and quite a few years as a teenager) cooking on a personal and professional level. After High School, I went to Johnson & Wales School of Culinary Arts in Providence, Rhode Island, where I attained my Bachelor's Degree in Culinary Arts with a double concentration in Advanced Culinary Studies and Sustainability. Since then, I have worked a myriad of jobs in the kitchen. From dishwasher, to prep cook and line chef at both a five star restaurant and a restaurant owned by a Michelin Star recipient in Denver, and even the founding of my own food truck. All throughout, I have done my best to absorb and retain every scrap of knowledge I encountered. And this is what I hope to bring to you: my experience, my flavors, and my own take on both classical and modern dishes. With that goal in mind, I present to you a humble offering of my philosophy, a collection of recipes, and a helpful reference for the more common terminology, abbreviations, and skills used in the pursuit of culinary delight. While I may not know everything, I do know quite a lot. And I hope that after you have utilized my book, you will too. Thank you for reading my book, and Happy Adventuring!

▶ @Cooking_Plus

M LvlUpCookbook@gmail.com

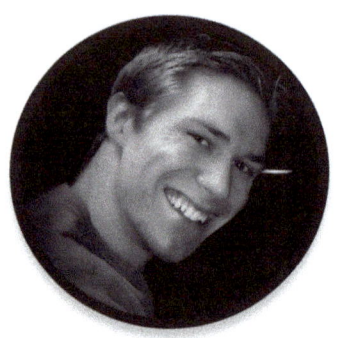

Sterling Vanderhoof

My name is Sterling Vanderhoof, a professional artist and fervent gamer. My journey has taken me from the gallery walls and award-winning paintings to designing my own card game and now, cooking up something entirely new.

This cookbook is where nostalgia meets imagination—a love letter to pixelated adventures and late-night snacks.

Whether I'm painting a canvas or designing a game, I'm always chasing the spark behind the story—the magic hidden in plain sight. Cooking, like art, is a kind of alchemy. And this book is my latest quest.

⬜ sterlingvanderhoof.art

▶ @VanderPrima

⬛ sterlingvanderhoof_art

M svanderhoof2@gmail.com

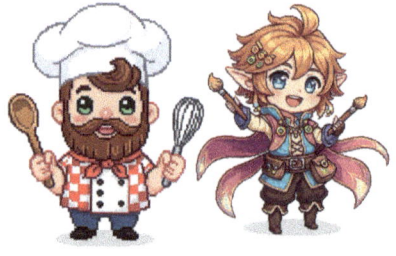